PET/CT for Inflammatory Diseases

Hiroshi Toyama • Yaming Li
Jun Hatazawa • Guang Huang
Kazuo Kubota
Editors

PET/CT for Inflammatory Diseases

Basic Sciences, Typical Cases, and Review

Springer

Editors
Hiroshi Toyama
Department of Radiology
Fujita Health University
Toyoake
Aichi
Japan

Yaming Li
Department of Nuclear Medicine
The First Hospital of China Medical University
Shenyang
Liaoning
China

Jun Hatazawa
Joint Research Division for the Quantum Cancer
Therapy, Research Center for Nuclear Physics
Professor Emeritus, Osaka University
Suita
Osaka
Japan

Guang Huang
Shanghai University of Medicine & Health
Sciences
Shanghai
China

Kazuo Kubota
Department of Radiology
Southern TOHOKU General Hospital
Koriyama
Fukushima
Japan

ISBN 978-981-15-0809-7 ISBN 978-981-15-0810-3 (eBook)
https://doi.org/10.1007/978-981-15-0810-3

This Springer imprint is published by the registered company Springer Nature Singapore Pte Ltd.
The registered company address is: 152 Beach Road, #21-01/04 Gateway East, Singapore 189721, Singapore

Foreword

In 2013, when I was the president of the Japanese Society of Nuclear Medicine, an inter-society agreement (MOU) was signed between the Japanese Society of Nuclear Medicine and the Chinese Society of Nuclear Medicine organized by the president, Prof. Gang Huang. After that, according to this MOU, Prof. Jun Hatazawa, my successor president, and Prof. Yaming Li, successor to Prof. Huang, have been carrying out exchange project that is unparalleled in the history of Japanese and Chinese nuclear medicine. The exchange has been becoming active year by year these 5 years.

The project accomplished many presentations of both sides at the conference. In addition, we visited each other's nuclear medicine facilities for a short time to deepen our relationship. From an academic point of view, collaborators were collecting and examining cases based on a common understanding of the theme of FDG PET inflammatory diseases. As an excellent result of symposium for this trial in 2017 Asia Oceania Congress of Nuclear Medicine and Biology (AOCNMB 2017), the publication of this textbook was planned by Dr. Hiroshi Toyama and Dr. Yaming Li with support of Springer Co. This textbook is well organized from basic science (Chap. 1) to clinical cases based on etiologies of infectious/inflammatory diseases (Chaps. 2–8). This book is written by veterans and young nuclear medicine physicians representing both countries, and I believe this textbook is a good reference for nuclear medicine physicians and researchers. This book is a testament to the fact that Japan-China nuclear medicine exchanges have been carried out substantially.

I would like to pay tribute for the efforts of Dr. Hiroshi Toyama and Dr. Yaming Li who have deepened nuclear medicine exchanges between China and Japan.

Tomio Inoue
Shonan Kamakura General Hospital, Iryohojin
Okinawa Tokushukai Kamakura
Kanagawa, Japan

Preface

On behalf of the organizing committee of Japan-China Nuclear Medicine Exchange Program and Japanese Society of Nuclear Medicine and as one of the editors, I am pleased to publish the textbook entitled *PET/CT for Inflammatory Disease: Basic Sciences, Typical Case Series, and Review* from Springer Co.

The contents of this book consist of eight chapters. In Chap. 1, overview of the basic science of PET imaging for inflammatory diseases is written. From Chaps. 2 to 8, typical case reports and review using PET imaging are written in each category of inflammatory disease.

Regarding the opportunity for publication of this book, for the first step, we have discussed the international joint research regarding ^{18}F-FDG PET/CT imaging for diagnosis of inflammatory disease at the task force meeting of Japan-China Nuclear Medicine Exchange Program on November 4, 2016, at the 56th Annual Meeting of Japanese Society of Nuclear Medicine in Nagoya. For the second step, we, Japanese and Chinese, discussed about PET imaging for inflammatory diseases at the eighth Sino-Japan Nuclear Medicine Exchange Seminar in 2017 Asian Nuclear Medicine Academic Forum on May 13, chaired by the Asian School of Nuclear Medicine (ASNM) Dean, Prof. Guan Huang. For the third step, the Japan-China Nuclear Medicine joint symposium entitled "FDG PET for Inflammatory Disease" was carried out at the 57th Annual Scientific Meeting of the Japanese Society of Nuclear Medicine and the 12th Asia Oceania Congress of Nuclear Medicine and Biology in Yokohama, Japan, October 7, 2017, headed by President Tomio Inoue, MD, PhD, professor and chairman, Yokohama City University Graduate School of Medicine. Several Japanese and Chinese physicians presented and discussed about various inflammatory diseases using PET imaging. Based on these consecutive steps, we have decided to publish the textbook regarding PET for inflammatory disease as a commemoration of the fifth anniversary of Japan-China Nuclear Medicine Exchange Program. I am really proud for publishing this book based on many people' s efforts and supports from both Japan and China sides. Finally, I appreciate Dr. Mototora Kai, secretary general of the ASNM, people of Sino-Japan Nuclear Medicine Exchange Association, Japan-China Nuclear Medicine Exchange Committee, and Springer Co.

Toyoake, Aichi, Japan Hiroshi Toyama

Preface

In China, both the numbers of PET/CT installation and the numbers of clinical examination are increasing in recent years. According to the national survey made by the CSNM in 2017, more than 90% of cases examined by PET/CT in China were due to diagnosing, efficacy evaluation of treatment, or prognosis evaluation of tumors.

PET/CT imaging is an important representative of molecular imaging. With one whole body imaging, lesions in tissues and organs examination can be detected with high sensitivity. However, the potential and feasibility of its application in non-tumor diseases need to be further explored and expanded.

The incidence of inflammatory and infectious diseases is high, but the clinical manifestations are often non-specific. Thus, its clinical diagnosis is very challenging. PET/CT imaging, as a highly sensitive whole body imaging, has great prospects for its application in the diagnosis. However, the application of PET/CT imaging in these diseases is rarely included in the relevant guidelines, and high-level evidence-based medical evidence is still needed in this regard. Based on the status quo, China and Japan have jointly carried out a multicenter study on the application value of PET/CT imaging in unexplained fever. To investigate the diagnostic value of ^{18}F-FDG-PET/CT for FUO and IUO and the imaging characteristics of PET/CT in the diseases of different etiology, the results of ^{18}F-FDG-PET/CT examinations of 376 FUO/IUO patients in 12 hospitals in China were analyzed. The clinicians were also surveyed to evaluate the significance of PET/CT in the diagnosis of FUO/IUO. The results showed that among 376 patients, infectious diseases accounted for 33.0%, rheumatism for 32.4%, malignant tumors for 19.1%, miscellaneous factors for 6.6%, and unexplained for 8.8%. According to the clinical questionnaire, 77.4% of patients provided additional diagnostic information, and 89.6% of patients benefited from.

^{18}F-FDG-PET/CT is a valuable tool for clinical diagnosis of FUO/IUO. Its application in inflammatory and infectious diseases requires in-depth research and exploration. This book describes the application, basic knowledge, and typical lesions of PET/CT imaging in inflammatory diseases. It can provide help for the accurate and effective application of PET/CT imaging in inflammatory diseases, provide objective basis for the diagnosis and treatment of those patients, and further promote the wider application of related diagnostic techniques in China.

I sincerely thank Professor Hatazawa and Professor Toyama of Japan for their efforts on organization and guidance on the edition of this book. I sincerely thank all the authors from Japan and China who participate in the writing of this book.

Shenyang, Liaoning, China Yaming Li

Preface

On behalf of all the contributors to publish this textbook, I would like to express sincere gratitude to Prof. Tomio Inoue and Prof. Huang Gang who initiated the China-Japan Exchange Collaboration Program in nuclear medicine since 2011. The Program was expanding every year. Physicians, technologists, researchers, and nurses bilaterally joined more and more in any occasions of the workshop and on-site education/training in the hospitals. Under the leadership by Prof. Yaming Li, Prof. Hiroshi Toyama, and Dr. Kazuo Kubota, we came to this book, a harvest of our friendship and academic achievement.

In the 14th International Conference on Radiopharmaceutical Therapy (ICRT) held in Nanjing on August 21–24, 2019, I learned the origin of thyroid therapy conducted by Dr. Saul Hertz, Thyroid Clinic of Massachusetts General Hospital, in 1942 by means of Iodine-131 to treat hyperthyroidism and later thyroid cancer. His daughter presented the old history of radioactive iodine use for therapy by the founders of the radiopharmaceutical therapy.

This book focuses on diagnosis of "inflammation," an alternative value of FDG PET/CT. FDG applications to benign and malignant diseases are quite similar to the application of Iodine-131. It will significantly contribute to understanding of FDG PET/CT in the clinical practices and will further facilitate more cancer-specific PET tracers than ever.

Based on this achievement by clinicians and researchers in China and Japan, we together go forward to improve our specialty and to foster nuclear medicine professionals for the next generation.

Suita, Osaka, Japan | Jun Hatazawa

Preface

PET Imaging and Inflammation

Positron emission tomography–computed tomography is an advanced medical device, which is a successful clinical application of the molecular imaging technique and a good tool for the transition to clinical application from molecular biology research. Moreover, PET/CT is the true carrier of clinical medicine from experience to precision medicine. The application of ^{18}F-FDG PET (PET/CT) in tumor diagnosis, staging, and efficacy prediction and evaluation has become a clinical routine. The application of PET (PET/CT) in brain science and neuropsychiatric diseases has become another highland for the development of molecular imaging technology in the future. Many domestic and foreign scholars use PET (PET/CT) to visualize a variety of physiological, biochemical, and pathophysiological processes in humans. It is like a guiding light in the ocean of transformation of medicine, leading the course of future development of medicine.

The inflammatory reaction is a complex pathophysiological reaction of human tissues and organs to various physical, chemical, immunological, or microbial damages and is the most important adaptive process for the body defense. The inflammatory reaction could be caused by various external and internal inflammatory factors, including biological factors, physicochemical factors, and immune responses. The physiological and pathological processes of the inflammatory response mainly include alteration, exudation, and proliferation. With the development of modern molecular biology techniques, the physiological and pathological processes of inflammatory reactions have evolved from descriptive structural change of the tissues under optical microscope to the interpretation of the change and regulation of different cells and different biomolecules during the process of inflammatory reaction. Molecular imaging technology accurately and objectively visualizes the changes of different biomarkers in the inflammatory response process, helping clinical accurate diagnosis and guiding precise treatment.

^{18}F-deoxyglucose (2-deoxy-2-^{18}F-fluoro-D-glucose, ^{18}F-FDG) is the most widely used PET imaging agent. ^{18}F-FDG is a glucose analog, which will be phosphorylated to ^{18}F-FDG-6-PO4 by hexokinase and remains trapped in the cells. ^{18}F-FDG is mainly used in the clinical diagnosis, staging, and efficacy evaluation of tumor. Inflammatory cells such as macrophages will undergo "breath excitement" when functioning, and macrophages require high uptake of glucose, resulting in increased uptake of ^{18}F-FDG in the inflammatory lesions; therefore the PET imaging result will be positive [1, 2]. ^{18}F-FDG PET/CT has become a clinical routine in the search for infections in unexplained fever. Macrophages uptake glucose highly, and the molecular signaling and mechanism that induce changes in the inflammatory response process have become a hotspot in the study of inflammation and metabolism.

^{111}In-8 hydroxyquinoline (^{111}In-oxine) and 99mTc-6-methyl propylenediamine (99mTc-HMPAO)-labeled leukocytes have been widely used clinically in SPECT imaging and have obtained positive value. However, PET imaging of labeled leukocytes is still in the clinical research stage, including molecular probes labeled with different nuclides such as ^{18}F, ^{64}Cu, and 89Zr [3]. ^{68}Ga-pentixafor is used for synovial angiogenesis imaging of rheumatoid arthritis [4]. The ligand of CXCR4 and ^{68}Ga-pentixafor utilizing the specificity of CXCR4 as a radiotracer for CXCR4 expression could be used for chronic inflammation imaging of bone [5]; ^{18}F-PEG-folate for rheumatoid arthritis active imaging; and ^{124}I-FIAU for bacterial infection imaging [6].

Inflammation can also directly or indirectly lead to a variety of diseases, including atherosclerosis, autoimmune diseases, and Alzheimer's disease. ^{18}F-NaF PET-CT could be used to evaluate the microcalcifications and its levels in atherosclerotic plaques, and it is the first non-invasive imaging method to identify and locate ruptured plagues and high-risk coronary atherosclerotic plaques [7]. Other imaging agents capable of visualizing atherosclerotic plaques and predicting ruptured plaques include targeted macrophage inflammatory imaging (somatostatin receptor analog SSTR, ^{11}C-choline, ^{68}Ga-pentixafor, ^{11}C-PK11195) and inflammation and neovascular imaging agent integrin $\alpha V\beta 3$ [8, 9]. TSPO PET can be used to assess neuroinflammation and play an important role in the assessment of disease progression, prognosis, and efficacy of multiple sclerosis [10, 11].

Inflammation molecular imaging technique could provide real-time information that plays an important role in disease diagnosis, prognosis, treatment, reaction monitoring, and understanding the nature of diseases. Targeted imaging agents with different biomarkers used in PET/CT or PET/MR will also contribute to the visualization and quantitative diagnosis of inflammatory diseases. As people have a better understanding of the inflammatory response of various disease types, researchers will look for more sensitive and more specific biomarkers and develop them into new inflammatory imaging probes.

As an important monograph of PET/CT in the exploration of inflammation and mechanism, this book will provide a valuable reference for clinical medicine and basic inflammation research. I sincerely appreciate all the experts who have dedicated their time and effort to this book: your enriched experience and wisdom will enhance the value of this book.

Shanghai, China Guang Huang

References

1. Hong YH, Kong EJ. (18F)Fluoro-deoxy-D-glucose uptake of knee joints in the aspect of age-related osteoarthritis: a case-control study. BMC Musculoskelet Disord. 2013;14:141. https://doi.org/10.1186/1471-2474-14-141.
2. Kubota R, Yamada S, Kubota K, Ishiwata K, Tamahashi N, Ido T. Intratumoral distribution of fluorine-18-fluorodeoxyglucose in vivo: high accumulation in macrophages and granulation tissues studied by microautoradiography. J Nucl Med. 1992;33:1972–80.
3. Sollini M, Berchiolli R, Kirienko M, Rossi A, Glaudemans A, Slart R, et al. PET/MRI in Infection and Inflammation. Semin Nucl Med. 2018;48:225–41. https://doi.org/10.1053/j.semnuclmed.2018.02.003.
4. Zhu Z, Yin Y, Zheng K, Li F, Chen X, Zhang F, et al. Evaluation of synovial angiogenesis in patients with rheumatoid arthritis using (6)(8)Ga-PRGD2 PET/CT: a prospective proof-of-concept cohort study. Ann Rheum Dis. 2014;73:1269–72. https://doi.org/10.1136/annrheumdis-2013-204820.
5. Bouter C, Meller B, Sahlmann CO, Staab W, Wester HJ, Kropf S, et al. (68)Ga-Pentixafor PET/CT imaging of chemokine receptor CXCR4 in chronic infection of the bone: first insights. J Nucl Med. 2018;59:320–6. https://doi.org/10.2967/jnumed.117.193854.
6. Diaz LA, Jr., Foss CA, Thornton K, Nimmagadda S, Endres CJ, Uzuner O, et al. Imaging of musculoskeletal bacterial infections by [124I]FIAU-PET/CT. PLoS One. 2007;2:e1007. https://doi.org/10.1371/journal.pone.0001007.
7. Joshi NV, Vesey AT, Williams MC, Shah AS, Calvert PA, Craighead FH, et al. ^{18}F-fluoride positron emission tomography for identification of ruptured and high-risk coronary atherosclerotic plaques: a prospective clinical trial. Lancet. 2014;383:705–13. https://doi.org/10.1016/S0140-6736(13)61754-7.

8. Alie N, Eldib M, Fayad ZA, Mani V. Inflammation, atherosclerosis, and coronary artery disease: PET/CT for the evaluation of atherosclerosis and inflammation. Clin Med Insights Cardiol. 2014;8:13–21. https://doi.org/10.4137/CMC.S17063.
9. Evans NR, Tarkin JM, Chowdhury MM, Warburton EA, Rudd JH. PET Imaging of atherosclerotic disease: advancing plaque assessment from anatomy to pathophysiology. Curr Atheroscler Rep. 2016;18:30. https://doi.org/10.1007/s11883-016-0584-3.
10. Yang ZL, Zhang LJ. PET/MRI of central nervous system: current status and future perspective. Eur Radiol. 2016;26:3534–41. https://doi.org/10.1007/s00330-015-4202-5.
11. Rocchi L, Niccolini F, Politis M. Recent imaging advances in neurology. J Neurol. 2015;262:2182–94. https://doi.org/10.1007/s00415-015-7711-x.

Contents

Basic Science of PET Imaging for Inflammatory Diseases

1

Kazuo Kubota, Mikako Ogawa, Bin Ji, Tadashi Watabe, Ming-Rong Zhang, Hiromi Suzuki, Makoto Sawada, Kodai Nishi, and Takashi Kudo

1.1 Mechanisms of FDG Accumulation in Inflammation

Kazuo Kubota

Abstract FDG-PET/CT has recently emerged as a useful tool for the evaluation of inflammatory diseases too, in addition to that of malignant diseases. The imaging is based on active glucose utilization by inflammatory tissue. Autoradiography studies have demonstrated high FDG uptake in macrophages, granulocytes, fibroblasts, and granulation tissue. Especially, activated macrophages are responsible for the elevated FDG uptake in some types of inflammation. According to one study, after activation by lipopolysaccharide of cultured macrophages, the [^{14}C]2DG uptake by the cells doubled, reaching the level seen in glioblastoma cells. In activated macrophages, increase in the expression of total GLUT1 and redistributions from the intracellular compartments toward the cell surface have been reported. In one rheumatoid arthritis model, following stimulation by hypoxia or TNF-α, the highest elevation of the [^{3}H]FDG uptake was observed in the fibroblasts, followed by that in macrophages and neutrophils. As the fundamental mechanism of elevated glucose uptake in both cancer cells and inflammatory cells, activation of glucose metabolism as an adaptive response to a hypoxic environment has been reported, with transcription factor HIF-1α playing a key role. Inflammatory cells and cancer cells seem to share the same molecular mechanism of elevated glucose metabolism, lending support to the notion of usefulness of FDGPET/CT for the evaluation of inflammatory diseases, besides cancer.

Keywords: Macrophage, Neutrophil, Fibroblast, Granulation tissue, GLUT, HIF-1α, FDG

1.1.1 Introduction

Fluorine-18-labeled 2-deoxy-2-fluoro-glucose (FDG) is used as a radiopharmaceutical in PET for evaluating glucose metabolism, and accumulates in malignant tissues because of the enhanced glucose utilization by neoplastic cells. Because of the increased metabolic demand for glucose,

K. Kubota (✉)
Department of Radiology, Southern TOHOKU General Hospital, Koriyama, Fukushima, Japan
e-mail: kkubota@cpost.plala.or.jp

M. Ogawa
Laboratory of Bioanalysis and Molecular Imaging, Graduate School of Pharmaceutical Sciences, Hokkaido University, Sapporo, Hokkaido, Japan
e-mail: mogawa@pharm.hokudai.ac.jp

B. Ji
Department of Functional Brain Imaging Research (DOFI), National Institute of Radiological Sciences, National Institutes for Quantum and Radiological Science and Technology, Chiba, Japan
e-mail: Ji.bin@qst.go.jp

T. Watabe
Department of Nuclear Medicine and Tracer Kinetics, Osaka University Graduate School of Medicine, Osaka, Japan
e-mail: watabe@tracer.med.osaka-u.ac.jp

M.-R. Zhang
Department of Radiopharmaceuticals Development, National Institute of Radiological Sciences, National Institutes for Quantum and Radiological Science and Technology, Chiba, Japan
e-mail: zhang.ming-rong@qst.go.jp

H. Suzuki · M. Sawada
Division of Stress Adaptation and Protection, Department of Brain Function, Research Institute of Environmental Medicine, Nagoya University, Nagoya, Aichi, Japan
e-mail: hiromi_s@riem.nagoya-u.ac.jp; msawada@riem.nagoya-u.ac.jp

K. Nishi · T. Kudo
Department of Radioisotope Medicine, Atomic Bomb Disease Institute, Nagasaki University, Nagasaki, Japan
e-mail: koudai@nagasaki-u.ac.jp; tkudo123@nagasaki-u.ac.jp

H. Toyama et al. (eds.), *PET/CT for Inflammatory Diseases*, https://doi.org/10.1007/978-981-15-0810-3_1

elevated activity of hexokinase and elevated expression of glucose transporter have been shown in tumor tissues [1]. Various applications of FDG-PET have been extensively studied in the field of clinical oncology, and the imaging modality, now used worldwide, is recognized as a powerful diagnostic modality for cancer [2, 3]. In 1989, elevated FDG uptake was reported in two patients with abdominal abscesses [4]. This was followed by reports of FDG uptake in brain abscess [5], tuberculosis, aspergillosis, sarcoidosis, and so on. In addition, early postoperative scarring and early inflammatory reactions after radiotherapy were also reported to show increased FDG uptake. Thus, elevation in glucose metabolism is not only specific for cancer but also seen in inflammation. Because FDG uptake is seen in benign inflammatory diseases as well, the accuracy of FDG-PET for the diagnosis of cancer is not 100% [6].

1.1.2 FDG Uptake by Inflammatory Tissues and Cells

Although the metabolic fate of FDG is well known, its cellular distribution within tumors or sites of inflammation has not yet been described. To clarify the mechanisms of FDG uptake by inflammatory and tumor tissues, we performed autoradiographic studies. To demonstrate the cellular localization of FDG and [^{3}H]2DG uptake by tumors in vivo, C3H/He mice with subcutaneously transplanted FM3A tumors were studied 1 h after intravenous injection of FDG or [^{3}H]2DG. Newly formed granulation tissue around tumors and macrophages, which had massively infiltrated the marginal areas surrounding the necrotic areas of the tumor, showed a higher FDG uptake than the viable tumor cells. A maximum of 24% of the glucose utilization was derived from the non-neoplastic tissues in these tumors (Fig. 1.1). The strong accumulation of FDG in these tumors was thought to represent both the high metabolic activity of the viable tumor cells and that of the tumor-associated inflammatory cells, especially activated macrophages. These results indicate that not only glucose uptake by the tumor cells but also that by non-neoplastic cellular elements which appear in association with the growth or necrosis of tumor cells should be considered for a precise analysis of FDG uptake in tumors, especially after radiotherapy (Fig. 1.2) [7, 8].

FDG uptake by inflammatory tissues was investigated by Yamada et al. [9]. A rat model of chemically induced inflammation using turpentine oil was used. A time-course study of the FDG tissue distribution showed that the uptake of FDG

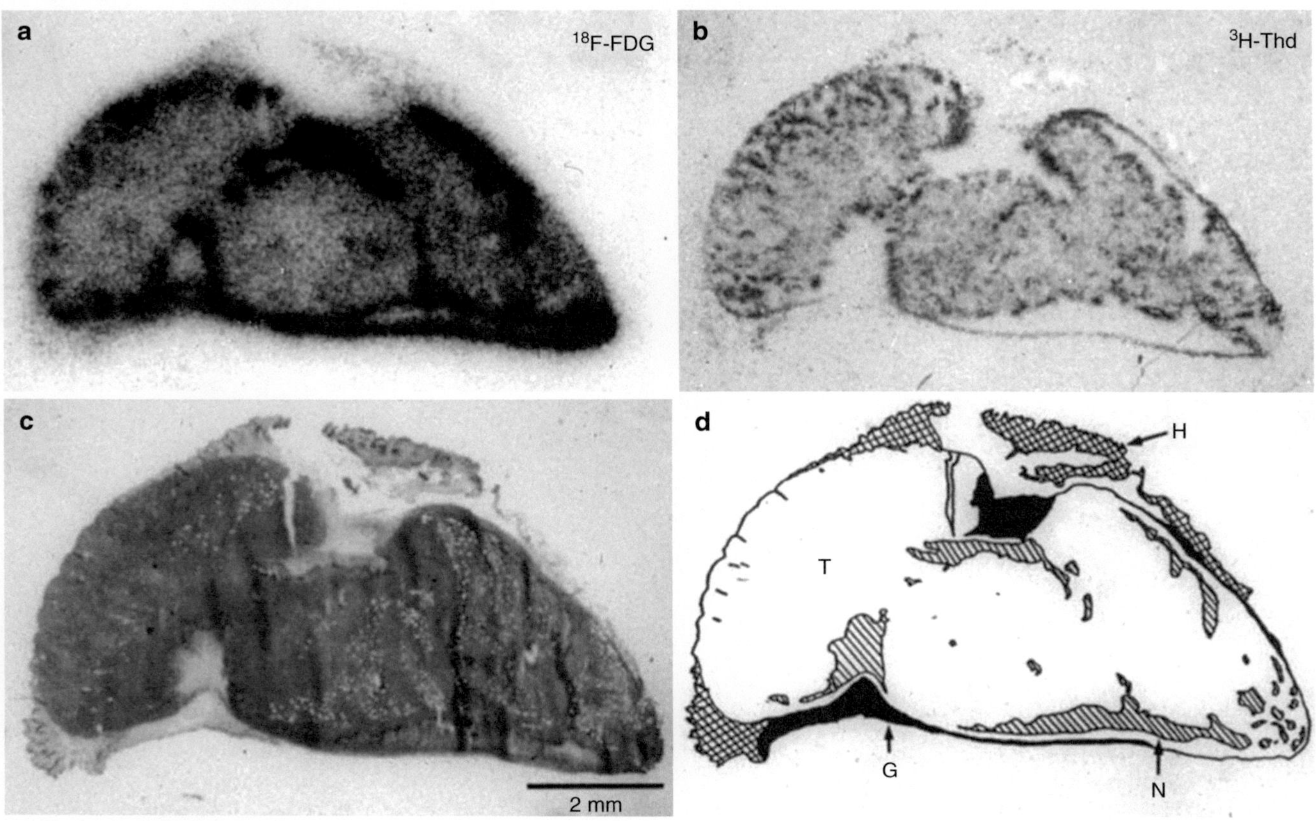

Fig. 1.1 A combination of double-tracer macro-autoradiograms and microscopy. Images of 18F-FDG distribution (**a**) and 3HThd (**b**), a photomicrograph of the tissue specimen (**c**) and an illustration of the micrograph (**d**). *T* tumor calls, *G* granulation tissue, *N* necrosis, *H* host normal tissue. Scale bar: 2 mm. Newly formed granulation tissue around the tumor and macrophages infiltrating the periphery of the necrotic areas of the tumor showed higher uptakes of FDG than the viable tumor cells. (From Ref. [7])

in inflammatory tissue increased gradually until 60 min, followed by a steady decrease thereafter. A longitudinal study showed that the uptake increased progressively after the start of inflammation, peaking at 4 days after the inoculation, and then gradually decreased (Fig. 1.3). These findings suggested that FDG uptake may reach a maximum during the subacute phase of inflammation, and then slightly decreases during the chronic phase of inflammation. An autoradiography study showed a high FDG uptake in the abscess wall, consisting of an inflammatory cell layer and granulation tissue. At the cellular level, the highest radioactivity was found in the marginal zone that contained young fibroblasts, endothelial cells of vessels, and phagocytes consisting of neutrophils and macrophages, followed by that in the neutrophil layer and the granulation tissue layer (Fig. 1.4). FDG uptake by inflammatory tissue seems to represent the activity of immune cells and fibroblasts mobilized to the lesion.

Mochizuki et al. [10] compared the FDG uptake by experimental hepatoma and by tissue with experimental infection with *Staphylococcus aureus*. The expressions of GLUT1 and GLUT3 were also studied in both the tumor and infected tissue by immunostaining. Uptake by the tumor tissue was significantly higher than that by the infected tissue. Both the tumor and infected tissue showed strong expression of GLUT1 and GLUT 3, although the expression level of GLUT1 was significantly higher in the tumor than in the infected tissue. GLUT1 may be responsible for FDG uptake in both tumor tissue and infected tissue.

Zhao et al. [11] compared the two models of inflammation: BCG-induced granuloma simulating sarcoidosis and

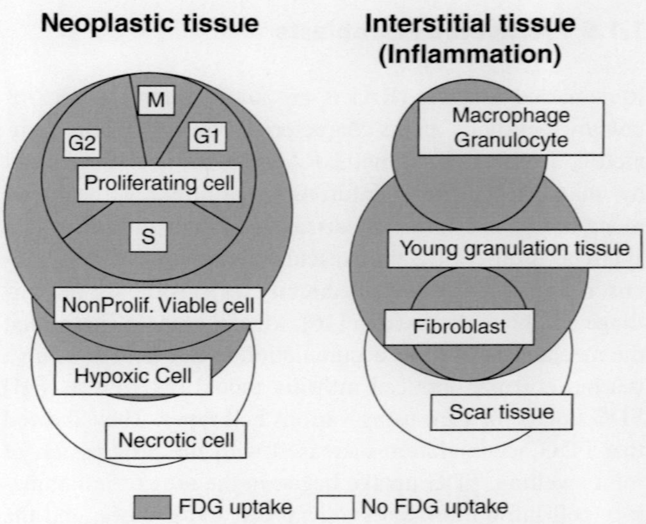

Fig. 1.2 A model of FDG accumulation in various cellular elements in a tumor. (Modified from Ref. [8])

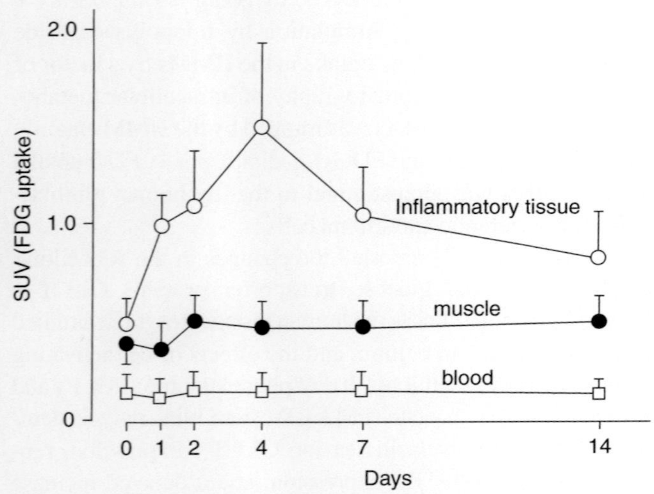

Fig. 1.3 FDG uptake changes along with the age of inflammation. FDG uptake by inflammatory tissue, muscle, and blood are plotted against the days after inoculation of turpentine oil. The highest uptake by inflammatory tissue was observed on day 4, which represented the subacute phase histologically ($n = 5$, each point). (From Ref. [9])

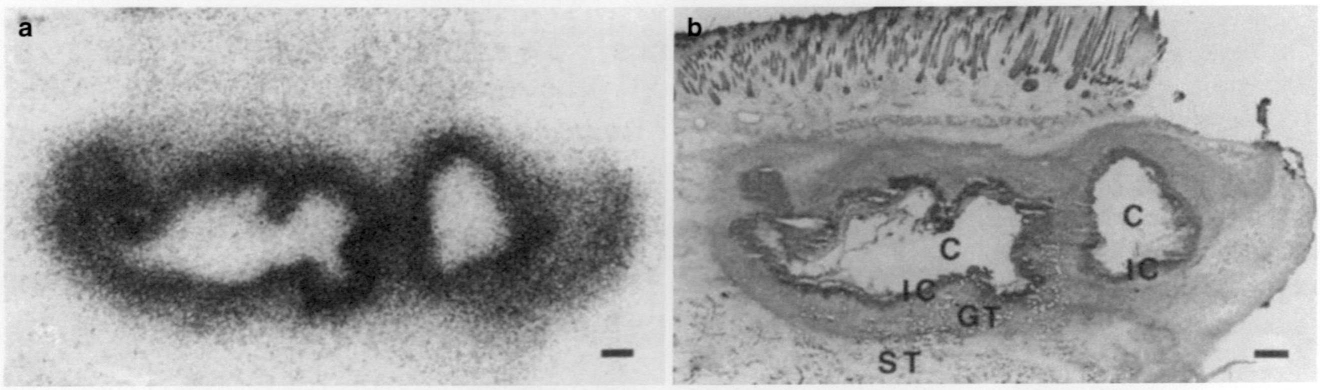

Fig. 1.4 Macro-autoradiogram (**a**) and the corresponding section (**b**) of inflammatory tissue 4 days after inoculation of turpentine oil. The center (C), surrounded by inflammatory cells (IC), thick granulation tissue (GT), and edematous subcutaneous tissue (ST). Scale bar 0.4 mm. (From Ref. [9])

turpentine oil-induced inflammation. FDG uptake by the granuloma was significantly higher than that by the tissue with chemical-induced inflammation. Their results explained the very high FDG uptake in sarcoidosis, equivalent to the uptake in cancer. However, the main objective of their study was not to compare the models of inflammation, but to compare the uptakes of ^{14}C-methionine, ^{18}F-fluorothymidine, and FDG. ^{14}C-methionine showed the best results for discrimination between tumor and inflammation.

1.1.3 Activated Macrophages and GLUT

Deichen et al. [12] studied the uptake of FDG in isolated human monocyte-macrophages (HMMs) in vitro. FDG uptake by the HMMs increased significantly with the duration of culture, the percent ID/100 μg being 7.5% ± 0.9% (% ID/100 μg) on day 14. Stimulation by lipopolysaccharide further enhanced the FDG uptake in the HMMs by a factor of 2. Radio-thin layer chromatography of intracellular metabolites revealed that the FDG was trapped by the HMMs mainly as FDG-6-phosphate and FDG-1,6-diphosphate. FDG uptake by the HMMs was almost equal to that by human glioblastoma and pancreatic carcinoma cells.

Malide et al. [13] reported the changes in the subcellular localization of the glucose transporter proteins GLUT-1, GLUT-3, and GLUT-5 as the human monocytes differentiated into macrophages in culture, and the effects of the activating agents *N*-formyl-methionyl-leucylphenylalanine (fMLP) and phorbol myristate acetate (PMA). Western blot analysis demonstrated progressively increasing GLUT-1 expression, rapidly decreasing GLUT-3 expression, and a delayed increase of the GLUT-5 expression during the differentiation process. Confocal microscopy revealed that each isoform exhibited a unique subcellular distribution and cell-activation response. GLUT-1 was localized primarily at the cell surface, but was also detected in the perinuclear region, in a pattern characteristic of recycling endosomes. Activation with fMLP induced similar GLUT-1 and GLUT-5 redistributions from the intracellular compartments toward the cell surface. Addition of PMA elicited a similar translocation of GLUT-1, but GLUT-5 was redistributed from the plasma membrane to a distinct intracellular compartment that appeared connected to the cell surface. These results suggest specific subcellular targeting of each transporter isoform and differential regulation of their trafficking pathways in cultured macrophages.

1.1.4 Activated Neutrophils

Not only macrophages but also neutrophil granulocytes play a key role in the pathogenesis of various types of inflammation. Jones et al. [14] studied [^{3}H]DG uptake in neutrophils isolated from human peripheral blood. They found elevated uptake of [^{3}H]DG by neutrophils, both after priming with tumor necrotic factor-alpha (TNF-α) and after activation with fMLP. It was not correlated with the respiratory burst or secretory activity, but may reflect the polarization and migrational status of these cells. Their study suggested that as far as neutrophils are concerned, priming is the cellular event predominantly responsible for the FDG uptake. Ishimori et al. [15] studied immunocompetent BALB/c mice and nude mice administered an intravenous injection of 10 mg/kg of concanavalin A (Con A). After the injection, the Con A-activated lymphocytes actively took up FDG both in vitro and in vivo, and FDG specifically accumulated in the tissues showing Con A-mediated acute inflammation in the immunocompetent mice.

1.1.5 Activated Fibroblasts

Rheumatoid arthritis (RA) is an autoimmune disorder of unknown etiology and is characterized by systematic, symmetric, and erosive synovitis. RA synovitis is characterized by massive leukocyte infiltration, proliferative synovial membranes, and neovascularization, which give rise to a synovial proliferative fibrovascular tissue known as a pannus. Formation of pannus is directly responsible for the cartilage and bone destruction [16]. Matsui et al. [17] reported the mechanism of FDG accumulation in RA in vivo using a murine collagen-induced arthritis model, as well as [^{3}H] FDG uptake in vitro using various cell types. They showed that FDG accumulation increased with the progression of joint swelling. FDG uptake began in the area of inflammatory cell infiltration and synovial cell hyperplasia, and the areas showing strong FDG uptake often coincided with the areas where mixed cellular patterns of macrophages and fibroblasts as well as bone destruction by mature osteoclasts were visible. These findings indicated that FDG accumulation reflected the characteristic changes of pathological progression, such as pannus formation and bone destruction. Based on the findings of in vitro experiments, Matsui et al. suggested that the cell types responsible for FDG uptake were mostly proliferating fibroblasts, with lesser contributions from activated macrophages. FDG uptake by fibroblasts was enhanced in the presence of cytokine stimulation and hypoxia within a joint. Hypoxia is a known feature of the microenvironment in inflamed joints [18]. Recently, Garcia-Carbonell et al. directly compared fibroblast-like synoviocytes (FLS) from RA patients and osteoarthritis patients [19]. In vitro experiments have shown that the FLS from RA patients were dependent on glycolysis rather than on oxidative phosphorylation, and this difference was more pronounced than that for the FLS from osteoarthritis patients. The expression of GLUT-1 messenger RNA was correlated with the functions of the FLS from the RA patients. These studies showed the importance of fibroblasts in the inflammation in RA.

1.1.6 Contribution of HIF-1α

Recently, the processes, at the molecular level, occurring in association with hypoxia and glucose metabolism within tumor and inflammatory tissues have been described. Cramer et al. reported that activation of hypoxia-inducible factor one-alpha (HIF-1α) is essential for myeloid cell infiltration and activation in vivo [20]. They showed that HIF-1α is essential for regulation of the glycolytic capacity of myeloid cells; when HIF-1α is knocked out, the cellular ATP pool decreases drastically. This metabolic defect results in a profound impairment of myeloid cell aggregation, motility, invasiveness, and bacterial killing at sites of inflammation where the tissue environment is hypoxic. Thus, HIF-1α has a direct regulatory effect on both the survival and functioning of cells in inflammatory microenvironments. Furthermore, the enhanced glycolysis in activated macrophages results in elevation of the FDG uptake. Regarding the molecular mechanisms responsible for the regulation of glycolysis, HIF-1α affects both glucose transporter and hexokinase expressions in tumors and inflamed tissues.

The significance of hypoxia in tumor pathophysiology has also been described by Denko [21]. Usually, proliferation of cancer cells is faster than the growth of capillaries, resulting in inadequate perfusion and hypoxia within the tumor. Activation of HIF-1α in the hypoxic tumor shifts the energy metabolism from oxidative phosphorylation to anaerobic glycolysis, saves oxygen, and avoids massive cell death. As a result of the elevated glucose metabolism, FDG-PET serves as a useful imaging modality for cancer patients.

1.1.7 Conclusion

Dominant inflammatory cells activated and responsible for FDG uptake in inflammatory diseases may differ depending upon the disease. All inflammatory cells and cancer cells seem to share the same molecular mechanism of elevated glucose metabolism, lending support to the idea of the usefulness of FDGPET/CT also for the evaluation of inflammatory diseases, besides cancer. Although a guideline [22] has been proposed, use of FDGPET/CT for inflammatory diseases is still limited. I hope that this book will help spread knowledge about the application of FDGPET/CT for inflammatory diseases to improve patient management, representing an advance in the field of medicine.

Acknowledgement
I would like to thank Roko Kubota, PhD, and Susumu Yamada, MD, PhD, for their comments and contribution to our research works that reviewed here.

1.2 FDG PET Imaging of Inflammation in Atherosclerosis

Mikako Ogawa

Abstract A vulnerable plaque is characterized by a large lipid-rich atheromatous core, a thin fibrous cap, and infiltration by inflammatory cells (e.g., macrophages). The rupture of high-risk, vulnerable plaques can cause thrombosis, the main cause of acute myocardial infarction and stroke. Thus, the detection of vulnerable plaques is clinically important for risk stratification and early administration of treatment. Macrophages play a central role in the destabilization of atherosclerotic lesions. Macrophages are metabolically active; therefore, these plaques can be detected by FDG-PET. Thus far, numerous clinical and basic research studies have been performed to investigate the effectiveness of FDG-PET for the imaging of vulnerable plaques. In addition, it was revealed that the foam cell formation of macrophages affects the accumulation of FDG. Notably, FDG accumulates in pro-atherogenic M1 macrophages rather than anti-inflammatory M2 macrophages. Therefore, assessing the effect of drugs in individual patients is important to monitor the therapeutic effect. Moreover, numerous studies have shown that FDG-PET is useful in evaluating the therapeutic effect of drugs.

Keywords: Macrophage, Atherosclerosis, Vulnerable plaque, FDG-PET

1.2.1 Introduction

Atherosclerotic plaques are classified into two types: stable and vulnerable. Vulnerable plaques are easy to rupture and may cause stroke and heart attack. Therefore, the prompt detection and treatment of vulnerable plaques, prior to the manifestation of symptoms, is of crucial importance. Vulnerable plaques are characterized by a lipid-rich atheromatous core, which is infiltrated by macrophages. There is a correlation between the number of infiltrating macrophages and the severity of symptoms in acute myocardial infarction [23, 24]. In contrast, infiltration by macrophages is rarely observed in stable plaques.

Macrophages are active in energy metabolism. Therefore, FDG-PET is a promising tool for the detection of vulnerable plaques, depending on the extent of macrophage infiltration.

1.2.2 Uptake of FDG in Vulnerable Plaques

Thus far, numerous clinical and nonclinical studies have investigated the use of FDG for the imaging of vulnerable plaques. In 1994, Kubota et al. demonstrated that FDG accumulated more in macrophages than in tumor cells [25]. Therefore, it is assumed that vulnerable plaques can be detected depending on the rate of macrophage infiltration in the plaque. In the early 2000s, several clinical studies suggested that it is possible to detect atherosclerosis, according to the level of inflammation [26–28]. Notably, through histological analysis of symptomatic carotid artery plaques, Rudd et al. reported the co-localization of [^{3}H]FDG and macrophages [27].

The investigators examined the relationship between the degree of macrophage infiltration and accumulation of FDG in Watanabe heritable hyperlipidemic (WHHL) rabbits—an arteriosclerotic animal model—, and explored the possibility of detection of vulnerable plaques using FDG-PET [29]. The atherosclerotic plaques were detected by FDG-PET (Fig. 1.5). In WHHL rabbits, thickening of the intima and infiltration by macrophages was observed in all individuals. We examined the degree of macrophage filtration via histological analysis. The results showed that the FDG uptake and number of macrophages in the atherosclerotic lesions were strongly correlated (Fig. 1.6). However, there was no correlation between the degree of macrophage infiltration and that of intimal thickening. These results suggested that macrophages are responsible for the accumulation of FDG in atherosclerotic lesions, and vulnerable plaques may be detected through FDG-PET.

Studies in humans have shown that the uptake of FDG into vulnerable plaques correlates with the infiltration by macrophages [30, 31]. Immunohistochemical staining of macrophage marker CD68 revealed a strong correlation with FDG accumulation. It has also been reported that the incorporation of Matrix Metalloproteinase-1—an enzyme involved in the destabilization of plaques—and FDG are strongly related [32]. Tahara et al. reported correlations between the accumulation of FDG and waist circumference, hypertension, insulin resistance, lowering of high-density lipoprotein cholesterol, etc. [33]. A recent study showed a correlation of FDG accumulation with C-reactive protein [34]. The results of these studies indicate the prospect for the use of FDG-PET in arteriosclerosis-related diseases.

1.2.3 Foam Cell Formation and FDG Uptake

Foam cell formation is responsible for the vulnerability of plaques. Macrophages are recruited from blood monocytes that enter through the endothelium (Fig. 1.7). Scavenger receptors on macrophages mediate the uptake of oxidized low-density lipoprotein (LDL) and cause the accumulation of LDL-derived cholesterol and foam cell formation. Foam cells release several proteases and cytokines, which lead to rupture of the plaques. We evaluated the effects of foam cell formation on the uptake of FDG [35]. Macrophages were isolated from the peritoneum cavity of mice, and foam cells

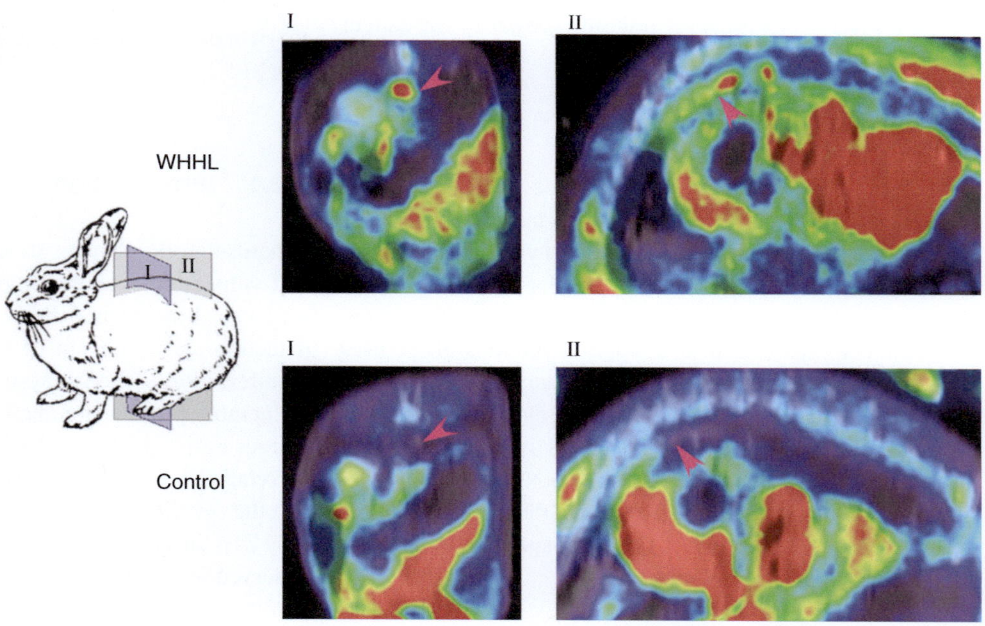

Fig. 1.5 Fused PET-CT images of WHHL and control rabbits. The WHHL rabbit is an animal model of atherosclerosis. The pink arrowheads show the aortas. The aorta was clearly imaged using FDG in WHHL rabbits

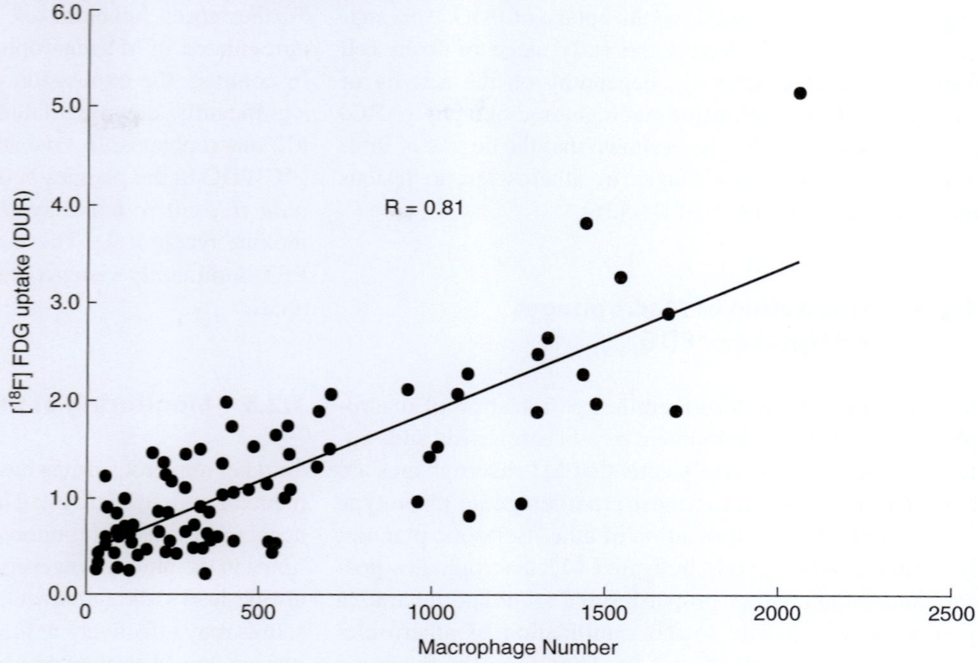

$$\text{DUR} = \frac{\text{tissue activity (Bq) / tissue weight (mg)}}{\text{injected RI activity (Bq) / animal body weight (kg)}}$$

Fig. 1.6 Correlation between the uptake of FDG and the number of macrophages in the aortic segments of WHHL rabbits. The uptake of FDG was well correlated with the degree of macrophage infiltration. *DUR* differential uptake ratio

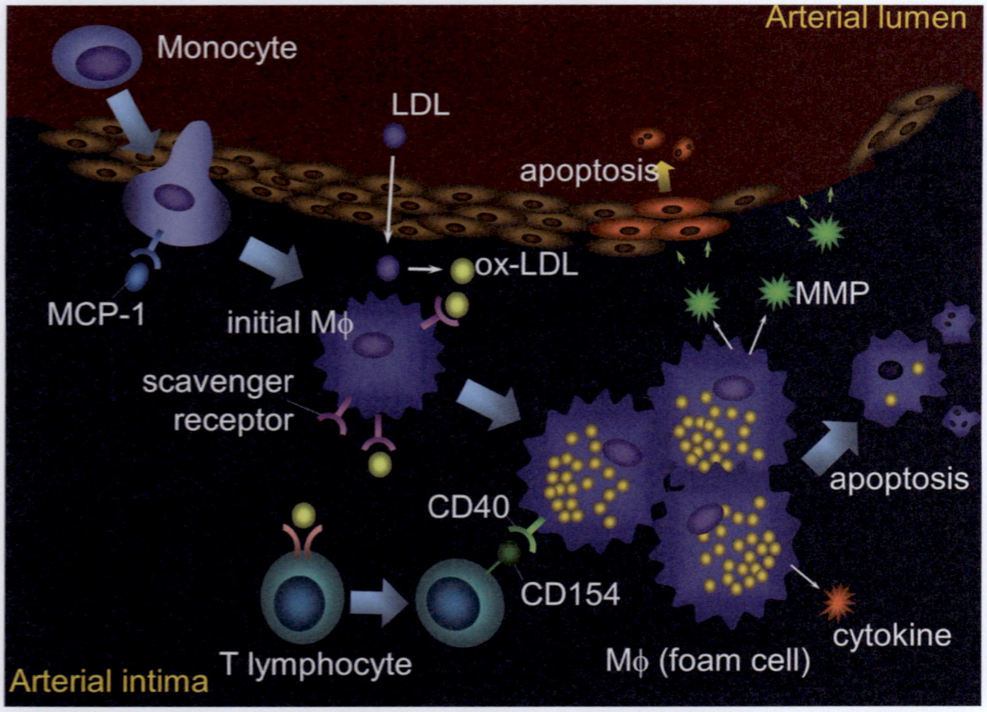

Fig. 1.7 Scheme of the development of vulnerable atherosclerotic plaques. Monocytes differentiate into macrophages, and foam cells are formed through stimulation of a scavenger receptor by oxidized low-density lipoprotein (ox-LDL)

were induced by acetylated LDL. The accumulation of FDG was increased via foam cell formation. However, the uptake was decreased to the level of control, following the complete differentiation into foam cells. The activity of hexokinase was changed in parallel with the uptake of FDG, i.e., higher activity was observed 24 h after acetylated-LDL loading versus the control condition. Of note, the observed changes in glucose-6-phosphatase activity and glucose transporter 1 expression were not parallel to the uptake of FDG. This suggests that FDG-PET detects the early stage of foam cell formation in atherosclerosis, depending on the activity of hexokinase. Moreover, using microautoradiography (ARG) in WHHL rabbits, it has been shown that the degree of infiltration by foamy macrophages in atherosclerotic lesions relates to the uptake of [^{3}H]FDG [36].

1.2.4 Polarization of Macrophages and Uptake of FDG

Recent studies have described that polarization of macrophages affects the development of atherosclerosis and rupture of plaques. Classically activated M1 macrophages are considered to possess the most proatherogenic phenotype and promote the destabilization of atherosclerotic plaques. In contrast, alternatively activated M2 macrophages possess anti-inflammatory properties and stimulate reparative processes, which lead to the stabilization of atherosclerotic plaques [37, 38] (Fig. 1.8). Therefore, the detection of M1 macrophages may assist in predicting cardiovascular events with greater accuracy. In our investigation, M1 macrophages showed a 2.6-fold increased uptake of [^{3}H]FDG versus M2 macrophages [39]. Glucose transporter (GLUT)-1 and GLUT-3, which are major isoforms of a glucose transporter in macrophages, were significantly upregulated in M1 macrophages versus M2 macrophages.

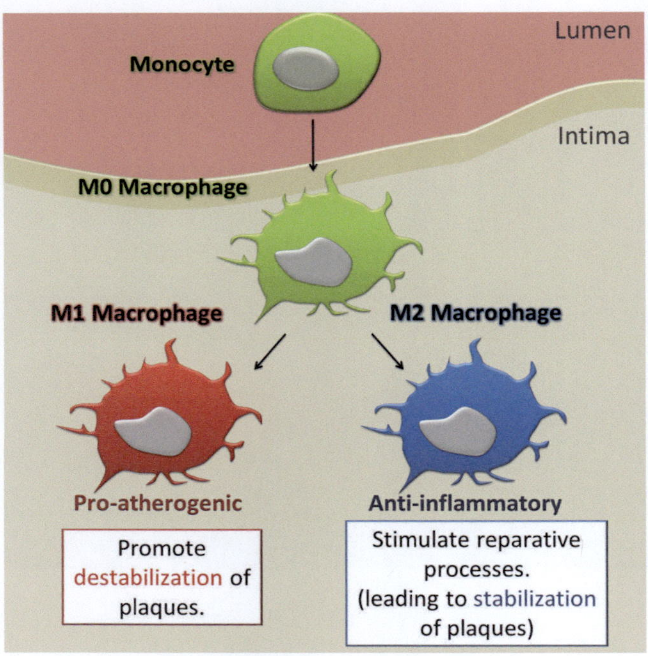

Fig. 1.8 Polarization of macrophages in vulnerable atherosclerotic plaques. M1 macrophages promote the destabilization of plaques, whereas M2 macrophages lead to the stabilization of plaques

Furthermore, hexokinases 1 and 2 were significantly upregulated in M1 macrophages versus M2 macrophages. In contrast, the expression of glucose-6-phosphatase was significantly downregulated in M1 macrophages versus M2 macrophages. In vivo studies showed accumulation of [^{14}C]FDG in the plaques and elevation of M1 markers (i.e., *inducible nitric oxide synthase*, interleukin-1b, and chemokine receptor 7). These results suggest that [^{18}F]FDG-PET dominantly visualizes the M1 macrophage-infiltrated areas.

1.2.5 Monitoring of the Therapeutic Effect

To date, numerous drugs have been developed for the treatment of atherosclerosis. The therapeutic effects of these agents are usually monitored by determining the levels of lipids in the blood. However, lipid-lowering therapy does not always lead to the stabilization of vulnerable plaques. Several statins may effectively reduce the levels of cholesterol in the plasma; however, they do not decrease the degree of macrophage infiltration [40, 41]. Thus, merely monitoring the levels of lipids in the plasma is not sufficient to determine the therapeutic effect of drugs. Macrophage infiltration plays an essential role in the rupture of plaques. Therefore, the administration of pharmacological therapy that reduces macrophage infiltration is required to stabilize the vulnerable plaques. Considering the individual differences in the stabilization of plaques induced by such drugs, monitoring the therapeutic effect in each individual plaque is important to accurately assess the effect.

Using probucol as a therapeutic drug in WHHL rabbits, we investigated the usefulness of FDG-PET for the monitoring of therapies that target vascular inflammation. In a number of animal studies, the lipid-lowering effect of probucol was moderate, and the drug did not decrease the levels of cholesterol in the plasma [42, 43]. However, probucol can reduce the macrophage-rich plaques even in advanced atherosclerotic lesions [43]. In the present study, the uptake of FDG was significantly decreased in the probucol group versus the pretreatment period (Fig. 1.9). However, there was no difference in the levels of cholesterol in the plasma between the probucol and control groups [44]. A large number of macrophages was observed at the initiation of the study. Nevertheless, treatment with probucol for 6 months resulted in diminished macrophage infiltration (Fig. 1.10). Notably, the ratio of the intima to the whole cross-sectional area was not affected by treatment with probucol. Hence, the observed decrease in the uptake of FDG was attributed to the decrease in the number of infiltrating macrophages. Collectively, these studies showed that the therapeutic effect of probucol was successfully monitored by FDG-PET independently of the cholesterol-lowering effect.

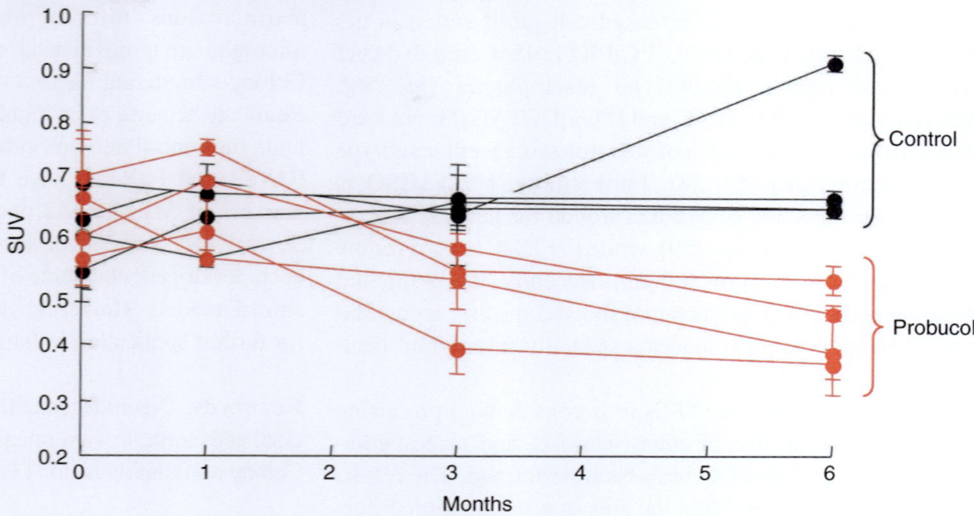

Fig. 1.9 Time course of the uptake of FDG in the aortas of WHHL rabbits over the treatment period. After 3 months of treatment with probucol, the uptake of FDG (SUV) decreased in all treated rabbits. In contrast, the SUV remained constant or increased in control rabbits

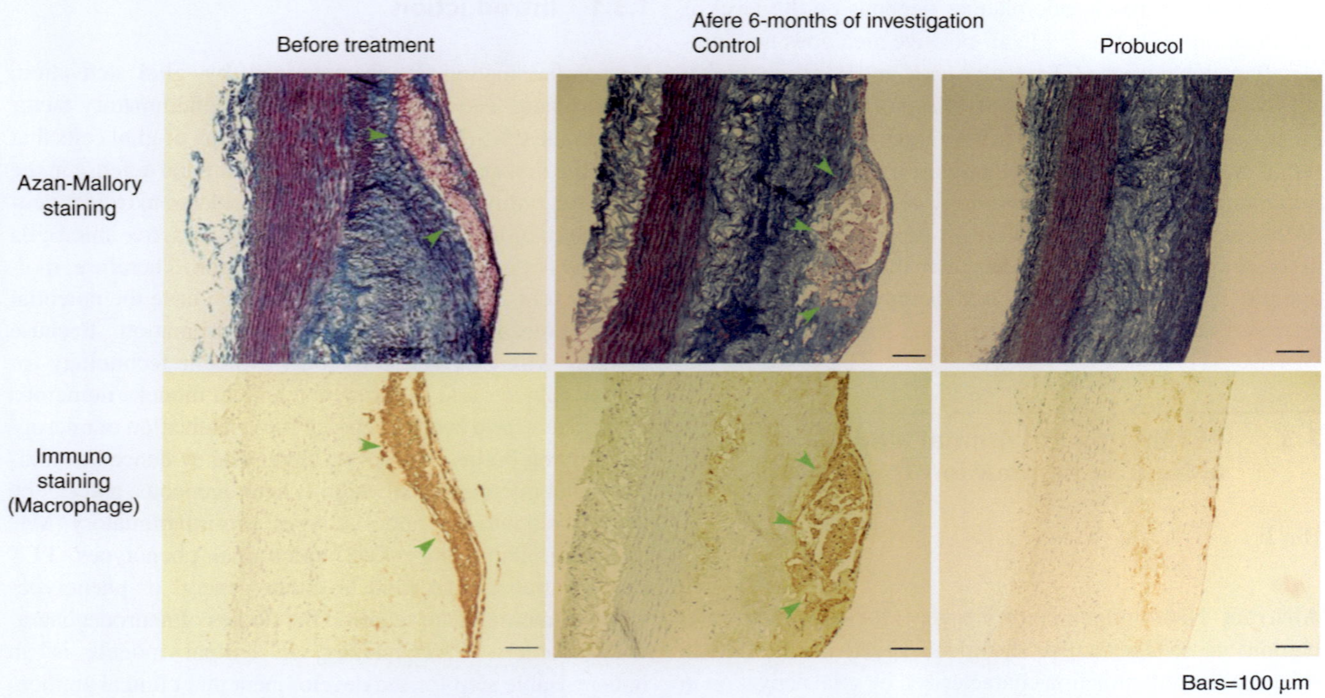

Fig. 1.10 Typical histological images of Azan–Mallory-stained and macrophage immunohistochemically stained slices. Green arrow heads indicate macrophages. Treatment with probucol resulted in diminished macrophage infiltration

These results demonstrated the usefulness of FDG-PET for drug development, and numerous clinical studies have been performed [45–49]. Tahara et al. conducted one of the initial clinical trials, showing that the therapeutic effect of simvastatin was successfully monitored by FDG-PET [50]. In 2011, the results of the first clinical multicenter study investigating the efficacy of dalcetrapib against atherosclerotic disease via a novel noninvasive multimodality imaging technique (dal-PLAQUE) were reported. Of note, FDG-PET was used to evaluate the level of vascular inflammation [51]. Moreover, in the dal-PLAQUE study, the relationship between serum inflammatory biomarkers and plaque inflammation was also assessed using FDG-PET [52].

1.2.6 Comparison with Other PET Tracers

Recently, several PET imaging tracers—apart from FDG—have been reported for the imaging of vulnerable plaques. For example, [^{11}C]choline and [^{18}F]fluoromethylcholine are used for the detection of increased cell proliferation in the plaques [53, 54]. In addition, [^{11}C]PK11195 is used to detect translocator protein (TSPO) on macrophages [55, 56]. Moreover, [^{68}Ga]DOTATOC and [^{68}Ga]DOTATATE are used to determine the expression of somatostatin receptor subtype 2 on macrophages [57, 58]. Furthermore, [^{18}F]FMISO is used for the detection of hypoxia around the neovascularization area near the plaques [59], while [^{18}F]NaF is used for the detection of calcification [60–63]. Recently, the β-amyloid imaging agent [^{18}F]Flutemetamol showed specific accumulation in human carotid plaques, especially in amyloid beta-positive areas [64].

Among these tracers, [^{18}F]NaF is considered a promising probe for the detection of atherosclerosis, and several comparison studies with FDG have been performed. The results of these studies showed that the area of accumulation differs between FDG and [^{18}F]NaF [65–67]. The accumulation of [^{18}F]NaF in atherosclerotic plaques depends on the level of calcification [68]. The [^{18}F]NaF-positive area does not completely match with the CT-positive area, and it is thought that [^{18}F]NaF accumulates in the early stage of calcification (i.e., microcalcification) [60, 69]. Since target molecules are different among these tracers, comparison study should be important to elucidate the specificity of these tracers for the different stages of atherosclerosis progression. This may assist in understanding the mechanism of plaque progression and provide important insight into therapy aimed toward the stabilization of plaques.

1.3 PET Imaging in Animal Model of Neuroinflammation 1

Bin Ji

Abstract Neuroinflammation is a general event in acute and chronic neurodegenerative disorders. Based on the critical role of neuroinflammation characterized by glial activation in neuropathogenesis, in vivo imaging with positron emission tomography (PET) is required in clinical and preclinical studies for the purposes of elucidation of pathogenesis and novel treatment development, because it is commonly available in human and experimental animal models. As a most widely used imaging biomarker for neuroinflammation, 18 kDa translocator protein (TSPO) imaging has been performed in a large number clinical and preclinical studies. Neuropathology-associated TSPO induction has been generally detected in various neurodegenerative animal models with acute and chronic neuroinflammation. However, studies with human subjects showed confusing results likely due to ineffectiveness of the tracers used or impediment of non-microglial TSPO expression in human diseased brains. Based on the above reasons, recently, alternative molecular targets for microglia imaging instead of TSPO have been proposed. Colony-stimulating factor 1 receptor (CSF1R) is a promising candidate because of its highly specific expression in microglia in the central nervous system (CNS). Purinergic receptors P2X7R and P2Y12R have been proposed as imaging biomarkers of M1 and M2 phenotype microglia, respectively. Several PET tracers for these non-TSPO biomarkers have been developed, and some of them showed positive results in animal models. However, more exploratory work is needed for further application in human subjects.

Keywords: Neurodegenerative disorders, Neuroinflammation, Glial activation, In vivo imaging, 18 kDa translocator (TSPO), Colony-stimulating factor 1 receptor (CSF1R)

1.3.1 Introduction

Neuroinflammation is characterized by glial activation, which would lead to an increase in the inflammatory factor level in the CNS. Microglia are a collection of glial cells that act as the first and main form of active immune defense in the CNS. Accordingly, its activation is considered to trigger neuroinflammation, and PET tracers bound to active microglia are used for imaging of neuroinflammation. Therefore, molecules exclusively expressed in microglia have the potential to be molecular targets for neuroinflammation. Because imaging with PET is a commonly available technology for human subjects and experimental animal models, numerous PET tracers have been developed for visualization of microglia in living brains. Moreover, increasing evidence has indicated that microglial activation is heterogeneous, and can be categorized into two opposite types: pro-inflammatory (M1) and anti-inflammatory (M2) microglial phenotypes. PET imaging tracers that bind to either general or phenotype-specific microglia are required for studies of neurodegenerative disorders. PET imaging in animal models is an indispensable step for the development and clinical application of PET tracers, as it will provide predictive evidence for tracer utility in human subjects. More importantly, it can easily provide a direct comparison between PET images and histopathology, which is usually difficult in human studies. PET imaging in animal models would supplement the weak points of human studies and provide interpretation for imaging in human subjects.

1.3.2 Current Standard of Neuroinflammation Imaging

18 kDa Translocator protein (TSPO) is a housekeeping protein in microglia and is greatly induced in active microglia in

response to neural injury. PET tracers with high affinity for TSPO are the most widely used for neuroinflammation imaging. Tracers have been developed for TSPO imaging for several decades, including typical first-generation tracer ^{11}C-PK11195 and second-generation tracer ^{11}C-DAA1106 [70]. Major parts of these tracers enable the visualization of microglial activation in acute neuroinflammation models triggered by acute events like traumatic brain injury, ischemia, and excitotoxic damages. A longitudinal PET imaging study has shown a continuing increased TSPO PET tracer uptake in a mouse model of mesial temporal lobe epilepsy induced by unilaterally intracranial kainic acid injection. The radioactivity uptake reached a peak at 7 days, mostly related to microglial activation. After 14 days, reactive astrocytes provided a major binding site for TSPO tracer [71]. The finding of phase-dependent TSPO expression in subtypes of glial cells might contribute to the identification of optimal treatment windows in further clinical studies [71]. Chronic neuroinflammation is usually observed in many chronic neurodegenerative disorders such as Alzheimer's disease (AD), amyotrophic lateral sclerosis (ALS), and non-AD tauopathies. Most animal models of chronic neurodegenerative disorders are genetically modified mouse models. Authors have clearly demonstrated glial activation in response to accumulation of amyloid aggregates and treatment with the aid of TSPO-PET, indicating the utility of neuroinflammation imaging in monitoring of pathogenesis (Fig. 1.11). Amyloid accumulation is the earliest pathological change in the brain with AD, followed by tau aggregation and glial activation. Glial activation is predominantly concentrated around neuritic plaques, not diffuse plaques [72]. More clinical studies have reported increased TSPO tracer accumulation in temporoparietal, entorhinal, and cingulate cortex rather than frontal cortex with rich diffuse plaques and poor neuritic plaques, partially supporting such observation, while a considerable number of studies failed to detect an increase in TSPO

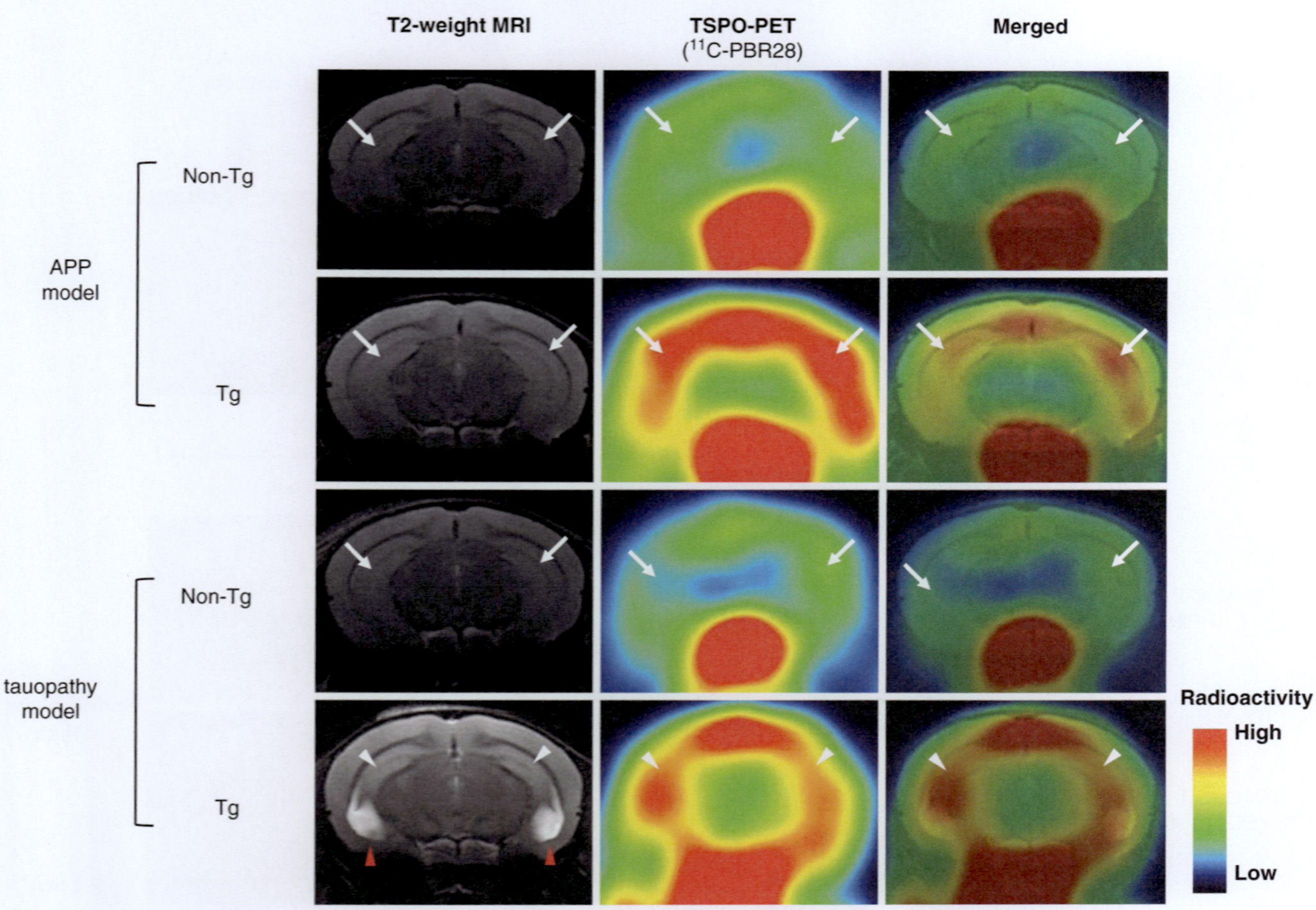

Fig. 1.11 TSPO-PET in AD mouse models mimicking amyloid and tau pathologies. Representative merged coronal brain images of T2-weighted MR, TSPO-PET and merged images showed that tracer binding was greatly increased in transgenic mice (Tg) of APP and tauopathy models mimicking amyloid (22-month-old) and tau (12-month-old) pathologies, respectively, compared with respective age-matched non-transgenic littermate mice (non-Tg). No obvious brain atrophy was observed in hippocampi of APP model as well as non-Tg mice (white arrows), while tauopathy model showed overtly atrophic hippocampi (white arrowheads). Red arrowheads indicated enlarged ventricles due to the hippocampal atrophy. Unpublished data

expression level [73]. The amyloid plaques accumulated in the amyloid precursor protein (APP) model are dense-core plaques, around which there are abundant activated glial cells and TSPO expression, indicating a similar glial response between neuritic and dense core plaques. However, immunohistochemical analysis showed that active astrocytes have provided the majority of binding sites for TSPO tracer in the APP model [74], while microglia around neuritic plaques expressed abundant TSPO [75]. This distinction between species concerning glial characteristics might be attributable to neurodegenerative tau pathologies, which exist in AD but are uncommon in the APP model. In vivo TSPO imaging also demonstrated increased TSPO expression accompanied by tau-related atrophic brain in another model of AD mimicking the tau-related pathologies (Fig. 1.11) [72, 76]. Considering that predominant microglial TSPO expression and age-dependent brain atrophy in these tauopathy models mimicking tau-related pathologies are consistent with the condition in AD patient brains, neuroinflammation imaging in tauopathy models might well reflect the actual situation of pathologies in human subjects. Based on the fact that in vivo imaging for amyloid and tau, as well as TSPO have been available for clinical and preclinical studies, multiple tracer imaging enables the clarification of the mutual relationship between these AD-related pathologies. For example, longitudinal in vivo imagings with TSPO-PET (^{18}F-FEDAA1106) and amyloid-PET (^{11}C-PiB) have captured the increased level of neuroinflammation triggered by Aβ immunotherapy, which greatly reduced amyloid accumulation in an identical APP model over the course of treatment (Fig. 1.12) [77]. TSPO-PET in combination with tau-PET (^{11}C-PBB3) in two tauopathy models showed that neuroinflammation was induced by two different tau aggregates (PBB3-positive and -negative) and thereby accelerated tau-mediated neuron damage via a distinct molecular mechanism [78]. These studies provide experimental evidence for neuroinflammation-targeting therapeutic strategy. Similarly, TSPO tracer signals were also increased in lesioned brain regions in a

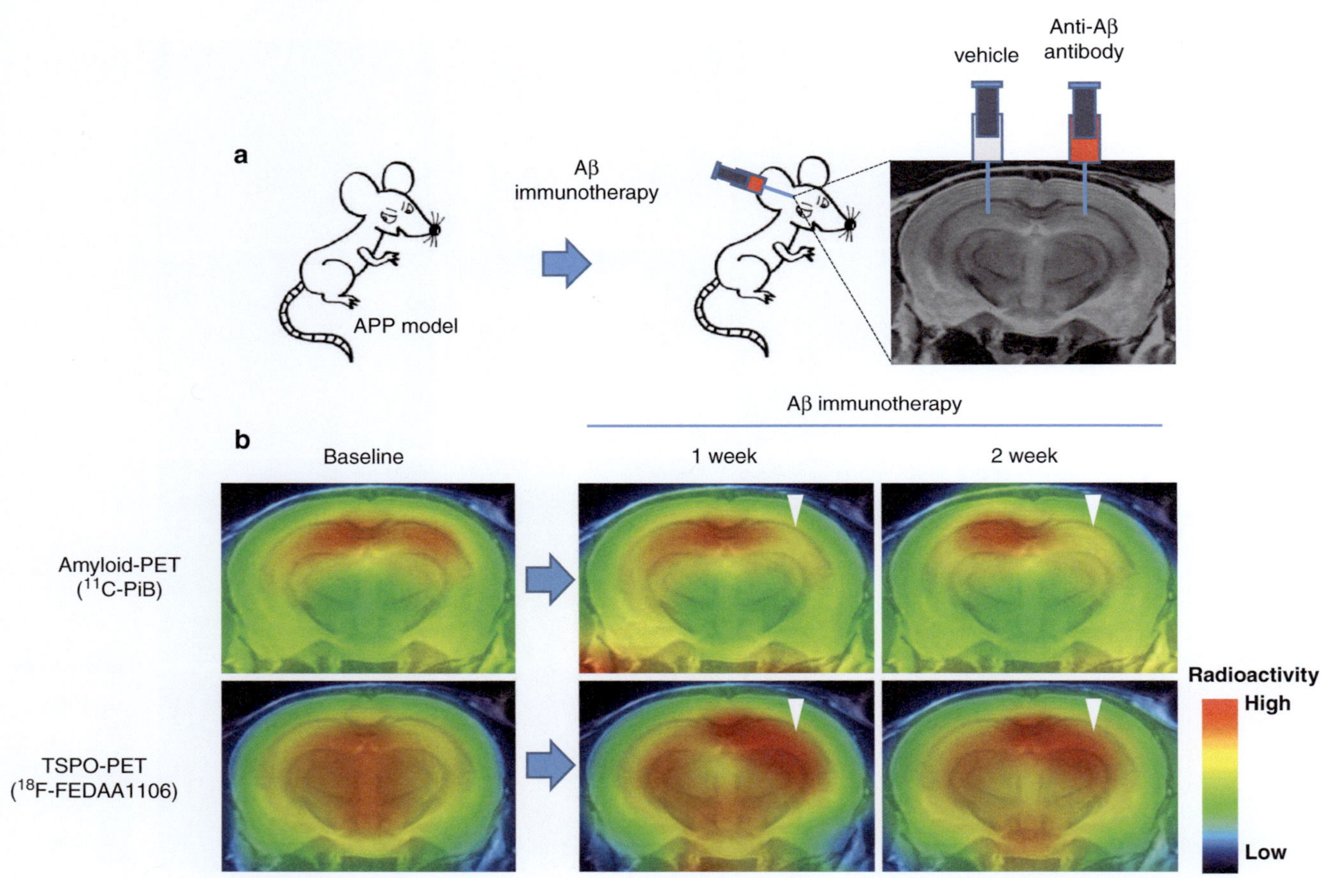

Fig. 1.12 Monitoring of anti-Aβ effect and neuroinflammation in amyloid immunotherapy. (**a**) Aβ immunotherapy was performed in APP model mice by intracranial injection of a therapeutic anti-Aβ antibody into the right hippocampus, and equivalent amount of vehicle was injected into the contralateral hippocampus as control. (**b**) APP model mice received repeated PET scans before (baseline) and after (1- and 2-week) treatment. Representative images of amyloid- and TSPO-PET merged with MRI brain template in an APP mouse showed that Aβ immunotherapy greatly reduced amyloid accumulation (amyloid-PET) and induced an increase in TSPO expression (TSPO-PET) around the region treated by antibody (white arrowheads), but not vehicle. (Data were modified from ref. [3])

mouse model of ALS, being consistent with microglial immunostaining [79]. In contrast, the results from Parkinson's disease (PD) animal models look more complicated. PD animal models are relatively easy to prepare by treating the animals with neurotoxins such as methamphetamine and 6-hydroxydompaine (6-OHDA). Methamphetamine-induced degeneration of dopaminergic neuron terminals did not trigger TSPO-positive gliosis [74], while 6-OHDA induced degeneration of dopaminergic neurons in either striatum or substantia nigra and increased the TSPO tracer signal [80]. Interestingly, most of the clinical PET studies found no increase in the level of TSPO expression in the striatal regions of PD patients [73, 81, 82] despite severe dopaminergic degeneration in these regions, supporting the proposal that TSPO imaging is inapplicable to monitoring the degeneration of nonmyelinated nerve [74].

Quantitative PET studies require that the input function, representing cumulative availability of authentic radiotracer in arterial plasma, is measured in case of the absence of ideal reference tissue. Because of the constitutive expression of TSPO in the whole brain, blood collection is needed for calculating the binding potential. However, this usually faces technical difficulties in the actual operation for the small mouse body. So the brain regions without pathological changes, such as cerebellum in rTg4510 mouse [76, 78] or striatum in PS19 mouse [72], are used as reference tissue when reference-tissue models are used. Although it will lead to underestimation of the binding potential due to constitutive low-level TSPO expression in reference regions, such analysis can provide relatively stable results compared to the percentage of injection dose, which is greatly affected by body weight, metabolic capacity, or other factors. Another issue is a concern for the partial volume effect due to the small volume of the region of interesting (ROI) in the case of mouse. This makes it difficult to correctly measure the radioactivity in certain subregions of mouse brain. The use of rat and nonhuman primate models is an alternative, but selectable neurodegenerative models are limited compared to mouse, as most models with pathologies of chronic neurodegenerative disorders, such as AD, ALS, and non-AD tauopathies [83, 84], are genetically modified murine models. Despite the fact that TSPO-PET successfully captured neuroinflammation in various animal models with acute and chronic neuroinflammation, the results in patients with chronic neuroinflammation seemed more complicated [73, 81]. One of the reasons is that a TSPO polymorphism (rs6971) greatly influences the affinity of a large majority of TSPO tracers in a tracer-dependent manner [85]. Another possible reason is the differing cellular distribution of TSPO expression. Recent studies have shown that TSPO expression is not limited to microglia. Other brain components, for example, astrocytes and vascular endothelial cells, also express TSPO. Some studies have demonstrated dominant induction of TSPO expression in active astrocytes in a neuropathological type-dependent and phase-dependent manner [71, 74]. Vascular expression of TSPO is also a factor that disturbs microglial TSPO imaging. Although no study has quantitatively measured the influence of vascular TSPO on tracer binding, inclusion of the additional vascular component in the modified reference-tissue model amplified the binding potential in AD more than in control by decreasing tracer binding to the vasculature in the disease cohort or was better correlated to brain TSPO mRNA [86, 87]. As few studies have focused on changes in vascular TSPO expression in diseased brains, determining which is responsible for the changes in TSPO tracer binding in diseased brains is a complicated issue. Further studies in combination with postmortem analyses or microglial TSPO-specific or vascular TSPO-specific knockout animals are desirable.

1.3.3 Alternative Molecular Targets for Microglia Imaging

CSF1R is a novel imaging biomarker for microglia by its exclusive expression in microglia in the CNS [88]. Recently, Horti et al. reported a newly developed PET tracer, ^{11}C-CPPC, for CSF1R imaging. ^{11}C-CPPC showed high initial brain uptake and rapid washout from brain in normal rodent brain, and increased accumulation in inflammatory brains of rodent and nonhuman primate models including LPS-injection and AD mouse models. In vitro autoradiogram showed higher binding in postmortem brains with AD compared to healthy control [88]. These results support the concept that CSF1R is a suitable molecular target for microglia imaging. However, ^{11}C-CPPC binding is increased in whole brain regions, and is not limited to regions with lesions as exemplified by cerebellum in AD model and intracranial LPS injection model, and immunohistochemistry for active microglia and CSF1R expression to support imaging results was not provided. Another reported CSF1R imaging tracer, ^{11}C-AZ683, showed high affinity for CSF1R (Ki = 8 nM) and >250-fold selectivity over other kinases tested, but low brain uptake in rodents and nonhuman primates limited its utility in living brains [89]. Further examinations and improvements will be required for their clinical application. It is still unclear which microglia phenotypes predominantly express CSF1R because of the lack of data from immunohistochemical and biochemical analyses of the various neurodegenerative models.

P2X7R and P2Y12R were considered to be predominantly expressed in M1 and M2 microglia phenotypes, respectively [90]. In vitro autoradiographic analysis with ^{11}C-SMW139 showed high specific binding to viral vector-mediated human P2X7R expressed in rat brain, but no increase in binding was detected in postmortem brain with

AD compared to healthy control [91]. Specific binding of ^{11}C-GSK1482160 is also detectable in P2X7R-overexpressing samples under in vitro condition [92]. However, more evidence is required for both of the above two P2X7R tracers to prove their utilities in the living inflammatory brain. In vivo imaging with ^{18}F-JNJ-64413739 with high affinity and selectivity for P2X7R showed significant increase in tracer accumulation in the living LPS-induced neuroinflammatory brain, indicating its leading status among the current P2X7R tracers, while further work is needed to verify its utility in other types of neuroinflammation [93–95]. Villa et al. recently developed a carbon-11-labeled P2Y12R-binding compound. In vitro and ex vivo experiments with this radioactive compound showed increased binding in brain sections of mice treated with anti-inflammatory stimuli and decreased binding to brain sections of a murine stroke model and of a stroke patient [96]. Immunohistochemistry and immunoblotting also supported the viewpoints that P2Y12R is a biomarker for M2 phenotype microglia [90, 96].

1.4 PET Imaging in Animal Models of Neuroinflammation 2

Tadashi Watabe

Abstract Neuroinflammation is defined as inflammatory responses in the brain and spinal cord, and microglia and astrocytes are the mainly involved cells. Translocator protein (TSPO) has been the major target used in positron emission tomography (PET) to detect neuroinflammation with glial activation. In a preclinical study conducted in small animal models of brain ischemia and traumatic brain injury, a second-generation TSPO tracer [^{18}F]DPA-714 PET was used for the evaluation of glial activation; the TSPO uptake was validated by comparison with the immunohistochemical findings of co-staining for TSPO and a microglial/macrophage or astrocyte maker. TSPO expression has also been reported in a model of Alzheimer's disease, where TSPO-positive cells with two opposing roles were observed: neuroprotective astrocytes for reversible neuronal injury and detrimental microglia for irreversible neuronal injury. Recently, new targets have been identified in microglia, namely, cyclooxygenase-1 (COX-1) and purinergic receptor P2X7, which have been shown to be specifically expressed in the microglia. PET imaging targeting glial cells is a promising modality to characterize and monitor neuroinflammation longitudinally and with quantitative accuracy. The findings of preclinical models need to be confirmed in clinical studies beyond the limitation of animal model and the species differences between rodents and humans.

Keywords: Neuroinflammation, Glial activation, Translocator protein, Microglia, Astrocyte

1.4.1 Introduction

Neuroinflammation is defined as inflammatory responses in the brain and spinal cord [97]. It is observed in various types of brain diseases, including brain ischemia, traumatic brain injury, neurodegenerative disorders (Alzheimer's disease, Parkinson's disease, etc.), and neuropsychiatric disorders (schizophrenia, autism spectrum disorder, etc.) [98–101]. In the central nervous system, two major glial cells are involved in the process of neuroinflammation, namely, microglia and astrocytes [99]. To evaluate neuroinflammation in vivo, translocator protein (TSPO) has been the major target used in PET for the detection of neuroinflammation with glial activation [102]. In glial cells, especially microglia, expression of TSPO is minimal in the resting state, but upregulated in the activated state [103]. In previous studies, the first-generation TSPO-PET tracer, [^{11}C]PK-11195, was mainly used to evaluate glial activation in small animals as well as humans. However, the evaluation using [^{11}C]PK-11195 was found to be highly limited by the high nonspecific binding of the tracer [104, 105]; therefore, over the last 10 years, second-generation TSPO-PET tracers, such as [^{11}C]DPA-713 and [^{18}F]DPA-714, have been used because of their higher specific binding [104, 105]. Although the binding affinity in humans has been shown to vary due to polymorphism, TSPO PET has been employed as an effective tool to visualize and quantify the degree of neuroinflammation associated with glial activation in preclinical studies conducted using animal models, including rodents [106]. However, attention needs to be paid to the inflammatory cells taking up TSPO, as TSPO expression is not only observed in activated microglia/macrophages but also in reactive astrocytes [107].

1.4.2 Brain Ischemia Model

For preclinical studies using small animals, the middle cerebral artery occlusion (MACO) model was frequently used owing to its ease of handling for reperfusion and the abundance of accumulated evidence [108, 109]. Martin et al. evaluated the time-course of TSPO expression in the rat model of MCAO, in which transient focal ischemia was induced by 2-h intraluminal occlusion of the MCA, followed by reperfusion [110]. [^{18}F]DPA-714 PET showed significantly enhanced uptake on the ipsilateral side on days 7, 11, 15, and 21 after the induction of ischemia, with the peak observed on day 11. This finding corresponded to the immunohistochemical results of TSPO expression in the microglia/macrophages (TSPO + /CD11b-positive cells) in the ischemic area. The authors also reported an increase in the number of TSPO + /glial fibrillary acidic protein (GFAP)-positive cells in the lesioned area on day 21, with peaking of the number of such cells on day 30; this latter finding suggested the later involvement of reactive astrocytes showing TSPO expression. These results show that [^{18}F]DPA-714 provides accurate quantitative information about the time-course of TSPO expression in the glial cells in experimental stroke. Figure 1.13 shows the [^{11}C]DPA-713 PET images and results of immunohistochemistry using antibodies for CD11b and GFAP in the rat model of MCAO 4 days after transient ischemia for 1 h followed by reperfusion. The areas of enhanced uptake of [^{11}C]DPA-713 correspond to the areas showing high expression of CD11b, namely, areas containing a high number of activated microglia/macrophages. Immunohistochemistry showed reactive astrocytes, represented by cells showing GFAP expression, in the boundary of the ischemic area, which showed a low uptake of [^{11}C]DPA-713 on PET images. In regard to the clinical significance of the findings in relation to treatment, Martin A et al. reported that uptake of [^{11}C]DPA-713 in the ischemic lesion could be attenuated by administration of minocycline 1 h after the reperfusion [111]. Thus, TSPO PET can also be used for monitoring the response to immunomodulatory therapy after brain ischemia.

1.4.3 Traumatic Brain Injury Model

To evaluate traumatic brain injury (TBI) in small animals, a model of controlled cortical impact with a pneumatic impact device has been used for its high reproducibility and low mortality [112]. We reported two peaks of [^{18}F]DPA-714 uptake in this model, namely, on day 7 in the cortical area and on day 21 in the thalamus after induction of the focal brain injury [99]. The enhanced thalamic uptake was sustained until 14 weeks after induction of the TBI (Fig. 1.14). Immunohistochemical analysis on day 7 revealed TSPO staining mainly co-localized with amoeboid CD11b-positive microglia/macrophages, and weakly with GFAP-positive astrocytes in the cortex; however, TSPO immunoreactivity was scarcely observed in the thalamus. Giemsa staining on day 7 revealed mononuclear cells, such as phagocytic macrophages, in the cortical area, although these cells were not detected in the ipsilateral thalamus. In the macrophage depletion study performed 1 week post-injury, the TSPO uptake was decreased in the cortex, but enhanced in the thalamus, suggesting that the cortical uptake was mainly attributable to uptake by phagocytic macrophages recruited from the bloodstream, while the thalamic uptake was most likely attributable to uptake by resident microglia. Electron microscopy at 4 weeks post-TBI revealed morphologically activated microglia surrounding the degenerated axons and poorly myelinated neurons in the ipsilateral thalamus, indicating activation of the resident microglia and damage to the remaining neurons. TSPO expression was mainly evident in the activated microglia in the thalamus at 6 weeks post-injury. Thus, by using [^{18}F]DPA-714 PET, inflammatory migration could be detected from the cortex to the thalamus after focal brain injury. In addition, we also showed that depletion of myeloid-derived suppressor cells (MDSCs) was associated with enhanced cortical TSPO uptake on day 7 after the induction of focal brain injury, by both immunohistochemistry and cellular phenotype analysis [113]. This finding indicated that MDSCs may have strong immunosuppressive characteristics and limit inflammation and facilitate wound healing and recovery.

1.4.4 Alzheimer's Disease Model

Postmortem analyses of the brains of patients with Alzheimer's disease (AD) have revealed neuroinflammatory changes, namely, accumulation of activated microglia and astrocytes, around senile plaques and fibrillary tau lesions [114]. In this study, diffuse plaques in the brains of these patients were enveloped by a small number of Iba-1-positive microglia not expressing TSPO, while numerous microglia expressing both Iba-1 and TSPO were found to be in close contact with neuritic plaques. Thus, microglia expressing TSPO were recruited to fibrillar tau inclusions, but not to Aβ deposits unaccompanied by tau pathology. Jin et al. reported that TSPO expression was observed, mainly in the astrocytes, in amyloid precursor protein 23 (APP23) transgenic (Tg) mice which show minimal neuronal loss, while TSPO-positive microglia were observed in the tangle-like tau lesions of tau Tg mice which show remarkable neuronal loss. They concluded that TSPO-positive astrocytes have protective roles against reversible neuronal injury, while TSPO-positive microglia have detrimental effects for irreversible neuronal injury [115]. We evaluated TSPO expression in the APP23 Tg mice by immunohistochemistry (Fig. 1.15). TSPO immunoreactivity was observed around the amyloid beta (Aβ) plaques and in reactive astrocytes (GFAP-positive). CD11b-positive microglia were relatively few in number as compared to the number of GFAP-positive astrocytes, consistent with the findings reported by Jin B et al. However, it should be borne in mind that no significant increase in the uptake of [^{18}F]DPA-714 or of the amyloid tracer [^{11}C]PIB was detected by in vivo PET performed prior to the immunohistochemistry in the same mice. Maier F et al. reported that Aβ deposition was detectable earlier by histology than by amyloid PET in APP23 Tg mice, indicating the existence of a lower limit of sensitivity for the detection of Aβ or neuroinflammation by PET [116].

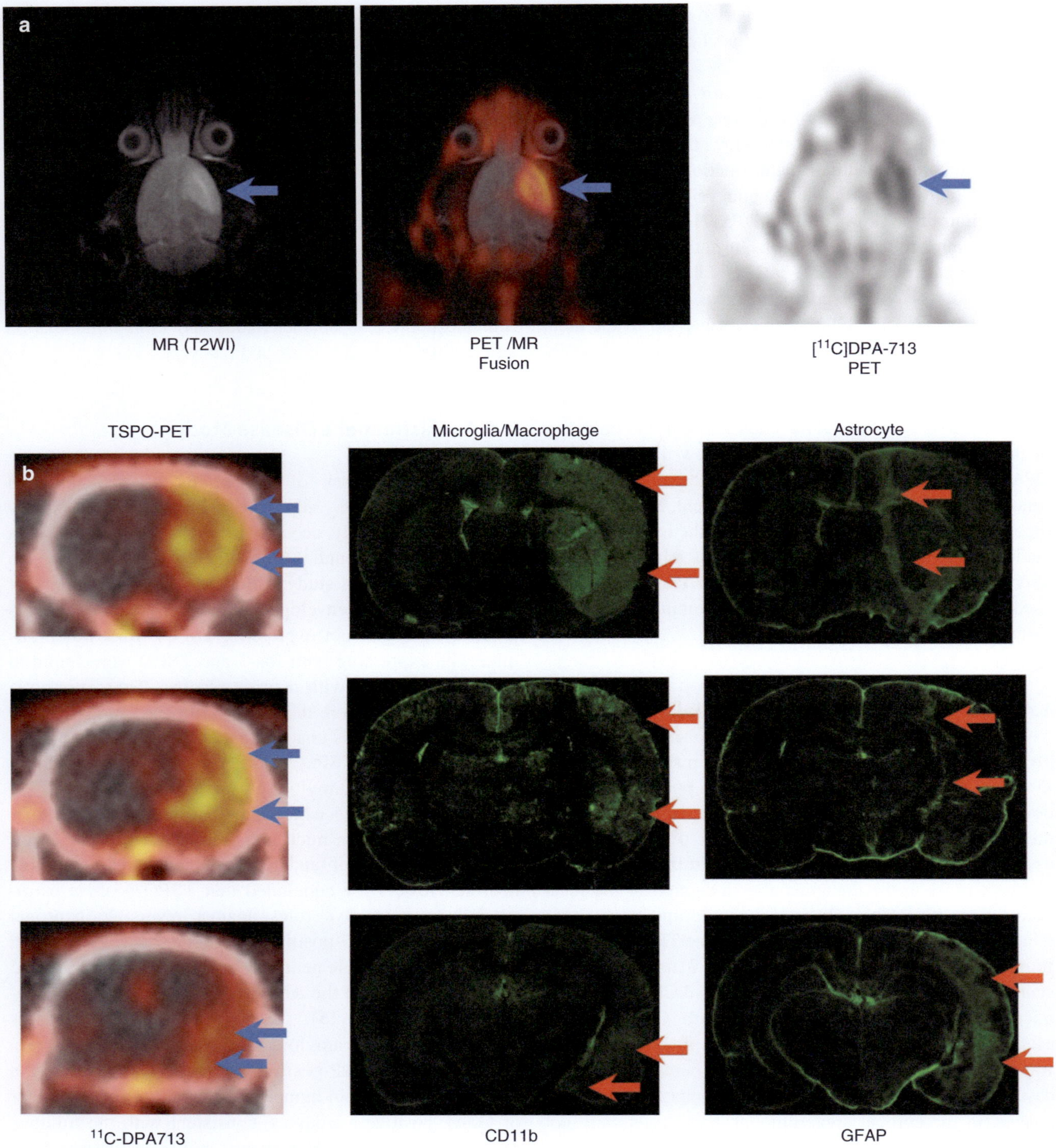

Fig. 1.13 (**a**) TSPO PET imaging of glial activation in the rat brain 4 days after 1-h occlusion of the middle cerebral artery (left: T2-weighted image (T2WI) of MRI, middle: PET/MRI fusion, right: [^{11}C]DPA-713 PET). High uptake was observed in the ischemic region corresponding to the hyperintensity lesion visualized on MRI (T2WI). (**b**) Comparison of TSPO PET and immunofluorescence images. Blue arrows indicate glial activation recognized on [^{11}C]DPA-713 PET and red arrows indicate CD11b expression in microglia/macrophages or GFAP expression in astrocytes

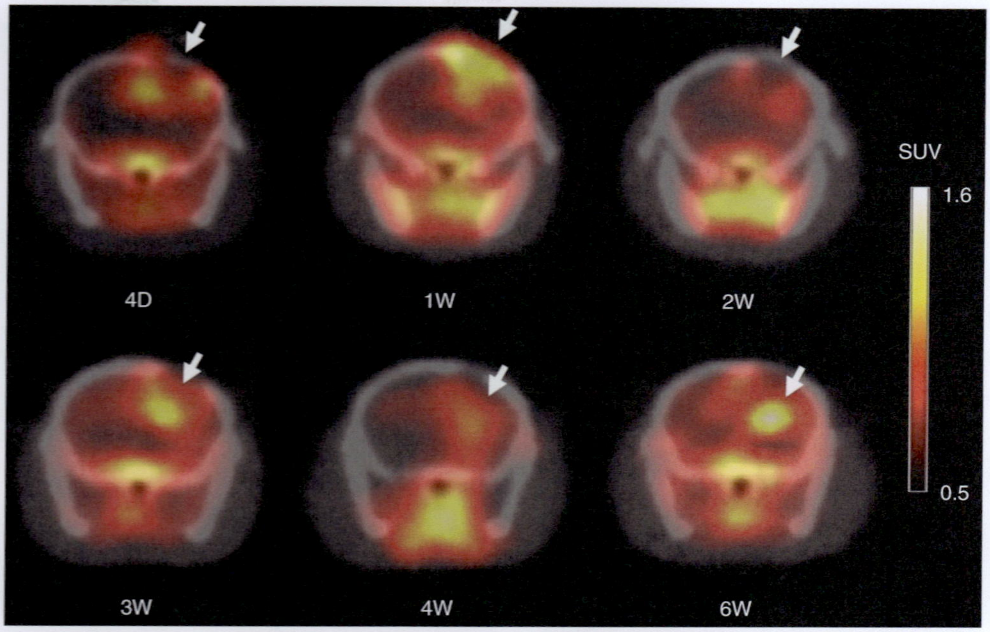

Fig. 1.14 [^{18}F]DPA-714 PET/CT images of mice after focal brain injury (static images obtained 20–30 min after radiotracer administration). Cortical uptake peaked at 1 week after induction of the injury and shifted to the ipsilateral thalamus after 3 weeks. Arrows indicate glial activation in the ipsilateral side

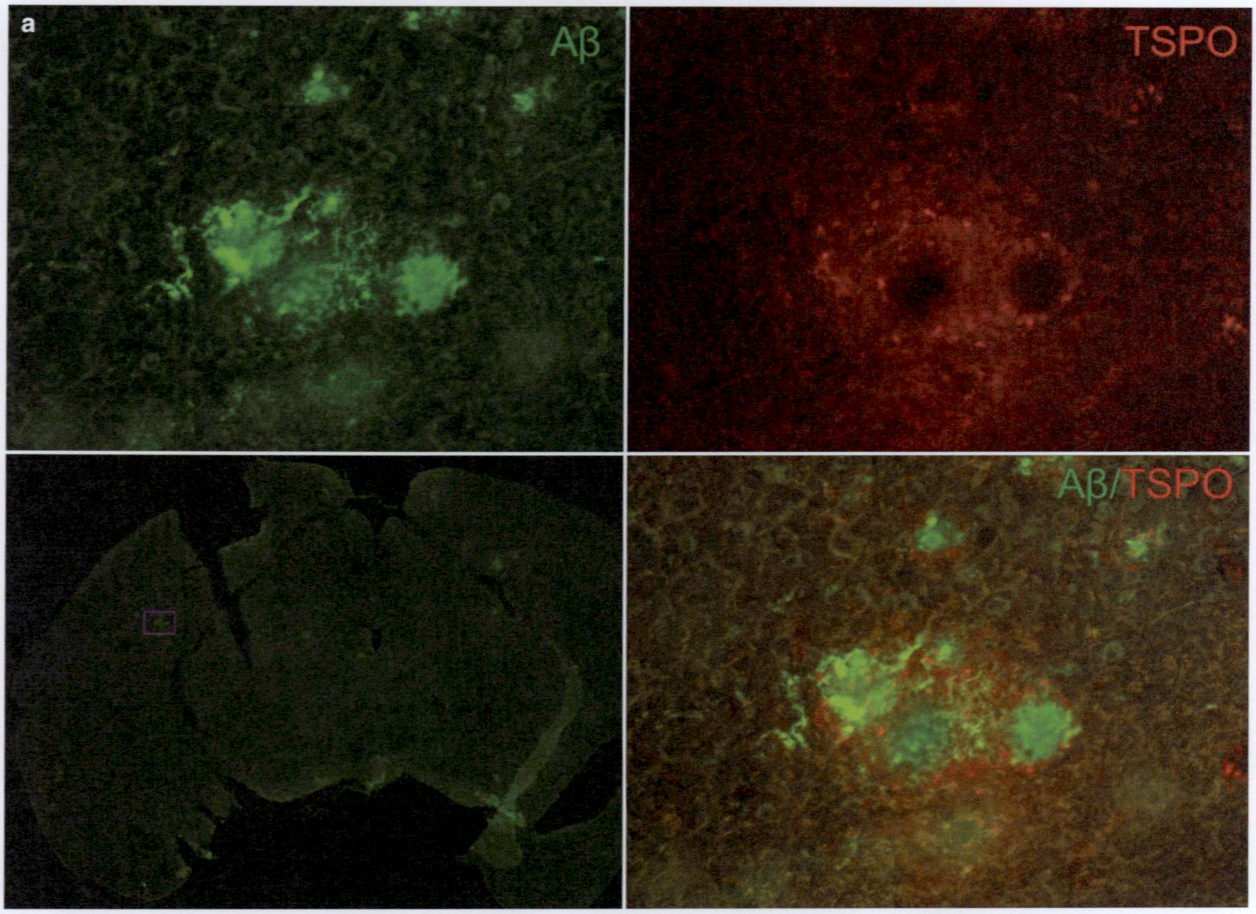

Fig. 1.15 Immunofluorescence images of APP23 Tg mice (15 months old) showing co-staining for (**a**) Aβ and TSPO, (**b**) GFAP and TSPO, and (**c**) CD11b and TSPO. Left lower figure indicates low-magnification images of the brain and the pink-colored square indicates the evaluated area under high magnification. TSPO expression is observed around the amyloid beta (Aβ) plaques, and GFAP-positive astrocytes show positive co-staining for TSPO. Microglia showing CD11b/TSPO co-staining are relatively few in number as compared to the number of astrocytes showing GFAP/TSPO co-staining. (**d**) [^{11}C]PIB PET images of APP23 Tg mice as compared to wild-type (WT) mice; amyloid deposition is observed in the cortical region and the hippocampus, whereas no significant accumulation is observed in the WT mice

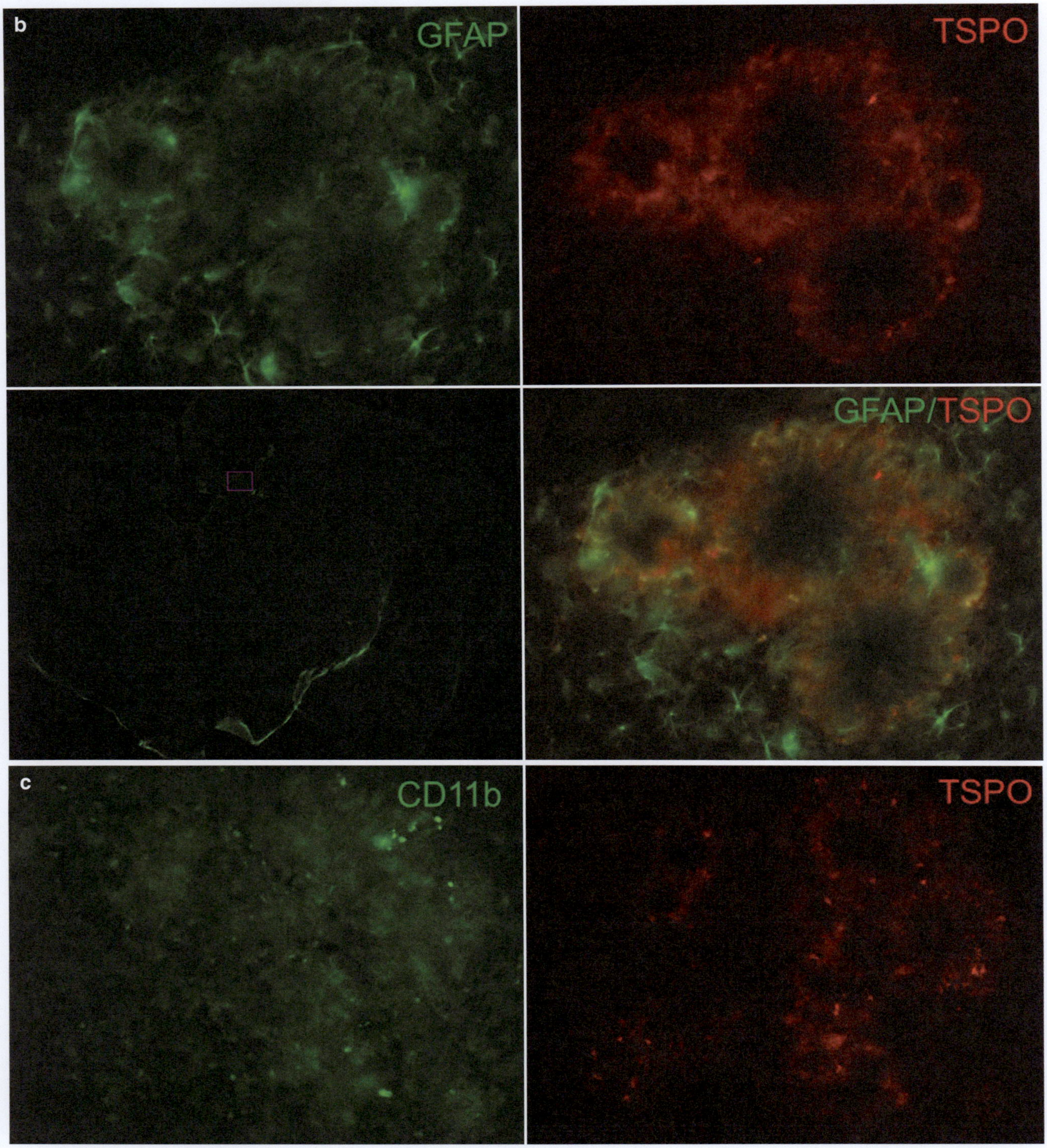

Fig. 1.15 (continued)

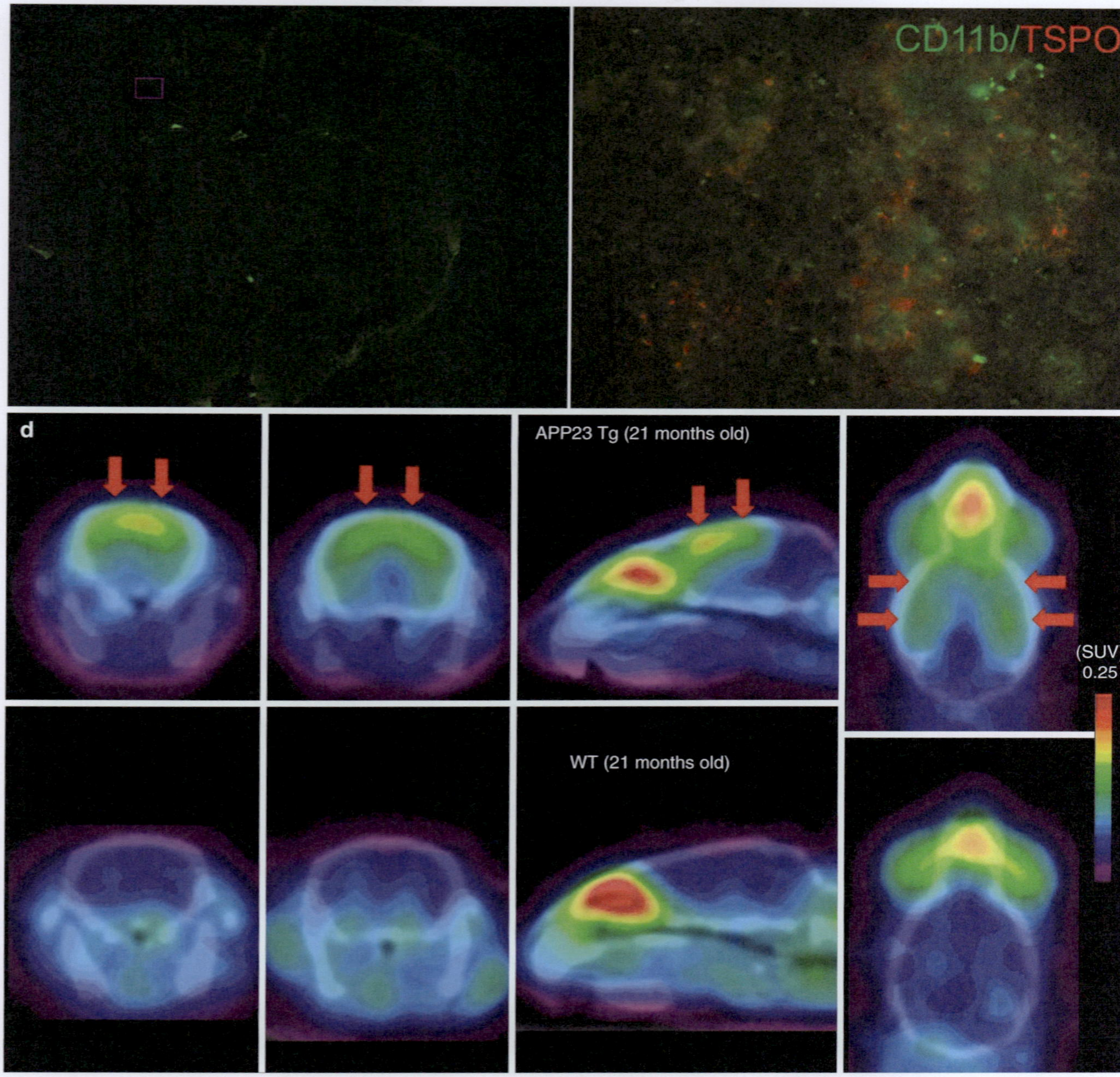

Fig. 1.15 (continued)

Shukuri et al. demonstrated that the expression of cyclooxygenase-1 (COX-1) in activated microglia and macrophages during neuroinflammation can be visualized by PET using [^{11}C]ketoprofen methyl ester (KTP-Me), with immunohistochemical confirmation [117]. One advantage of [^{11}C]KTP-Me PET as compared to TSPO PET is that COX-1 is expressed only in activated microglia and not in astrocytes. They also reported that expression of COX-1 could be detected in 16- to 24-month-old APP23 Tg mice, in accordance with the time of histopathologic appearance of abundant Aβ plaques and activated microglia [118]. They also reported the possibility of treating AD by inhibition of COX-1 activity, as a treatment target, with nonsteroidal anti-inflammatory drugs (NSAIDS). Besides TSPO, PET imaging of [^{11}C]KTP-Me could also be a useful tool for monitoring COX-1 activity in activated microglia in neuroinflammation.

1.4.5 Other Models of Neuroinflammation

Imamoto et al. showed that glial activation could be quantitatively imaged in the spinal cord of a rat model of neuropathic pain using [^{11}C]PK11195 PET [119]. It was suggested that high-resolution PET using TSPO-specific radioligands is useful for imaging to assess the role of glial activation, including neuroinflammatory processes, in the spinal cord. Belolli et al. reported increased enhanced TSPO uptake in a mouse model of multiple sclerosis induced by experimental autoimmune encephalomyelitis (EAE), with neuropathological confirmation of activated microglia [120]. They concluded that combined use of TSPO-PET and MRI could provide complementary evidence of the ongoing disease process.

Evaluation of neuroinflammation by PET in neuropsychiatric disorders, such as schizophrenia and autism spectrum disorder, has been limited to clinical studies, possibly due to the difficulty in establishing appropriate animal models mimicking the pathological condition of the patients.

1.4.6 New PET Tracer for Neuroinflammation

As mentioned in Sect. 1.4.4, TSPO-positive glial cells have both neurotoxic and neuroprotective effects. Two phenotypes of microglia have been recognized, namely, neurotoxic "M1" and neuroprotective "M2," although it cannot be clearly separated as M1 or M2 [121]. TSPO-positive microglia that accelerate tau deposition and neuronal deterioration are likely to be M1-polarized. When considering the treatment strategy for neurodegenerative disorders, it is important to detect the detrimental glial cells to suppress their function. Expression of the P2X7 receptor (purinergic receptor) has been reported to be observed in M1-polarized microglia, which could be a promising target for the detection of deleterious neuroinflammation [122]. In contrast, expression of the P2Y12 receptor has been reported to be observed in the M2-like microglia [123]. Recently, a PET radioligand for the P2X7 receptor was synthesized and its efficacy was evaluated in preclinical models. Finally, reproducible and dose-dependent receptor occupancy studies with a P2X7 receptor antagonist were performed using [^{18}F]JNJ-54175446 in rhesus monkeys and humans [124, 125]. The usefulness of PET radioligands for the P2X7 receptor is not only limited to the diagnosis of neuroinflammation. [^{18}F]PTTP, which is also a radioligand targeting the P2X7 receptor, has been shown to be potentially useful for the quantification of peripheral inflammation targeting macrophages and to distinguish inflammation from certain solid tumors [126]. Other targets in microglia, such as sphingosine-1-phosphate receptor 1 (S1P1) or receptor for advanced glycation end products (RAGE), are also promising, but only in the preliminary stage of investigation at this moment [127].

1.4.7 Conclusion

Findings of PET imaging in animal models of neuroinflammation are summarized in this article. In preclinical studies, the pathology can be confirmed by immunohistochemistry or cellular phenotype analysis, as well as by comparison of the PET results. PET imaging targeting TSPO, COX-1, or P2X7 is a promising modality to characterize and monitor neuroinflammation longitudinally and with quantitative accuracy. However, it needs to be borne in mind that preclinical models do not always reflect the pathologies of the heterogeneous characteristics of patients in clinical practice. In addition, we should consider the species differences between rodents and humans. Any findings in preclinical models should be confirmed in clinical situations, which is one of the goals of translational research.

Acknowledgements
I would like to thank my collaborators: Dr. Sanae Hosomi (Department of Traumatology and Acute Critical Medicine) for the TBI study and Dr. Naoyuki Sato (Department of Clinical Gene Therapy) for the AD study.

1.5 PET Imaging of Inflammation in the Peripheral System with [^{18}F]FEDAC, a Radioligand for Translocator Protein (18 kDa)

Ming-Rong Zhang

Abstract Translocator protein (18 kDa; TSPO) has a broad array of functions, such as regulation of cholesterol transport, steroid hormone synthesis, porphyrin and heme transport, apoptosis, cell proliferation, anion transport, mitochondrial function regulation, immunomodulation, and inflammation. TSPO is widely expressed in peripheral tissues, including the adrenal gland, kidney, lung, and heart. Because of its pharmacological actions related to inflammation, TSPO has become a useful biomarker for monitoring inflammation using positron emission tomography (PET) with a specific radiotracer. Herein, the author reviews the results of PET imaging with a TSPO-specific radiotracer [^{18}F]FEDAC to noninvasively visualize and quantify TSPO in the peripheral tissues and monitor various inflammatory diseases, such as lung inflammation, nonalcoholic fatty liver disease, liver damage, liver fibrosis, multiple sclerosis, and rheumatic arthritis, in animal models. [^{18}F]FEDAC-PET is a powerful tool for imaging TSPO and monitoring the progress of various inflammatory diseases of the peripheral system.

Keywords: Translocator protein (18 kDa), Lung inflammation, Nonalcoholic fatty liver disease, Liver damage, Liver fibrosis, Multiple sclerosis, Rheumatic arthritis

1.5.1 Introduction

Translocator protein (18 kDa; TSPO) is the critical component of a multimeric 140–200-kDa complex located in the outer mitochondrial membrane and enriched in the outer/inner mitochondrial membrane contact sites [128]. TSPO has broad functions related to the regulation of cholesterol transport, steroid hormone synthesis, porphyrin and heme transport, apoptosis, cell proliferation, anion transport, mitochondrial function regulation, immunomodulation, and inflammation [128]. TSPO is widely distributed in the peripheral tissues, and the mRNA levels of TSPO are high in the adrenal glands, kidneys, spleen, skeletal muscle, heart, and lungs, and are low in the liver and brain. TSPO expression in blood cells has also been reported, in which phagocytic cells, including monocytes and polymorphonuclear neutrophils, show significantly higher TSPO expression than lymphocytes. It has been demonstrated that TSPO expression increases in inflammatory cells during the occurrence and progression of inflammation. Thus, TSPO has become a useful biomarker for monitoring inflammation using PET with a TSPO-specific radiotracer [128].

Since 2002, we have developed more than 10 PET radiotracers for the imaging of TSPO in preclinical studies and have translated four new TSPO radiotracers to clinical studies in our institute: [^{11}C]DAA1106 [129–131], [^{18}F]FEDAA1106 [132–134], [^{11}C]AC-5216 [135, 136], and [^{18}F]FEDAC [137–139]. Here, the author reviews their results from PET with [^{18}F]FEDAC to noninvasively visualize TSPO in the peripheral tissues [140] and monitor various inflammatory diseases, such as lung inflammation [141], nonalcoholic fatty liver disease [142], liver damage [143], liver fibrosis [144], multiple sclerosis [145], and rheumatic arthritis [146, 147], in animal models.

1.5.2 PET Imaging and Quantitative Analysis of TSPO in Rat Peripheral Tissues

Using small-animal PET with [^{18}F]FEDAC, we performed TSPO imaging to quantify TSPO density in rat peripheral tissues, including heart, lungs, and kidneys [140]. The in vivo distribution and kinetics of [^{18}F]FEDAC were first examined and measured in rat peripheral tissues. Using the in vivo pseudo-equilibrium method, TSPO binding parameters (TSPO density [B_{max}] and dissociation constant [K_D]) and receptor occupancy were estimated in the peripheral tissues.

PET study showed that the uptake of radioactivity was highly distributed in the lungs, heart, and kidneys, and the TSPO-enriched tissues could be clearly visualized after the injection of [^{18}F]FEDAC (Fig. 1.16). The kinetics of this radiotracer in the tissues was moderate, which is suitable for determining the in vivo binding parameters and receptor occupancy. The B_{max} values of TSPO in the heart, lung, and kidney were 393, 141, and 158 pmol/mL, respectively (Table 1.1). The K_D values of [^{18}F]FEDAC in the heart, lung, and kidney were 119, 36, and 123 nM, respectively. After pretreatment with 5 mg/kg Ro 5-4864 (a TSPO-selective ligand), about 90% of binding sites for TSPO in the heart and lung were occupied. In the kidneys, the TSPO binding was also completely inhibited by Ro 5-4864.

Through this study, we demonstrated that [^{18}F]FEDAC is a useful PET tracer for TSPO imaging and quantitative analysis of TSPO expression in peripheral tissues. Therefore, [^{18}F]FEDAC-PET can be used to study the TSPO function and evaluate the in vivo binding parameters and receptor occupancy of TSPO ligands. Subsequently, we used PET with [^{18}F]FEDAC to determine if TSPO increases in inflamed peripheral tissues of various animal models.

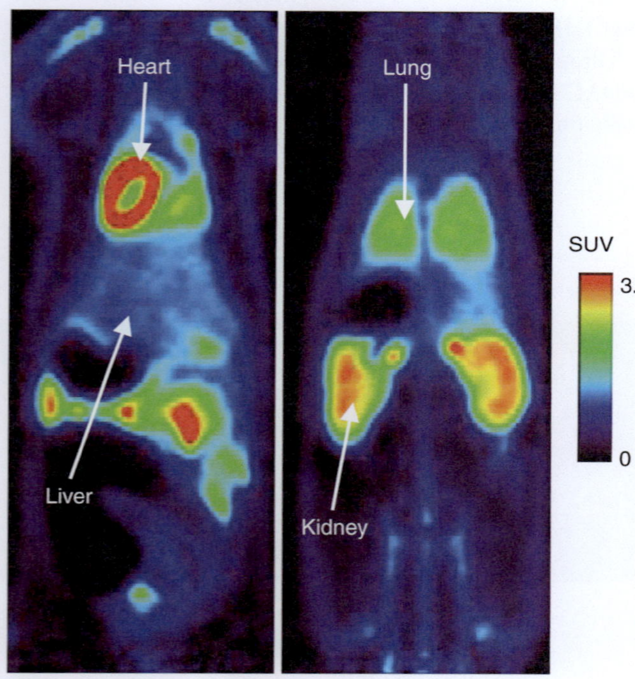

Fig. 1.16 Representative coronal PET images of [^{18}F]FEDAC in the isoflurane-anesthetized rat, which was placed in the prone position. PET images were generated by summating the whole scan (0–30 min)

Table 1.1 TSPO density (B_{max}) and dissociation constant (K_D) of [^{18}F]FEDAC measured by PET in peripheral tissues of living rats

Tissue	B_{max} (pmol/mL)	K_D (nM)
Heart	393 [323–529][a]	119 [89–180][a]
Lung	141 [112–205][a]	119 [26–61][a]
Kidney	158 [129–217][a]	123 [92–191][a]

[a]95% Confidence intervals ($n = 3$)

1.5.3 TSPO in Lung Inflammation

TSPO is highly expressed on the bronchial and bronchiole epithelium, submucosal glands in intrapulmonary bronchi, pneumocytes and alveolar macrophages in human lungs. We performed PET imaging of lung inflammation with [^{18}F]FEDAC and determined cellular sources that enrich TSPO in the lung [141]. We prepared an acute lung injury model by using intratracheal administration of lipopolysaccharide (LPS) to rats. PET with [^{18}F]FEDAC demonstrated that, in response to LPS treatment, the uptake of radioactivity increased in the lungs as the inflammation progressed (Fig. 1.17). Pretreatment with a TSPO-selective unlabeled ligand PK11195 significantly decreased the lung uptake of [^{18}F]FEDAC because of competitive binding to TSPO. TSPO expression was elevated in the inflamed lung section and its level responded to the [^{18}F]FEDAC uptake and severity of inflammation. The presence of TSPO was examined in the lung tissue using western blotting and immunohistochemical assays. The increase of TSPO expression was mainly found in the neutrophils and macrophages of inflamed lungs (Fig. 1.18).

Through this study, we demonstrated that PET with [^{18}F]FEDAC is a useful tool for imaging TSPO expression and evaluating the progression of lung inflammation.

1.5.4 TSPO in Nonalcoholic Fatty Liver Disease

Mitochondrial dysfunction is responsible for liver damage and disease progression in nonalcoholic fatty liver disease (NAFLD). TSPO, as a mitochondrial transmembrane protein, plays important roles in regulating mitochondrial function. We conducted PET with [^{18}F]FEDAC to explore if TSPO could be used as an imaging biomarker of noninvasive diagnosis and staging of NAFLD [142]. PET with [^{18}F]FEDAC, CT, autoradiography, histopathology, and gene analysis were performed to evaluate and quantify TSPO levels and NAFLD progression in methionine and choline-deficient diet-fed mice. The uptake of [^{18}F]FEDAC increased with disease progression from simple steatosis to nonalcoholic steatohepatitis (NASH) (Fig. 1.19). A strong correlation was observed between [^{18}F]FEDAC uptake ratio and NAFLD activity score in the liver. The specific binding of [^{18}F]FEDAC to TSPO in the NAFLD livers was demonstrated by competition experiments with the unlabeled TSPO-selective PK11195. Autoradiography and histopathology supported these PET imaging results. Further, there were greater mRNA levels of the functional macromolecular signaling complex composed of TSPO, compared to controls (Fig. 1.20).

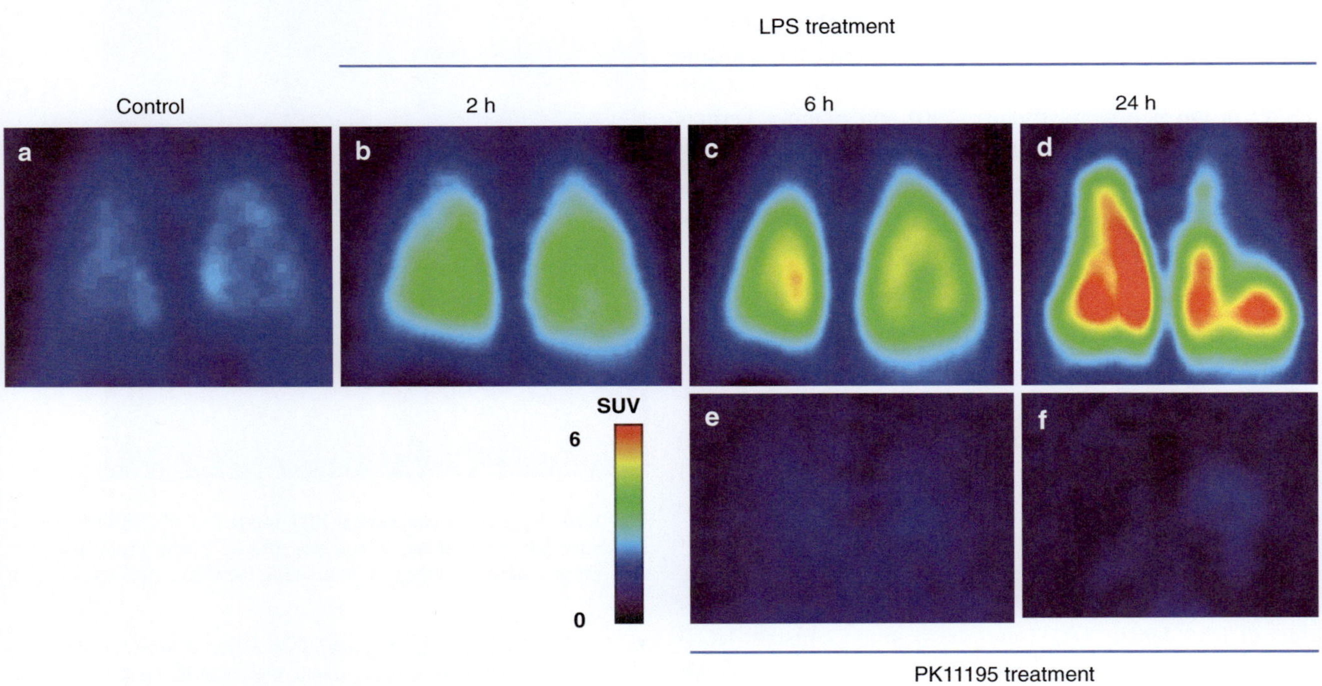

Fig. 1.17 Representative coronal PET lung images acquired between 0 and 30 min after injection of [^{18}F]FEDAC. (**a**) control; (**b**) LPS-2 h; (**c**) LPS-6 h; (**d**) LPS-24 h inducement; pretreatment with (**e**) PK11195 for LPS-6 h; (**f**) PK11195 for LPS-24 h

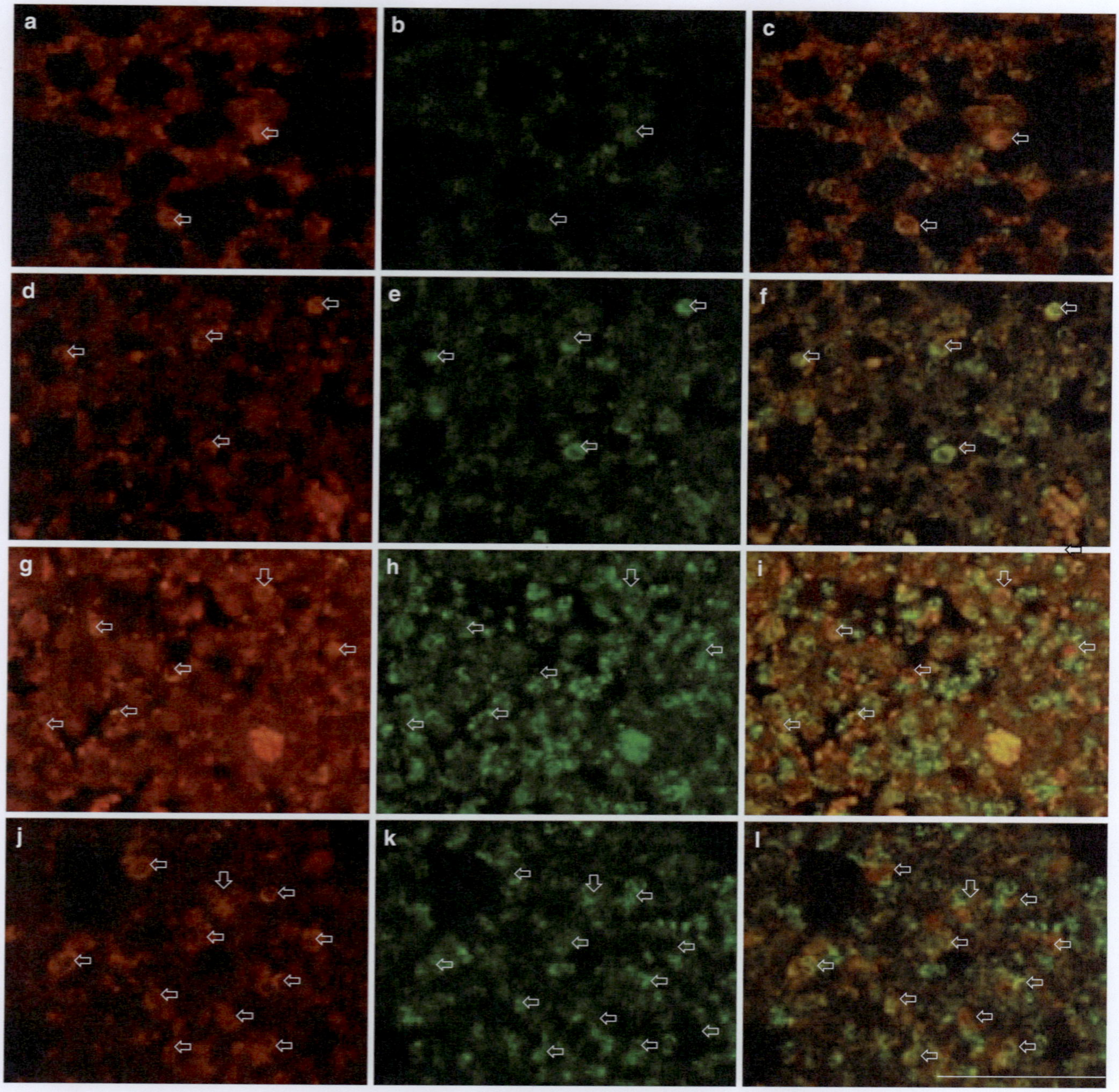

Fig. 1.18 Double immunofluorescence labeling of ED1 (red) and TSPO (green) displayed as a two-channel image. The images demonstrated temporal alterations of TSPO expression in macrophages at 2 h (**d–f**), 6 h (**g–i**), and 24 h (**j–l**) after LPS inducement, and in the control (**a–c**). Arrows indicate examples of cells doubly positive for ED1 and TSPO. (**a–c**) TSPO expression was observed in a few macrophages. (**d–f**) Several macrophages demonstrating TSPO immunoreactivity were observed in the alveolar spaces. (**g–i**, **j–l**) Numbers of macrophages with TSPO gradually increased over time. Scale bar: 20 μm

Through this study, we demonstrated that TSPO expression increased in NAFLD and was strongly correlated with NAFLD progression. TSPO as a specific molecular imaging biomarker could provide a novel tool for noninvasive, reliable, and quantitative diagnosis and staging of NAFLD.

1.5.5 TSPO in Liver Damage

Liver damage induced by drug toxicity is an important problem for both medical doctors and patients. In this study, we noninvasively visualized acute liver damage using PET with [^{18}F]FEDAC and determined cellular

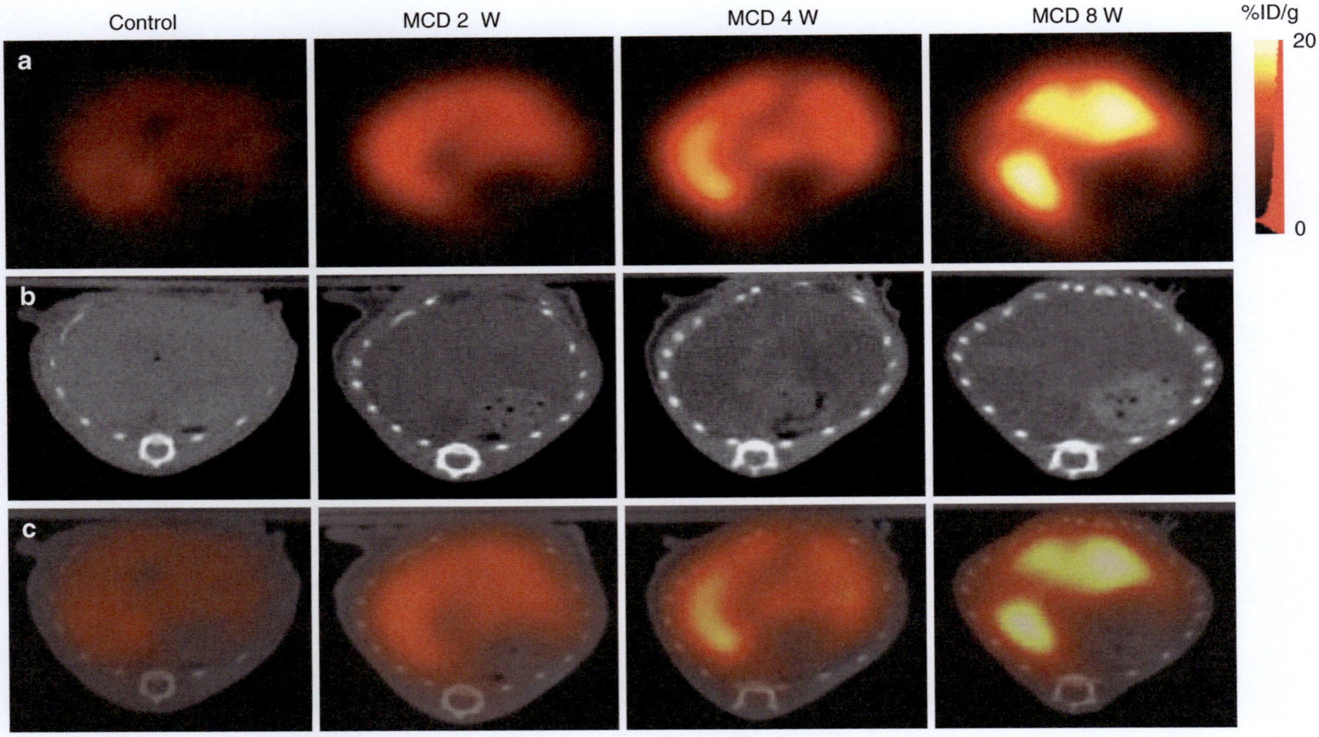

Fig. 1.19 Representative TSPO-PET/CT images of livers in MCD and control mice. (**a**) Summed TSPO-PET images of 0–30 min scanning in the 2, 4, 8 weeks MCD-fed mice and the 8 weeks normal-fed mice. [^{18}F] FEDAC-PET signal gradually increased compared to the controls. (**b**) Average unenhanced CT images. Decreased attenuation value in the parenchyma was presented in all stages of NALFD. (**c**) TSPO-PET/CT fusion images. More severe pathologic injures took place in the areas of higher radioactivity accumulation

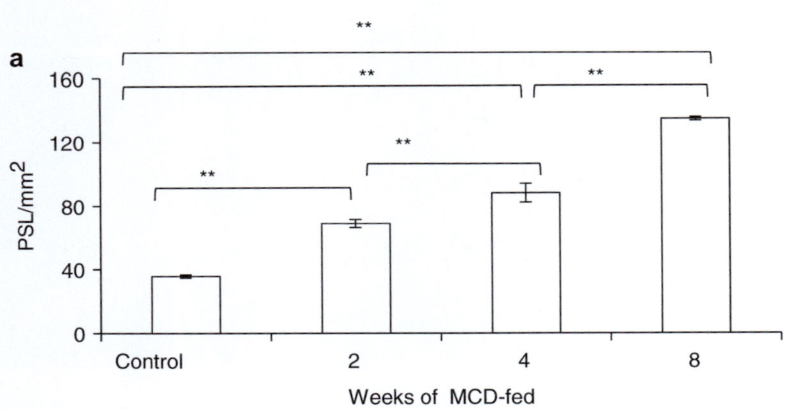

Fig. 1.20 Ex vivo autoradiography and immunohistochemistry in liver sections of MCD and control mice (n = 6, respectively). (**a**) Ex vivo autoradiography demonstrated that radioactivity gradually increased in the livers with the time of MCD feeding. (**b**) Representing autoradiographic images of liver sections. (**c**) Double immunohistochemistry including TSPO (blue) and CD11b (orange). Preferential localization of TSPO indicated in the liver lesion sites, CD11b/TSPO active macrophages and lymphocytes increased in the MCD livers (Scale bars = 500 μm). $**P < 0.01$

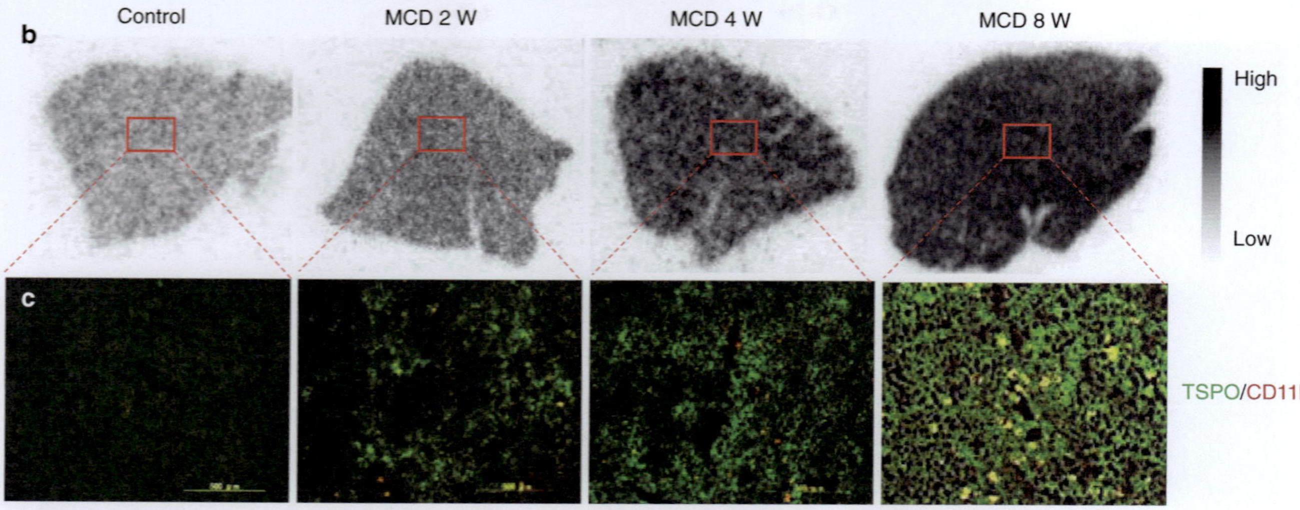

Fig. 1.20 (continued)

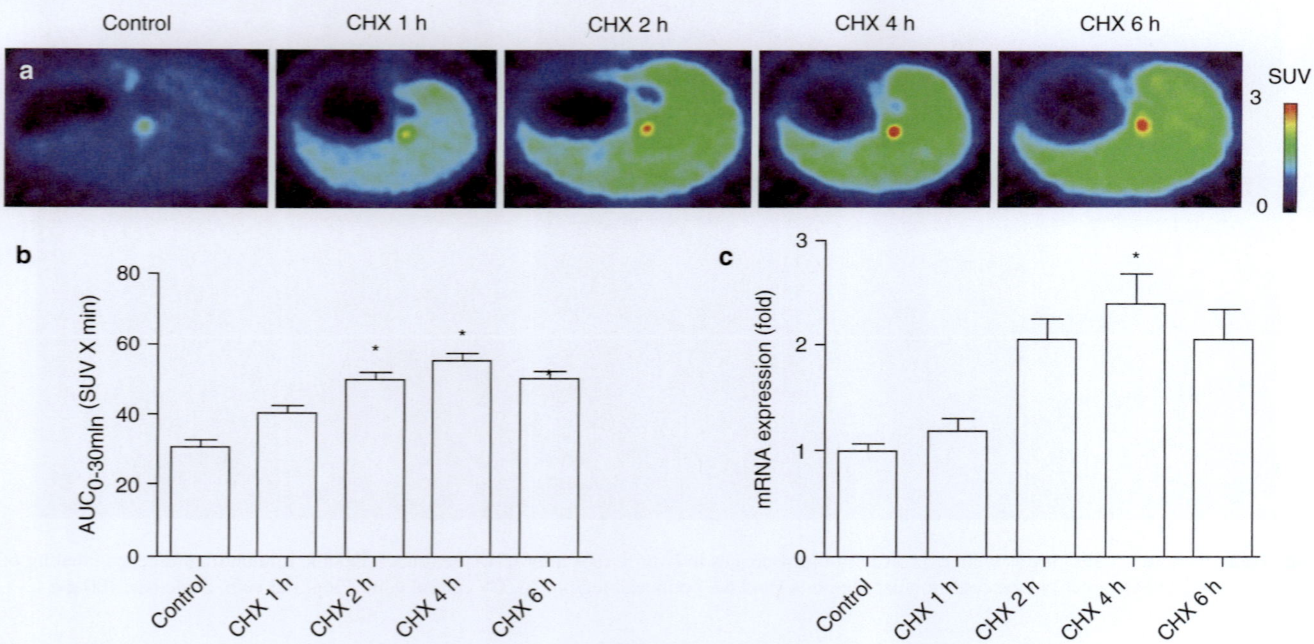

Fig. 1.21 Radioactivity and TSPO level in the livers of the control and CHX-treated rats. (**a**) Representative transverse PET liver images acquired between 0 and 30 min after injection of [^{18}F]FEDAC. (**b**) Values of areas under time-activity curves. The values ($AUC_{0\text{-}30\ min}$; SUV × min, mean ± SEM, $n = 4$) were calculated from the time-activity curves between 0 and 30 min after the injection. A significant difference ($P < 0.05$) was observed on the following comparisons, ∗: control vs. CHX 2 h, 4 h, and 6 h. (**c**) Effect of CHX treatment on the mRNA expression of TSPO. A significant difference ($P < 0.05$) was observed on the following comparisons, ∗: control vs. CHX treatment

sources enriching TSPO expression in the liver [143]. A mild acute liver damage model was prepared by a single intraperitoneal injection of cycloheximide (CHX) to rats. Treatment with CHX induced apoptosis and necrotic changes in hepatocytes with a slight neutrophil infiltration. The uptake of radioactivity in the rats' livers was measured with PET after injection of [^{18}F]FEDAC. PET with [^{18}F]FEDAC showed that the uptake of radioactivity increased in livers treated with CHX, compared to the controls (Fig. 1.21). The mRNA expression of TSPO was increased in the damaged livers compared to the controls, and the TSPO level was correlated with the [^{18}F]FEDAC uptake and severity of damage. TSPO expression in the damaged liver sections was mainly found in macrophages (Kupffer cells) and neutrophils, but not in hepatocytes (Fig. 1.22). The increase in expression of TSPO mRNA was induced by an increase in the numbers of macrophages and neutrophils with TSPO in the damaged livers.

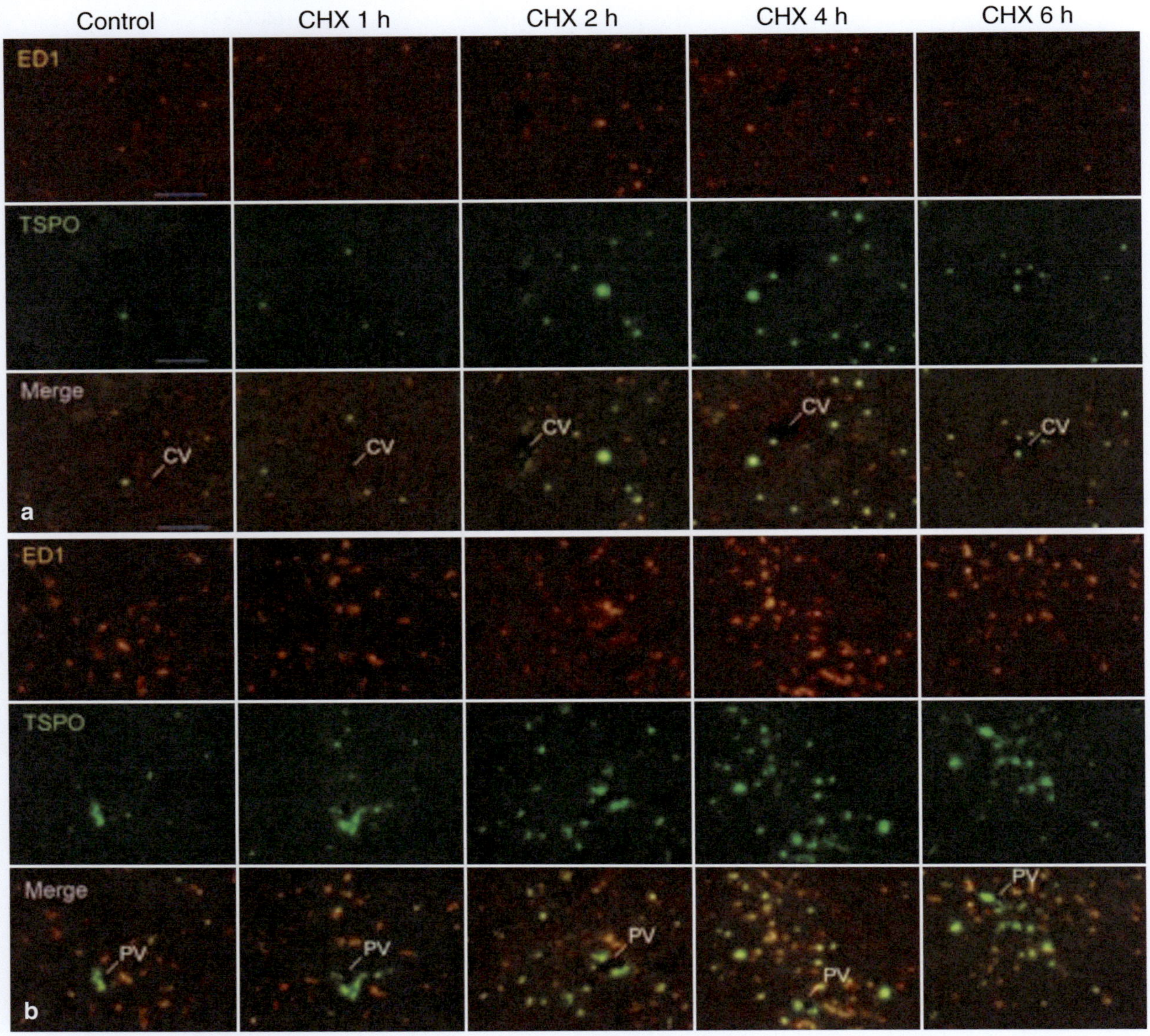

Fig. 1.22 Increased TSPO levels were expressed in macrophages in liver tissues after CHX treatment. Double immunofluorescence labeling of ED1 (red) and TSPO (green) in the centrilobular region (**a**) and the periportal region (**b**). *CV* central vein, *PV* portal vein. Scale bar: 100 μm

Through this study, we demonstrated that PET imaging with [^{18}F]FEDAC provided visible evidence that mild liver damage occurs through the enhanced TSPO signal in inflammatory cells, and that this method is a useful diagnostic tool in the early stages of acute liver damage.

1.5.6 TSPO in Liver Fibrosis

Liver fibrosis is the wound healing response to chronic liver injury, which is caused by various factors. In this study, we evaluated the utility of TSPO as a molecular imaging biomarker for monitoring the progression of liver fibrosis in response to cirrhosis [144]. To induce cirrhosis, carbon tetrachloride (CCl_4) was administered to rats and the subsequent liver fibrosis was assessed. PET with [^{18}F]FEDAC was used to noninvasively visualize liver fibrosis in vivo. PET scanning, immunohistochemical staining, ex vivo autoradiography, and quantitative reverse-transcription polymerase chain reaction were performed to elucidate the relationships among radioactivity uptake, TSPO level, and cellular source enriching TSPO expression in damaged livers. PET with [^{18}F]FEDAC showed that the uptake of radioactivity in livers significantly increased after 2, 4, 6, and 8 weeks of CCl_4 treatment (Fig. 1.23). Immunohistochemical analysis demonstrated that TSPO was primarily expressed in macrophages and liver stellate cells (HSCs). TSPO-expressing macrophages and HSCs increased with the progression of liver fibrosis (Fig. 1.24). The distribution of radioactivity from [^{18}F]FEDAC was strongly correlated with TSPO expression, and TSPO mRNA levels increased with the severity of liver damage.

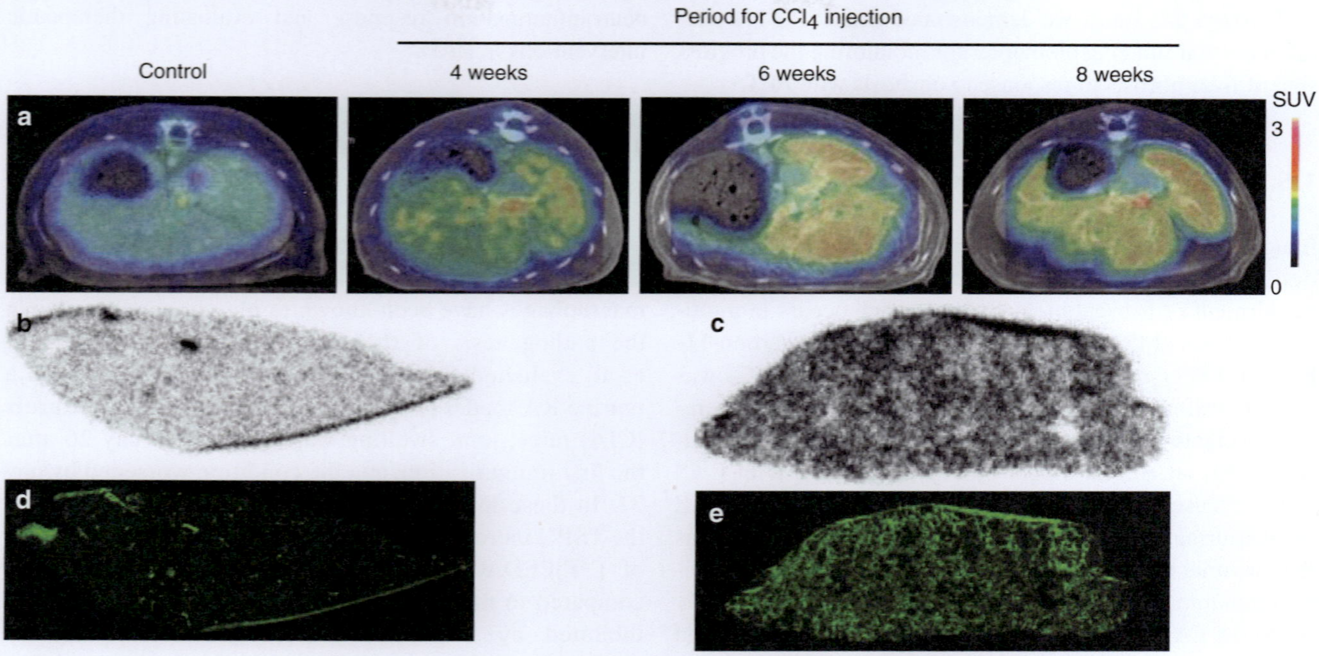

Fig. 1.23 Accumulation of radioactivity and TSPO level in the livers of control and CCl_4-treated rats. (**a**) Representative transverse PET/CT fusion images of rat livers. PET images were acquired between 0 and 30 min after injection of [^{18}F]FEDAC. (**b**) Autoradiographic image of liver section 1 h after injection of [^{18}F]FEDAC is shown for control rat. (**c**) Autoradiographic image is shown for rat treated with CCl_4 for 6 weeks. (**d**) Immunofluorescence staining of TSPO using the same sections as in (**a**) is shown for control rat. (**e**) Immunofluorescence staining and rats treated with CCl_4 for 6 weeks. The distribution of radioactivity from [^{18}F]FEDAC correlated well with the netlike appearance of TSPO expression in the hepatic lobules (**c**, **e**). Scale bar: 1 mm

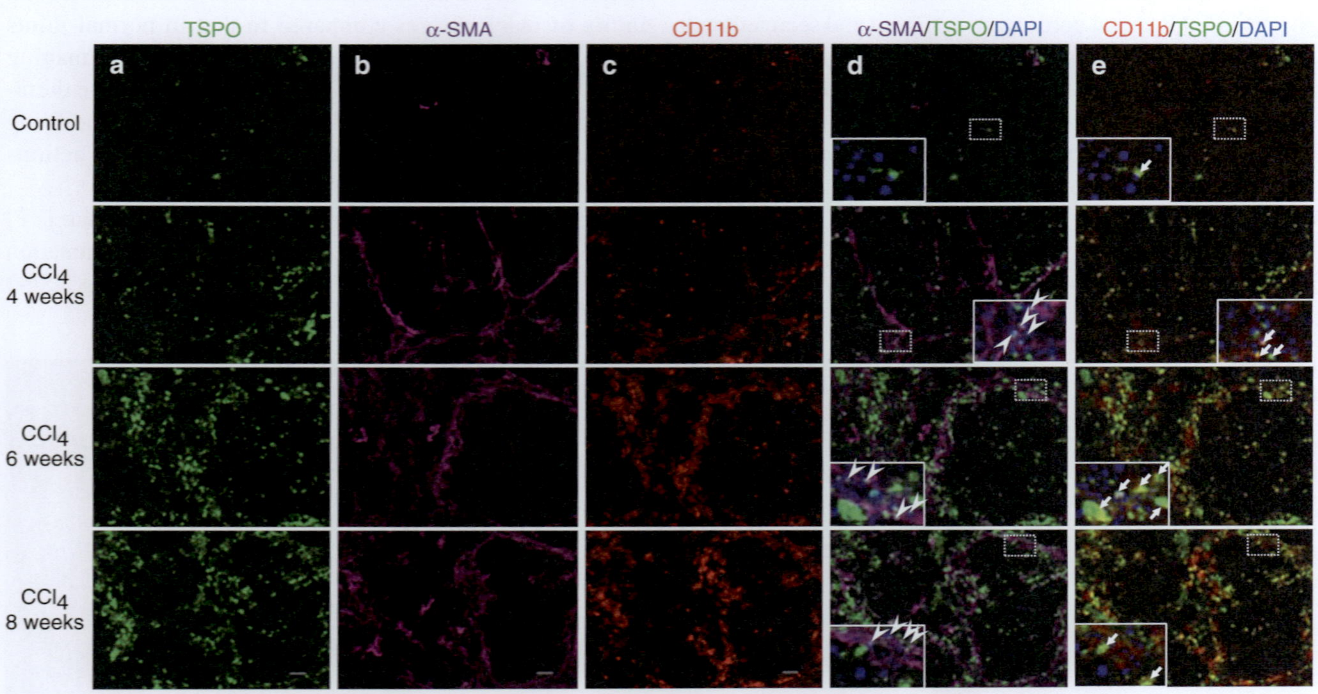

Fig. 1.24 Increased levels of TSPO expressed in HSCs and macrophages from liver tissues after CCl_4 treatment. Triple immunofluorescence labeling of TSPO (**a**, green), α-SMA (**b**, pink), CD11b (**c**, red), and DAPI (blue) in liver sections from control animals and animals treated with CCl_4 for 4, 6, or 8 weeks (**a–e**). (**d** and **e**) Show merged images of (**a**) and (**b**) and of (**a**) and (**c**), respectively. The dotted line square in each slide (**d**, **e**) is enlarged and shown in the inset with DAPI. Arrowheads point to TSPO double-stained HSCs (a-SMA-positive cells). Arrows point to TSPO double-stained macrophages (CD11b-positive cells). Scale bar: 50 μm

Through this study, we demonstrated that TSPO is a useful molecular imaging biomarker for monitoring the progression of liver fibrosis in response to cirrhosis with PET.

1.5.7 TSPO in Multiple Sclerosis

Imaging modalities have the potential to monitor inflammation in order to guide treatment before significant functional impairment or irreversible cellular damage occurs in multiple sclerosis (MS). In this study, [^{11}C]DAC, a carbon-11-labeled TSPO radiotracer derived from [^{18}F]FEDAC, was used to evaluate neuroinflammation and quantify the therapeutic effects of experimental autoimmune encephalomyelitis (EAE), an animal model of MS [145]. PET with [^{11}C]DAC was used to visually assess neuroinflammation in EAE by measuring TSPO expression in the spinal cords; there was the maximal uptake on day 11 and 20 EAE rats with significant inflammatory cell infiltration, compared to controls, day 0 and 60 EAE rats (Fig. 1.25). Biodistribution studies and in vitro autoradiography confirmed the PET imaging results. Doubling immunohistochemical studies demonstrated the infiltration and expansion of CD4+ T cells and CD11b+ microglia; CD68+ macrophages caused the increase in TSPO levels visualized by [^{11}C]DAC-PET. Furthermore, mRNA level analysis of the cytokines using quantitative reverse-transcription polymerase chain reaction revealed that TSPO+/CD4 T cells, TSPO+ microglia, and TSPO+ macrophages in EAE spinal cords were activated and secreted multiple pro-inflammation cytokines, which mediated the inflammation lesions of EAE. The EAE rats treated with an immunosuppressive agent FTY720 exhibited an absence of inflammatory cell infiltrates and displayed a faint radioactive signal, compared to the high accumulation in untreated EAE rats (Fig. 1.26).

Through this study, we demonstrated that [^{11}C]DAC-PET imaging is a useful tool for noninvasively monitoring the neuroinflammation response and evaluating therapeutic interventions in EAE.

1.5.8 TSPO in Rheumatic Arthritis

Rheumatoid arthritis (RA) is a chronic disease characterized by systemic inflammation that results in the destruction of multiple articular cartilages and bones. Activated macrophages have been known to play important roles in the pathogenesis of rheumatoid arthritis (RA). Cheon et al. evaluated the feasibility of [^{18}F]FEDAC-PET in a murine RA model [146]. In the collagen-induced arthritis (CIA) mice, joint swelling was apparent on day 26 after the first immunization, and the condition worsened by day 37. In these mice, the mRNA and protein expression of the TSPO increased in activated macrophages. The uptake of [^{18}F]FEDAC in activated macrophages was greater compared to the uptake in nonactivated cells, which was inhibited by PK11195. The [^{18}F]FEDAC uptake by arthritic joints increased early on (day 23), whereas [^{18}F]FDG uptake did not (Fig. 1.27). However, [^{18}F]FDG uptake by arthritic joints markedly increased at later stages (day 37) to a higher level than [^{18}F]FEDAC uptake. The [^{18}F]FEDAC uptake correlated weakly with the summed severity score, whereas the [^{18}F]FDG uptake correlated strongly with the summed severity score. Histologic sections of arthritic joints demonstrated an influx of macrophages compared to that in normal joints (Fig. 1.28). Moreover, these indicated that PET imaging using [^{18}F]FEDAC may be used as a predictor of the therapeutic effects caused by biological disease-modifying antirheumatic drugs that have anti-inflammatory actions to inhibit activated macrophages [147].

Through these results, it was demonstrated that [^{18}F]FEDAC enabled the visualization of active inflammation sites in arthritic joints in a CIA model by targeting TSPO

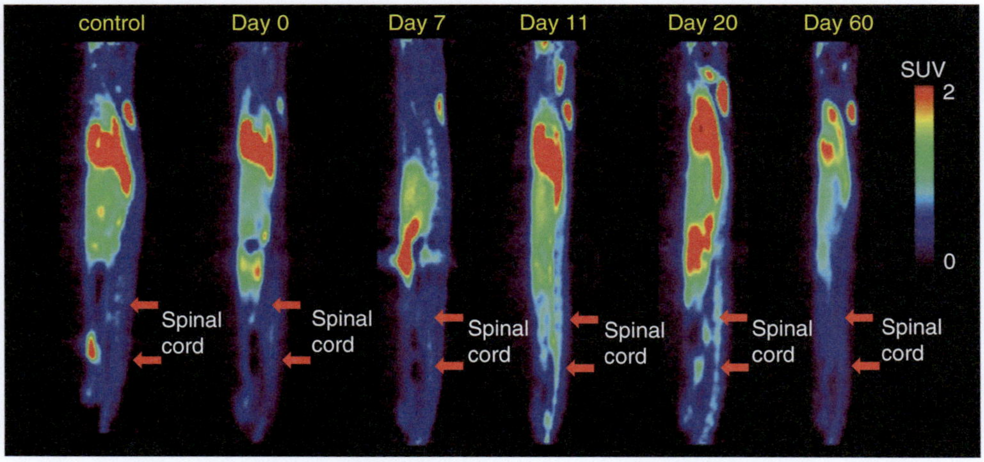

Fig. 1.25 Representative PET images acquired by summed whole scan duration of 0–30 min after [^{11}C]DAC injection. [^{11}C]DAC-PET signal increased significantly in day 7, 11, and 20 EAE spinal cords

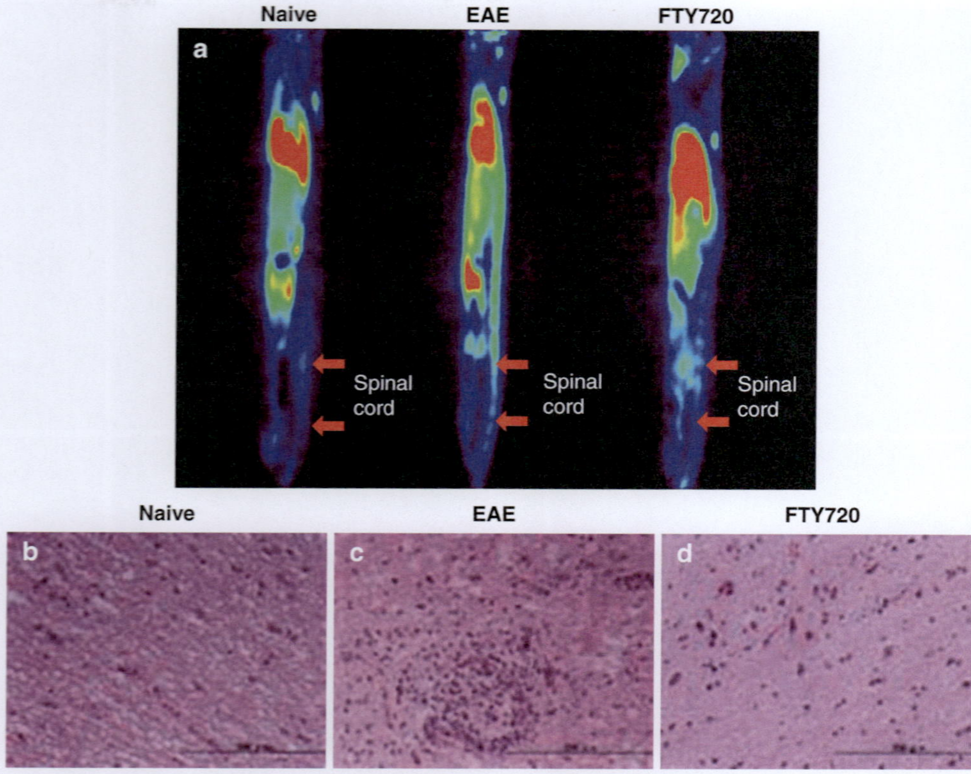

Fig. 1.26 Reduced uptake of [^{11}C]DAC in EAE by FTY720 treatment. (**a**) [^{11}C]DAC-PET scans were performed at 11 days EAE rats that treated or untreated with FTY720 ($n = 8$, respectively). Uptake of [^{11}C]DAC was clearly increased only in day 11 untreated rats, uptake in FTY720-treated rats remained low and unchanged, similar to naïve rats. Reduced uptake of [^{11}C]DAC reflected the inhibition of neuroinflammation in EAE by FTY720 treatment. (**b–d**) H&E staining of day 11 spinal sections indicated that rats with FTY720 treatment exhibited a complete absence of inflammatory cell infiltrates compared to the compressive inflammatory lesions in untreated rats

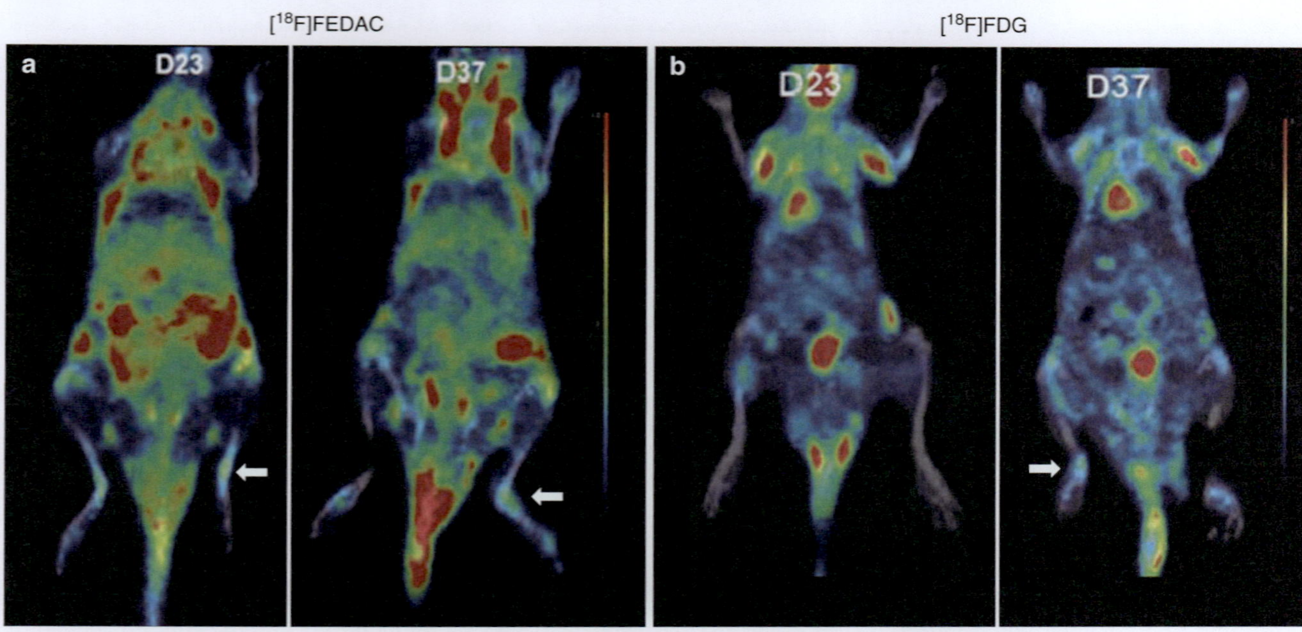

Fig. 1.27 (**a**) Coronal [^{18}F]FEDAC PET/CT section of same CIA mouse on days 23 and 37, showing increased uptake in front and hind paws. (**b**) Coronal section of [^{18}F]FDG PET/CT (**a**, **b**) in the same mouse. On day 23, uptake by joints was not observed before the onset of arthritis. On day 37, increased [^{18}F]FDG uptake was observed for all four arthritic joints

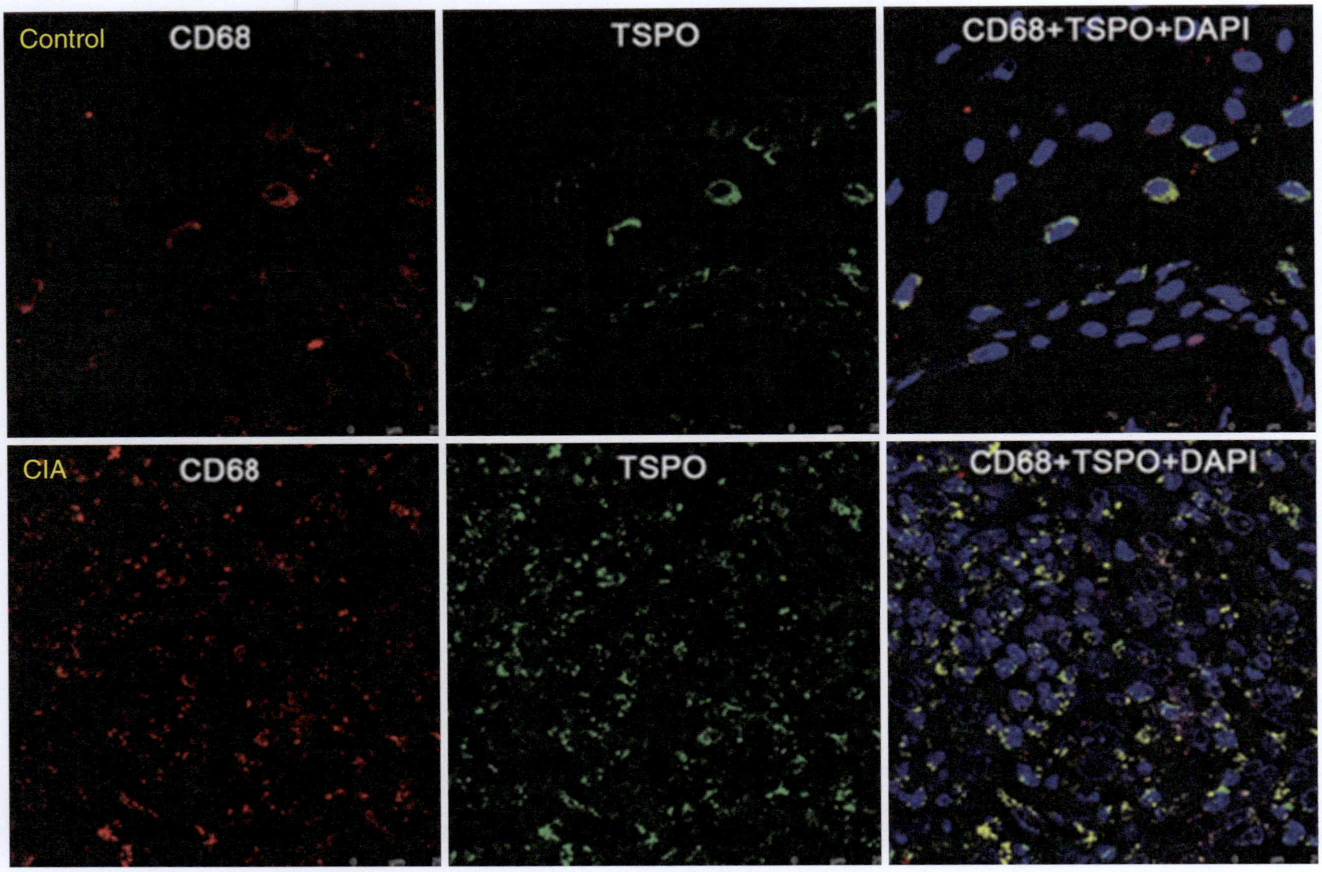

Fig. 1.28 Immunofluorescence staining for CD68 (red) and TSPO (green) in synovium of control and CIA joints. Merged images at far right show increased number and TSPO expression of CD68-positive macrophages, compared to controls

expression in activated macrophages. The results suggest the potential usefulness of [^{18}F]FEDAC-PET imaging in the early phase of RA.

1.5.9 Conclusion

[^{18}F]FEDAC-PET is a powerful tool for visualizing TSPO and monitoring the progress of various inflammatory diseases of the peripheral system. The present studies will contribute to determination of the pathogenic progress and will be of use in evaluating the therapeutic effects of anti-inflammatory drugs. In future studies, we will perform or are performing PET imaging with [^{18}F]FEDAC or other TSPO radiotracers to detect various inflammation in humans.

Acknowledgements
The author thanks Mr. Kumata, Ms. Hatori, Dr. Xie, Dr. Yanamoto, and Dr. Yamasaki in my group for their fruitful experiments and continuous outputs which contributed to this review.

1.6 Role of Microglia in Neuroinflammation

Hiromi Suzuki and Makoto Sawada

Abstract At present, common diseases of CNS were often chronic and progressive which could affect the patient's quality of life seriously. But the pathogenesis for most of them had not been fully understood and was no effective prevention or treatment. Certain pathological injury could cause cellular inflammatory response. Microglia, the first activated effector cells, played an important role in the immune defense process. Microglia had a two-way effect. On the one hand, activated microglia phagocytosed damaged cell debris and removed antigenic substances, and could release cytotoxic factors which would aggravate the injury of neuron. On the other hand, activated microglia may accumulate around damaged neurons and might induce neurotrophin-dependent protective activity. Therefore, to study the mechanism of microglia in the diseases of CNS and limit their effects on neuronal injury may help to retard the procession of some chronic disease and enhance the therapeutic effect of acute CNS diseases. Microglia are expected to become a new target for the treatment of neurodegenerative diseases and central nervous system diseases.

Keywords: Microglia, Subtype, Cytokine, Toxic change, Neuroprotection

Abbreviations

dbcAMP	dibutyryl cyclic AMP
GM-CSF	granulocyte-macrophage colony-stimulating factor
M-CSF	macrophage colony-stimulating factor
MHC	major histocompatibility complex
TGF	transforming growth factor

1.6.1 Introduction

Neurodegenerative diseases such as Alzheimer's disease and Parkinson's disease cause neuroinflammation including expression of MHC antigens and production of inflammatory cytokines. However, the condition changes greatly in relation to the onset and the formation of a pathological condition. Microglia, macrophage-like cells in the central nervous system (CNS), are multifunctional cells; they play important roles not only in the neuro-inflammation but also in the development, differentiation, and maintenance of neural cells via their phagocytic activity and production of enzymes, cytokines, and trophic factors [148].

1.6.2 Microglia Diversity

Microglial cells show a rather uniform distribution of cell numbers throughout the brain with only minor population in some brain regions. Their in situ morphologies, however, may vary markedly from elongated forms observed in apposition with neuronal fibers to spherical cell bodies with sometimes extremely elaborated branching. Human fetal microglia display heterogeneity in phenotype identified by CD68 [149]. This heterogeneity gave rise to the hypothesis that these cells are differentially conditioned by their microenvironment and, therefore, also display specific patterns of differential gene expression. For example, mRNAs of TNF-alpha, CD4, and Fc gamma receptor II are differentially expressed in microglia isolated from different area of the brain [150]. It has been reported that production of IL-12 [151] and histamine [152] are different in the subtypes of microglia. Furthermore, the subtypes of microglia show distinct acidification profiles by treatment with pepstatin A [153] and selective clearance of oligomeric beta-amyloid peptide [154]. The distinct phenotypes in activated forms of microglia might result from this heterogeneity.

Although the origin of microglia is still controversial, resident microglia is thought to be of mesodermal origin, being derived from a bone marrow precursor cell [155]. These cells or a lineage related to monocytes and macrophages may invade the CNS at an early embryonic stage to give rise eventually to typical process-bearing resident microglia [155]. Like macrophages in other tissues, the growth and activation of microglia is regulated by macrophage colony-stimulating factor (M-CSF) [156]. However, unlike macrophages, microglia are observed in macrophage-deficient mice [157–159], suggesting the possibility of the presence of M-CSF-independent populations.

Despite the postulate that microglia arise from blood monocytes, microglia appear to display phenotypes differing from macrophages. In vivo, microglia do not normally express MHC class I and II [160], CD14 [161], or scavenger receptor I and II [162]. Their appearance takes a ramified form [160]. In contrast, monocytes and macrophages express these surface antigens absent in microglia and their shape is ameboidal [160]. Like their in vivo counterparts, isolated microglia also differ from macrophages. Although cultured microglia are ameboidal, they can transform to a ramified form [163]. Microglial cell proliferation is induced by conditioned medium from astrocyte-enriched cultures [163]. Microglial production of interleukin (IL)-5 is stimulated by bioactive phorbol ester but not by interferon-γ, while the opposite is there for macrophages [164]. Microglia do not constitutively express IL-2 receptors under normal culture conditions, as do monocytes and macrophages [165]. Microglia express these receptors only after stimulation such as with lipopolysaccharide (LPS) [165]. IL-2 increases viability and proliferation of lipopolysaccharide-stimulated microglia [165], while macrophages respond to IL-2 by expressing IL-1, IL-6, and tumor necrosis factor α mRNAs, peroxide production, and microbicidal and tumoricidal activity [166, 167]. LPS, cyclosporin A, and FK506 downregulate expression of CD4 in microglia, but not in macrophages [168]. Finally, bone marrow chimera experiments have shown that resident microglia form highly stable pool of CNS cells displaying very little exchange with the bone marrow compartment [169–171]. These controversial observations suggest that microglia in the brain may be different from macrophages.

Recently, we identified two distinct subpopulations of microglia in the normal mouse brain: type I and type II. Both types had similar phagocytic activity, but they showed distinct phenotypes such as cell-surface markers, mRNA expression, and growth factor dependency. Type I, but not type II, microglia expressed the hallmarks of microglia such as CD14 and C3b receptor, and production of interleukin

1β. Type II microglia expresse surface markers for immature bone marrow cells, such as antigens against ER-MP12 and ER-MP20 antibodies, which are not detected in mature monocyte/macrophages. In addition, it also express one-tenth amount of mature cell markers compared to monocytes/macrophages. Therefore, type II microglia may arise from progenitor cells similar to immature bone marrow cells which migrate to the CNS during the early developmental stages then differentiate in the CNS; monocyte-differentiation out of bone marrow like extrathymic differentiation of T-cells [172]. This suggests that the two distinct type of microglia arise from distinct origins. In addition, type I microglia exhibited M-CSF-dependent growth, while the type II were M-CSF-independent. A previous report suggested that alveolar macrophages are GM-CSF- but not M-CSF-dependent [173]. These observations indicate that there are two distinct populations of microglia which are probably of different origins and have different functions in the brain.

1.6.3 Microglia and Neuroinflammation

The presence of oxidative stress and inflammatory activity is one of the significant pathological features of neuroinflammatory diseases [174, 175]. It has been shown that the levels of cytokines such as tumor necrosis factor (TNF)-α, interleukin (IL)-1β, and interferon (IFN)-γ are elevated in the substantia nigra of patients with Parkinson's disease [176]. Since microglia are a principal source of these cytokines, the data support microglial involvement in the pathogenesis of neuroinflammatory diseases. However, the role of activated microglia is controversial. For example, the characteristic pathological features of the Parkinson's disease brain are a selective and progressive loss of dopamine neurons of the substantia nigra and their terminals in the caudate-putamen, along with focal accumulation of activated microglia in the substantia nigra and caudate-putamen. The traditional view is that microglia act merely as scavengers and their activation is secondary to the neuronal damage. However, activated microglia have been observed in the limbic system and neocortex, where there are few or no degenerating neurons, in significantly higher numbers in PD brains than in brains from normal controls [177].

Activation of microglia has also been identified in the substantia nigra and/or striatum of parkinsonian animal models, such as l-methyl-4-phenyl-1,2,3,6-tetrahydropyridine (MPTP)-induced parkinsonism [178, 179]. The link between microglia activation and selective neuronal vulnerability has led many researchers to suggest that microglia activity participates in neuronal demise. In this respect, microglial cytotoxicity may contribute to or even promote neuronal damage. Activated microglia are capable of releasing numerous cytotoxic agents, including proteolytic enzymes, cytokines, complement proteins, reactive oxygen intermediates, NMDA-like toxins, and nitric oxide [148]. In fact, β-amyloid, the senile plaque-derived component found in Alzheimer's disease, appears to elicit neurotoxic responses through the activation of microglia [180]. However, this suggestion relies solely on in vitro data and as yet no evidence has been presented that indicates that activated microglia destroy neurons under in vivo conditions.

1.6.4 Existence of Nontoxic Activated Form of Microglia in the Brain

Recently we showed that highly activated microglia treated with LPS may have neurotrophic potential toward dopamine neurons in neonatal mice administered MPTP [181]. Tyrosine hydroxylase activity and the levels of dopamine and dihydroxyphenylacetic acid (DOPAC), as well as those of the pro-inflammatory cytokines IL-1β and IL-6, were elevated in the midbrain of LPS- and MPTP-treated neonatal mice. The viability of dopamine (A9) neurons was preserved in neonatal mice of the LPS-MPTP group compared with the MPTP group. In contrast, the viability of these neurons in aged mice dropped significantly. These results may suggest that activated microglia show different phenotypes; i.e., microglia activated by LPS in the neonatal brain may be neuroprotective for dopaminergic neurons in MPTP-treated mice, whereas in aged mice they may be neurotoxic for dopaminergic neurons. The dissociation between injury-induced microglial activation and neuronal degeneration in TNF receptor and colony-stimulating factor 1 (CSF-1) knockout mice suggests that microglial activation is not a determinate event in dopaminergic neuronal damage in brain. Furthermore, there is a growing body of evidence that microglia may play a beneficial role in ischemia by secreting factors (growth factors or cytokines) that promote survival of neurons. Therefore, activated microglia may produce not only neurotoxic effects but also neuroprotective ones, depending upon their environmental situation.

1.6.5 Direct Evidence of Neuroprotection by Microglia in the Brain

We have reported that exogenous microglia enter the brain parenchyma through the blood–brain barrier and migrate to ischemic hippocampal lesions when they are injected into the circulation. By applying this brain-targeted delivery technique, we investigated the effect of exogenous microglia on ischemic pyramidal neurons [182]. To this end, we isolated microglia from neonatal mixed brain cultures, labeled them with a fluorescent dye PKH26, and injected them into the artery of Mongolian gerbils subjected to ischemia reperfusion neuronal injury. PKH26-labeled microglia migrated to the ischemic hippocampal lesion and increased the survival of neurons, even when the cells were injected 24 h after the ischemic insult. Furthermore, stimulation of isolated microglia with IFN-γ enhanced the neuroprotective effect on the ischemic neurons.

Microglia also protected ischemia-induced learning disability. As migratory microglia increased the expression of brain-derived neurotrophic factor (BDNF) and glial cell line-derived neurotrophic factor (GDNF) in the ischemic hippocampus, they might induce neurotrophin-dependent protective activity in damaged neurons. These results represent the first experimental demonstration of neurotrophic effects of microglia on transient global ischemia in vivo. Since peripherally injected microglia exhibit specific affinity for ischemic brain lesions and protect against ischemic neuronal injury in the present model, we suggest that microglia may have the potential to be used as a candidate for cell therapy for CNS repair following transitory global ischemia and other neurodegenerative diseases.

1.6.6 Toxic Transformation of Microglia by Nef Protein Introduction

Nef, a multifunctional HIV protein, activates the Vav/Rac/p21-activated kinase (PAK) signaling pathway. Given the potential role of this pathway in the activation of the phagocyte NADPH oxidase, we have investigated the effect of the HIV-1 Nef protein on microglia superoxide production and toxicity for neurons [183]. Microglia were transduced with lentiviral expression vectors to produce a high level of Nef protein. Expression of Nef did not activate the NADPH oxidase by itself, but led to a massive enhancement of the responses to a variety of stimuli (Ca2+ ionophore, formyl peptide, endotoxin) and induction to produce a large amount of superoxide. These effects were not caused by upregulation of phagocyte NADPH oxidase subunits. Nef mutants lacking motifs involved in the interaction with plasma membrane and/or other cytosolic proteins failed to reproduce the effects of wild-type Nef, suggesting involvement of a certain signaling pathway in microglia for their trophic-toxic control. Our results suggest a key role for Rac activation in the priming for microglia toxic activation, which is enhanced by Nef introduction in the nontoxic form of microglia. Rac activation is not sufficient to induce the toxic form of microglia accompanied by stimulation of the phagocyte NADPH oxidase; however, it markedly enhances the NADPH oxidase response to other stimuli and might be involved in the trophic-toxic control of microglia.

1.6.7 CNS Cytokine Network

Cytokines are polypeptidic soluble factors that control the growth and differentiation of cells involved in immune and hematopoietic systems. These factors were initially considered to act on target cells in a cell-type and stage-specific manner. However, it has been shown that their biological actions are pleiotropic, complementary, and counteractive; each of them exerts multiple effects on different cells, and different factors can act on the same cell populations to induce similar or opposite effects. Moreover, production of several cytokines is controlled by other cytokines in a stimulatory or inhibitory manner, and, in some cases, acts as a cascade. These complex cytokine actions are therefore referred to as a cytokine network.

Recent evidence suggests that bidirectional communication occurs between cells of the nervous and immune systems. The basis for this communication is the release of cytokines by immune component cells, as well as hormone products of the neuroendocrine system. Cells resident within the CNS can synthesize, secrete, and respond to inflammatory cytokines not only contributing to the responses to injury or immunological challenge within the CNS but also regulating their own growth and differentiation potential. There are many similarities of cytokine actions between the immune system and the CNS. However, there are also several unique modes of cytokine action in the CNS (i.e., their target cells, inducing functions on the target cells such as other cytokine production, major histocompatibility complex (MHC) antigen induction, and cell growth control, and inducing agents of their production). Therefore, the actions and communication of cytokines in the CNS are designated as the CNS cytokine network [184].

Microglia are one of the most important cells in the CNS cytokine network. They produce a variety of cytokines, as well as their proliferation and other functions are regulated by cytokines. Astrocytes are another cell population important in the CNS cytokine network. There are many similar aspects of cytokine production and responses between microglia and astrocytes; however, the roles in the CNS cytokine network may differ between these cells; microglia may have an important function in the removal of dead cells or their remnants by phagocytosis in brain injury, while astrocytes provide structural and environmental support for neurons. There are no clear indications of the difference between the roles of microglia and astrocytes in the cytokine production and response.

Some of these cytokines control the growth, differentiation, and activation of cells in the CNS, and some modulate growth factor production, MHC antigen expression, and morphological changes. Their biological functions are mediated by specific receptors, some of which are expressed in the CNS, and cellular localization of cytokine receptors in the CNS has been demonstrated. Neuronal cells and oligodendrocytes as well as microglia and astrocytes expressed several cytokine receptors indicating that certain functions of these cells may also be controlled by some cytokines. However, to determine the involvement of cytokines in controlling the functions and development of CNS cells requires elucidating the functional relationships of cytokines and these cells.

There are two aspects of roles of the CNS cytokine network, one of which is regulation of growth and differentiation of neural cells, and production of cytokines in the CNS. Another aspect of the CNS cytokine network is its interaction with the immune system. Since the majority of cytokines are produced by immune cells, it is possible that immune cells may also control the growth and function of CNS cells. Therefore, the control of microglial growth by cytokines is an important method of regulation of CNS cells by peripheral immune cells. In addition to this, cytokines produced in the CNS can control immune cell functions. These communications may be important for brain-immune interactions, and some aspects may play crucial roles in certain pathological conditions such as AIDS-dementia complex and multiple sclerosis as well as several neurological diseases.

1.7 Application of Preclinical PET Imaging for Infectious Diseases

Kodai Nishi and Takashi Kudo

Abstract PET is a useful imaging tool for basic studies. Preclinical imaging studies such as small-animal PET allow the performance of imaging experiments using the same individuals, without sacrificing the animals. Some researchers who study infectious diseases are thus paying close attention to preclinical imaging techniques. Generally, pathogens are classified by their risk, as the biosafety level (BSL). When conducting research using high-BSL pathogens, special facilities are necessary for pathogen containment. At Nagasaki University, a small-animal imaging system was introduced into BSL-3 section, and various infectious disease imaging studies have been conducted, such as for severe fever with thrombocytopenia syndrome (SFTS), leishmaniasis, and so on. FDG and ^{67}Ga-citrate are widely used radiotracers for the clinical imaging that can detect inflammation due to infection. For animal imaging, ^{68}Ga-citrate is a PET tracer that is not yet approved for human imaging, and can be used instead of ^{67}Ga-citrate, which is single photon emission computed tomography (SPECT) tracer. Even without using special or unorthodox radiotracers, new knowledge and important information can be obtained from preclinical PET studies.

Keywords: Small animal imaging, Preclinical study, Infectious diseases, Biosafety level

1.7.1 Introduction

PET imaging has recently gained wide use not only in clinical stages but also in basic studies. Small-animal imaging uses the same technology as clinical imaging. Clinical research and problems can thus be introduced to preclinical research directly using small animals. Conversely, applying results obtained from preclinical studies to clinical imaging is also possible. Imaging has bridged the gap between basic studies and clinical research, and has become widely recognized as a tool for translational research.

In traditional animal experiments, relatively high numbers of animals are often required. One reason is that animals are sacrificed to remove organs or tissues for the purposes of observation and measurement. Another is the influence of individual differences. In particular, the four elements of pharmacokinetics (absorption, distribution, metabolism, and excretion) are known to be strongly affected by individual differences. The number of samples must therefore be increased for accurate statistical processing.

On the other hand, preclinical imaging experiments allow use of the same individual, performing the study and repeatedly acquiring data without killing the individual. This means that applying human imaging techniques to a small animal allows follow-up of changes over time in disease models in the same individual, clarifying changes according to the disease condition more precisely, as in daily practice in the clinical field. In addition, preclinical imaging is an effective technique not only for providing biological information but also for reducing the number of experimental animals.

In the area of research into infectious diseases, evaluation of pathogen infection, tracking disease state, and observation over time of individuals are very important, because infectious and inflammatory diseases change with the passage of time. For example, diseases may pass through stages of infection, pathogenesis, ingravescence, remission, and healing. When those stages of infectious disease are studied by sacrificing the animals, the number of animals required to obtain meaningful results will become extremely large due to the large interindi-

Table 1.2 BSL classification of representative pathogens

BSL	Virus	Bacteria	Fungi	Parasitic insect
2	*Dengue virus*	*C. botulinum*	*Aspergillus fumigatus*	*Balantidium coli*
	Hepatitis C virus	*C. jejuni, coli*	*Candida albicans*	*Leishmania*
	Norovirus	*E. coli*	*Cryptococcus neoformans*	*Echinococcus*
	Papillomavirus	*H. pylori*		*Anisakinae*
3	*SARS corona virus*	*F. tularensis*	*Blastomyces dermatitidis*	N/A
	West-Nile virus	*M. tuberculosis*	*Histoplasma capsulatum*	
	SFTS virus	*S. enterica*	*Penicillium marneffei*	
	New York virus	*R. japonica*		
4	*Lassa*	N/A	N/A	N/A
	Ebola			
	Marburg			

vidual variance of animals. Small animal PET imaging has therefore gained attention as a useful experimental method.

1.7.2 Imaging Laboratory for Infectious Diseases

To conduct imaging studies using infected model animals, a special laboratory is required. This is because researchers must be protected not only from radiation exposure but also from the risk of infection. Biosafety level (BSL) is a classification depending on the degree of pathogen risk. Table 1.2 shows representative pathogens sorted by BSL from the guidelines of the National Institute of Infectious Disease (NIID).

When dealing with high-risk pathogens, researchers need to use a biocontainment laboratory conforming to the World Health Organization (WHO) guidelines. When using imaging systems, measures must also be taken to avoid contamination by biohazards, such as installation in separated safety rooms, prevention of cross-contamination using sealed animal tubes, and so on [185]. In addition, researchers need to wear a Tyvek coverall, mask, rubber gloves and face guard (Fig. 1.29). Given the restrictions as described above, only limited numbers of facilities around the world are capable of performing imaging studies for infectious diseases, and relatively few studies have been conducted.

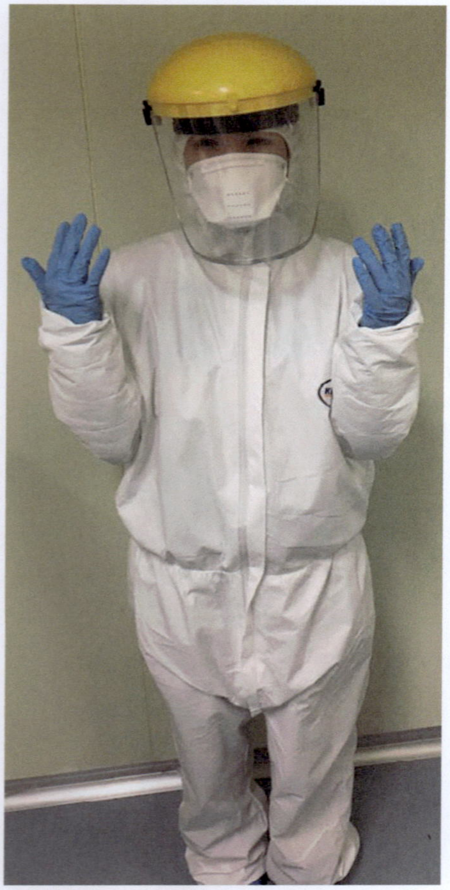

Fig. 1.29 An example of using protective clothing to prevent exposure of the skin and cover the face completely with the face guard

1.7.3 PET Imaging with Infectious Small Animals

In 2012, a small-animal imaging system was introduced to the BSL-3 section of the radioisotope center at Nagasaki University, making this the only facility in which researchers could perform imaging of infectious diseases requiring a high BSL in Japan. Since then, various infectious diseases imaging studies have been conducted.

Hayasaka et al. reported an FDG-PET study using mice infected with severe fever with thrombocytopenia syndrome (SFTS) virus, which is categorized as BSL-3. SFTS is a tick-borne infection that causes severe inflammation in the gastrointestinal tract [186]. In that study, SFTSV-infected mice were administered about 10 MBq of FDG intravenously via the tail vain. PET acquisition was performed for 30 min from 30 min after FDG injection. FDG uptake was found along the course of the intestine in the SFTS-infected mouse (Fig. 1.30) [187].

PET studies on SFTS have also been performed using ^{68}Ga tracer. Fuchigami et al. tried to visualize SFTS with ^{68}Ga-citrate [188]. Generally, ^{67}Ga-citrate is a radiotracer used for single-photon computed tomography (SPECT), and is widely used to detect tumors [189, 190], inflammation, and infectious diseases [190, 191]. Since ^{68}Ga-citrate is a PET tracer behaving exactly the same as ^{67}Ga-citrate, targets can be imaged quantitatively and with higher sensitivity. In that study, SFTSV-infected mice were administered about 5 MBq of ^{68}Ga-citrate intravenously via the tail vain. PET acquisition was performed for 1 h, starting 2 h after ^{68}Ga-citrate injection. As shown in Fig. 1.31, high accumulation of ^{68}Ga-citrate in the gastrointestinal tract was observed in SFTSV-infected mice, and the accumulation pattern of ^{68}Ga-citrate resembled that of FDG.

In addition, ^{68}Ga-citrate was used for PET imaging of leishmaniasis [188]. Leishmaniasis is a tropical disease caused by *Leishmania* parasites categorized as BSL-2, and *Leishmania* leads to strong localized inflammation [192]. *Leishmania* parasite-infected mice were administered about 4 MBq of ^{68}Ga-citrate intravenously via the tail vein. PET acquisition was performed for 1 h, starting 2 h after ^{68}Ga-citrate injection. As shown in Fig. 1.32, inflammation site-specific accumulation of ^{68}Ga-citrate was observed [188].

The examples given here are only a small selection of many studies underway at Nagasaki University. Infectious disease studies are more diverse than tumor studies, because infectious diseases have numerous diseases classified as tropical infections and emerging infectious diseases, and many issues have not been elucidated for each disease. FDG and ^{68}Ga-citrate used in the studies introduced this section are widely used general radiotracers that are easily obtained. Even without using special or unorthodox radiotracers, new knowledge can be obtained from preclinical PET studies.

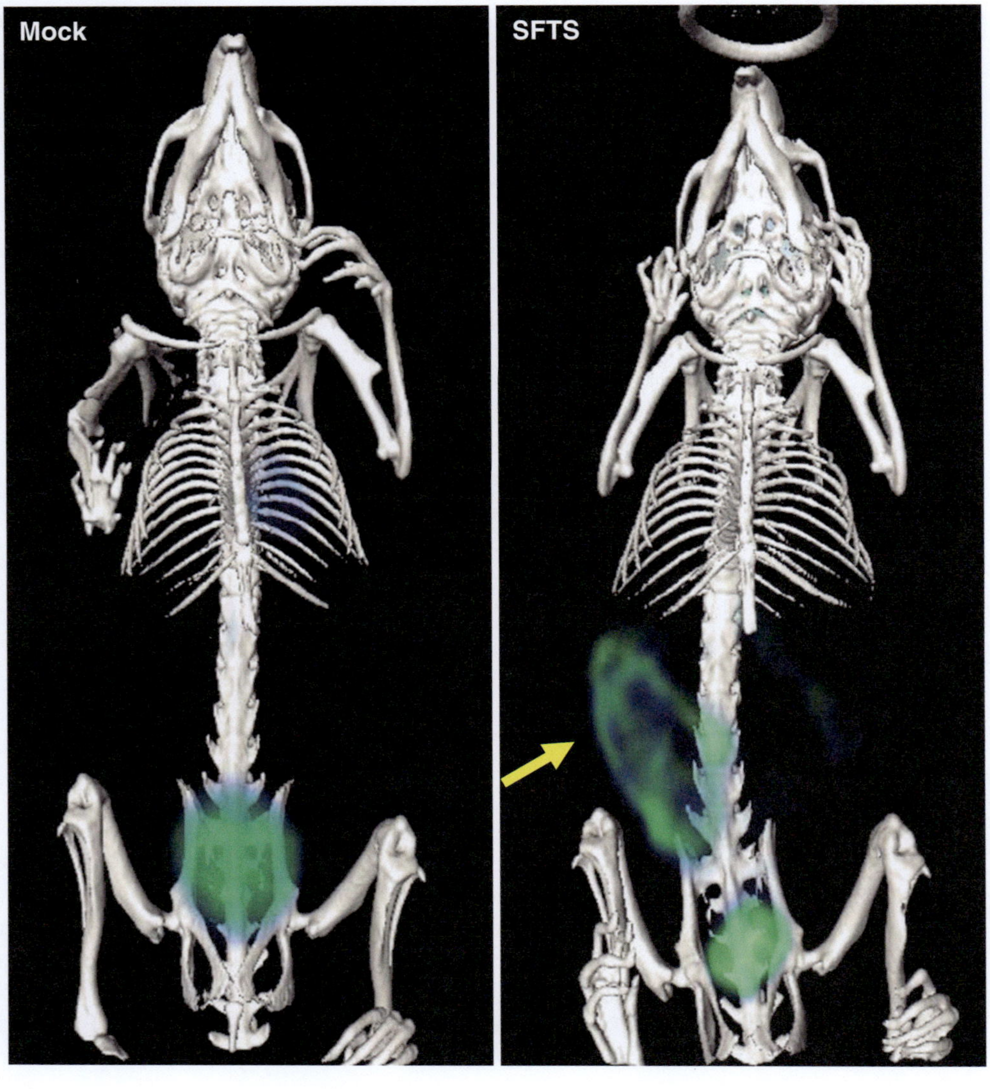

Fig. 1.30 FDG-PET/CT images of mice with or without SFTSV infection. In the mock-infected mouse, FDG accumulation is observed in the heart and bladder. On the other hand, in the SFTSV-infected mouse, FDG accumulates in the gastrointestinal tract (yellow arrow)

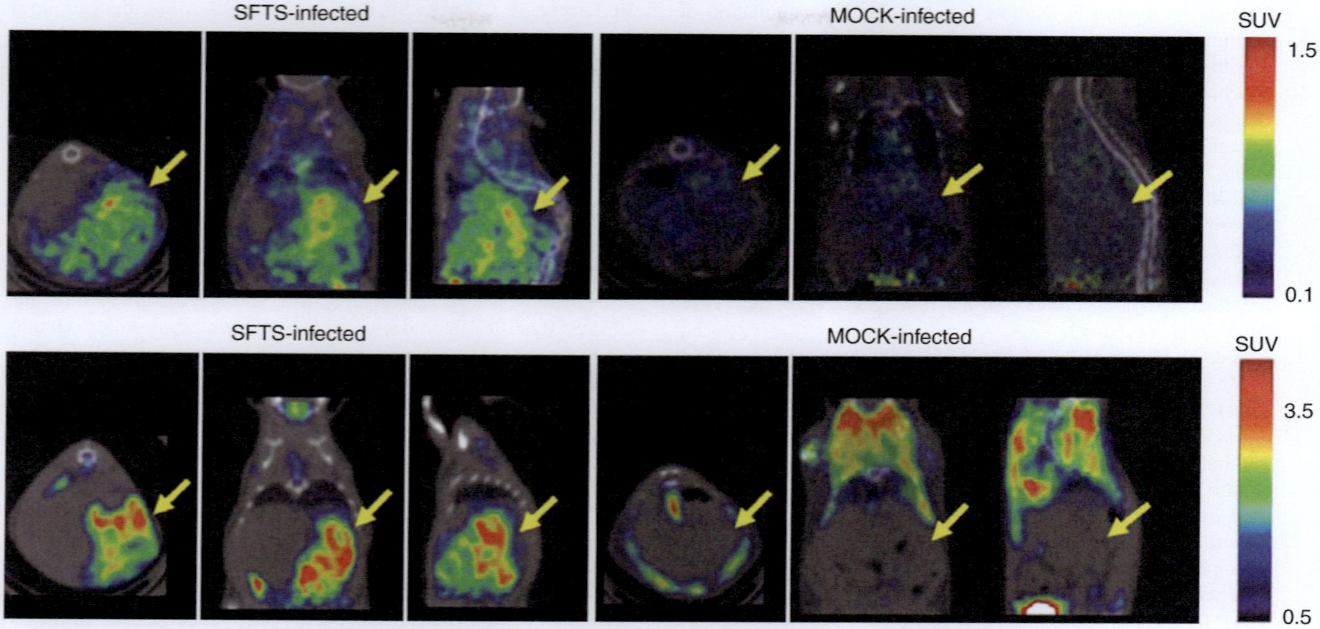

Fig. 1.31 Images from ^{68}Ga-citrate (**a**) and FDG (**b**) PET/CT of SFTSV-infected and mock-infected mice. Yellow arrows indicate the gastrointestinal tract

The pathological condition of the infected animal will change depending on species differences and the infected pathogen. Some models only have about 3 days between infection and death. When conducting imaging research into infectious diseases, investigation of the survival rate of model animals as a preliminary experiment and preparation of a survival curve is desirable. Also, breeding of model animals requires prevention of infection with other infectious diseases. Experiments using infected animals thus require some additional caution, as previously mentioned.

In conclusion, small animal imaging using preclinical PET bridges the gap between basic researches and clinical practices and works as an important tool for translational research in infectious disease.

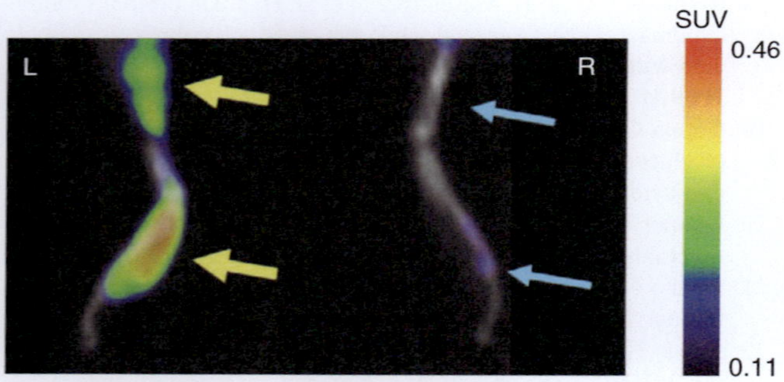

Fig. 1.32 PET/CT images of footpad regions in *L. major*-infected mice. A signal from the ^{68}Ga-citrate is observed at a site in the left leg (yellow arrows), with no signal in the contralateral leg (blue arrows)

Acknowledgement
The authors are grateful to the American Chemical Society (ACS) for allowing reuse of some images (Figs. 1.31 and 1.32) and a direct link to the ACS article: https://pubs.acs.org/doi/abs/10.1021/acsomega.7b00147.

References

1. Kubota K. From tumor biology to clinical PET: a review of positron emission tomography (PET) in oncology. Ann Nucl Med. 2001;15:471–86.
2. Fletcher JW, Djulbegovic B, Soares HP, et al. Recommendations on the use of 18F-FDG PET in oncology. J Nucl Med. 2008;49:480–508.
3. Boellaard R, Delgado-Bolton R, Oyen WJ, et al. FDG PET/CT: EANM procedure guidelines for tumour imaging: version 2.0. Eur J Nucl Med Mol Imaging. 2015;42:328–54.
4. Tahara T, Ichiya Y, Kuwabara Y, et al. High [18F]fluorodeoxyglucose uptake in abdominal abscess: a PET study. J Comput Assist Tomogr. 1989;13:829–31.
5. Sasaki M, Ichiya Y, Kuwabara Y, et al. Ring-like uptake of [18F] FDG in brain abscess: a PET study. J Comput Assist Tomogr. 1990;14:486–7.
6. Kubota K, Matsuzawa T, Fujiwara T, et al. Differential diagnosis of lung tumor with positron emission tomography: a prospective study. J Nucl Med. 1990;31:1927–33.
7. Kubota R, Yamada S, Kubota K, et al. Intratumoral distribution of fluorine-18-fluorodeoxyglucose in vivo: high accumulation in macrophages and granulation tissues studied by microautoradiography. J Nucl Med. 1992;33:1972–80.
8. Kubota K, Kubota R, Yamada S. FDG accumulation in tumor tissue. J Nucl Med. 1993;34:75–82.

9. Yamada S, Kubota K, Kubota R, et al. High accumulation of fluorine-18-fluorodeoxyglucose in turpentine-induced inflammatory tissue. J Nucl Med. 1995;36:1301–6.
10. Mochizuki T, Tsukamoto E, Kuge Y, et al. FDG uptake and glucose transporter subtype expressions in experimental tumor and inflammation models. J Nucl Med. 2001;42:1551–5.
11. Zhao S, Kuge Y, Masashi Kohanawa M, et al. Usefulness of 11C-Methionine for differentiating tumors from granulomas in experimental rat models: a comparison with 18F-FDG and 18F-FLT. J Nucl Med. 2008;49:135–41.
12. Deichen TJ, Prante O, Gack M, et al. Uptake of [18F]fluorodeoxyglucose in human monocyte-macrophages in vitro. Eur J Nucl Med. 2003;30:267–73.
13. Malide D, Davies-Hill TM, Levine M, et al. Distinct localization of GLUT-1, -3, and -5 in human monocyte-derived macrophages: effects of cell activation. Am J Phys. 1998;274(3):E516–26.
14. Jones HA, Cadwallader KA, White JF, et al. Dissociation between respiratory burst activity and deoxyglucose uptake in human neutrophil granulocytes: implications for interpretation of 18F-FDG PET images. J Nucl Med. 2002;43:652–7.
15. Ishimori T, Saga T, Mameda M, et al. Increased 18F-FDG uptake in a model of inflammation: Concanavalin A–mediated lymphocyte activation. J Nucl Med. 2002;43:658–63.
16. Lee DM, Weinblatt ME. Rheumatoid arthritis. Lancet. 2001;358:903–11.
17. Matsui T, Nakata N, Nagai S, et al. Inflammatory cytokines and hypoxia contribute to 18F-FDG uptake by cells involved in pannus formation in rheumatoid arthritis. J Nucl Med. 2009;50:920–6.
18. Roiniotis J, Dinh H, Masendycz P, et al. Hypoxia prolongs monocyte/macrophage survival and enhanced glycolysis is associated with their maturation under aerobic conditions. J Immunol. 2009;182:7974–81.
19. Garcia-Carbonell R, Divakaruni AS, Lodi A, et al. Critical role of glucose metabolism in rheumatoid arthritis fibroblast-like synoviocytes. Arthritis Rheumatol. 2016;68:1614–26.
20. Cramer T, Yamanishi Y, Clausen BE, et al. HIF-1α is essential for myeloid cell-mediated inflammation. Cell. 2003;112:645–57.
21. Denko NC. Hypoxia, HIF1 and glucose metabolism in the solid tumour. Nat Rev Cancer. 2008;8:705–13.
22. Jamar F, Buscombe J, Chiti A, et al. EANM/SNMI guideline for 18F-FDG use in inflammation and infection. J Nucl Med. 2013;54:647–58.
23. Lendon CL, Davies MJ, Born GV, et al. Atherosclerotic plaque caps are locally weakened when macrophages density is increased. Atherosclerosis. 1991;87:87–90.
24. MacNeill BD, Jang IK, Bouma BE, et al. Focal and multi-focal plaque macrophage distributions in patients with acute and stable presentations of coronary artery disease. J Am Coll Cardiol. 2004;44:972–9.
25. Kubota R, Kubota K, Yamada S, et al. Microautoradiographic study for the differentiation of intratumoral macrophages, granulation tissues and cancer cells by the dynamics of fluorine-18-fluorodeoxyglucose uptake. J Nucl Med. 1994;35:104–12.
26. Tatsumi M, Cohade C, Nakamoto Y, et al. Fluorodeoxyglucose uptake in the aortic wall at PET/CT: possible finding for active atherosclerosis. Radiology. 2003;229:831–7.
27. Rudd JH, Warburton EA, Fryer TD, et al. Imaging atherosclerotic plaque inflammation with [18F]-fluorodeoxyglucose positron emission tomography. Circulation. 2002;105:2708–11.
28. Yun M, Jang S, Cucchiara A, et al. 18F FDG uptake in the large arteries: a correlation study with the atherogenic risk factors. Semin Nucl Med. 2002;32:70–6.
29. Ogawa M, Ishino S, Mukai T, et al. (18)F-FDG accumulation in atherosclerotic plaques: immunohistochemical and PET imaging study. J Nucl Med. 2004;45:1245–50.
30. Graebe M, Pedersen SF, Borgwardt L, et al. Molecular pathology in vulnerable carotid plaques: correlation with [18]-fluorodeoxyglucose positron emission tomography (FDG-PET). Eur J Vasc Endovasc Surg. 2009;37:714–21.
31. Tawakol A, Migrino RQ, Bashian GG, et al. In vivo 18F-fluorodeoxyglucose positron emission tomography imaging provides a noninvasive measure of carotid plaque inflammation in patients. J Am Coll Cardiol. 2006;48:1818–24.
32. Wu YW, Kao HL, Chen MF, et al. Characterization of plaques using 18F-FDG PET/CT in patients with carotid atherosclerosis and correlation with matrix metalloproteinase-1. J Nucl Med. 2007;48:227–33.
33. Tahara N, Kai H, Yamagishi S, et al. Vascular inflammation evaluated by [18F]-fluorodeoxyglucose positron emission tomography is associated with the metabolic syndrome. J Am Coll Cardiol. 2007;49:1533–9.
34. Skeoch S, Williams H, Cristinacce P, et al. Evaluation of carotid plaque inflammation in patients with active rheumatoid arthritis using (18)F-fluorodeoxyglucose PET-CT and MRI: a pilot study. Lancet. 2015;385(Suppl 1):S91.
35. Ogawa M, Nakamura S, Saito Y, et al. What can be seen by 18F-FDG PET in atherosclerosis imaging? The effect of foam cell formation on 18F-FDG uptake to macrophages in vitro. J Nucl Med. 2012;53:55–8.
36. Ishino S, Ogawa M, Mori I, et al. 18F-FDG PET and intravascular ultrasonography (IVUS) images compared with histology of atherosclerotic plaques: 18F-FDG accumulates in foamy macrophages. Eur J Nucl Med Mol Imaging. 2014;41:624–33.
37. Colin S, Chinetti-Gbaguidi G, Staels B. Macrophage phenotypes in atherosclerosis. Immunol Rev. 2014;262:153–66.
38. Mantovani A, Garlanda C, Locati M. Macrophage diversity and polarization in atherosclerosis: a question of balance. Arterioscler Thromb Vasc Biol. 2009;29:1419–23.
39. Satomi T, Ogawa M, Mori I, et al. Comparison of contrast agents for atherosclerosis imaging using cultured macrophages: FDG versus ultrasmall superparamagnetic iron oxide. J Nucl Med. 2013;54:999–1004.
40. Shiomi M, Ito T, Hirouchi Y, et al. Fibromuscular cap composition is important for the stability of established atherosclerotic plaques in mature WHHL rabbits treated with statins. Atherosclerosis. 2001;157:75–84.
41. Fukumoto Y, Libby P, Rabkin E, et al. Statins alter smooth muscle cell accumulation and collagen content in established atheroma of watanabe heritable hyperlipidemic rabbits. Circulation. 2001;103:993–9.
42. Daugherty A, Zweifel BS, Schonfeld G. The effects of probucol on the progression of atherosclerosis in mature Watanabe heritable hyperlipidaemic rabbits. Br J Pharmacol. 1991;103:1013–8.
43. Steinberg D, Parthasarathy S, Carew TE. In vivo inhibition of foam cell development by probucol in Watanabe rabbits. Am J Cardiol. 1988;62:6B–12B.
44. Ogawa M, Magata Y, Kato T, et al. Application of 18F-FDG PET for monitoring the therapeutic effect of antiinflammatory drugs on stabilization of vulnerable atherosclerotic plaques. J Nucl Med. 2006;47:1845–50.
45. Pirro M, Simental-Mendia LE, Bianconi V, et al. Effect of statin therapy on arterial wall inflammation based on 18F-FDG PET/CT: a systematic review and meta-analysis of interventional studies. J Clin Med. 2019;8:118.
46. Moghbel M, Al-Zaghal A, Werner TJ, et al. The role of PET in evaluating atherosclerosis: a critical review. Semin Nucl Med. 2018;48:488–97.
47. Mehta NN, Torigian DA, Gelfand JM, et al. Quantification of atherosclerotic plaque activity and vascular inflammation using [18-F] fluorodeoxyglucose positron emission tomography/computed tomography (FDG-PET/CT). J Vis Exp. 2012;63:e3777.

48. Wu YW, Kao HL, Huang CL, et al. The effects of 3-month atorvastatin therapy on arterial inflammation, calcification, abdominal adipose tissue and circulating biomarkers. Eur J Nucl Med Mol Imaging. 2012;39:399–407.
49. Ishii H, Nishio M, Takahashi H, et al. Comparison of atorvastatin 5 and 20 mg/d for reducing F-18 fluorodeoxyglucose uptake in atherosclerotic plaques on positron emission tomography/computed tomography: a randomized, investigator-blinded, open-label, 6-month study in Japanese adults scheduled for percutaneous coronary intervention. Clin Ther. 2010;32:2337–47.
50. Tahara N, Kai H, Ishibashi M, et al. Simvastatin attenuates plaque inflammation: evaluation by fluorodeoxyglucose positron emission tomography. J Am Coll Cardiol. 2006;48:1825–31.
51. Fayad ZA, Mani V, Woodward M, et al. Safety and efficacy of dalcetrapib on atherosclerotic disease using novel non-invasive multimodality imaging (dal-PLAQUE): a randomised clinical trial. Lancet. 2011;378:1547–59.
52. Duivenvoorden R, Mani V, Woodward M, et al. Relationship of serum inflammatory biomarkers with plaque inflammation assessed by FDG PET/CT: the dal-PLAQUE study. JACC Cardiovasc Imaging. 2013;6:1087–94.
53. Hellberg S, Silvola JM, Kiugel M, et al. Type 2 diabetes enhances arterial uptake of choline in atherosclerotic mice: an imaging study with positron emission tomography tracer (1)(8) F-fluoromethylcholine. Cardiovasc Diabetol. 2016;15:26.
54. Kato K, Schober O, Ikeda M, et al. Evaluation and comparison of 11C-choline uptake and calcification in aortic and common carotid arterial walls with combined PET/CT. Eur J Nucl Med Mol Imaging. 2009;36:1622–8.
55. Ammirati E, Moroni F, Magnoni M, et al. Carotid artery plaque uptake of (11)C-PK11195 inversely correlates with circulating monocytes and classical CD14(++)CD16(−) monocytes expressing HLA-DR. Int J Cardiol Heart Vasc. 2018;21:32–5.
56. Gaemperli O, Shalhoub J, Owen DR, et al. Imaging intraplaque inflammation in carotid atherosclerosis with 11C-PK11195 positron emission tomography/computed tomography. Eur Heart J. 2012;33:1902–10.
57. Lee R, Kim J, Paeng JC, et al. Measurement of (68)Ga-DOTATOC uptake in the thoracic aorta and its correlation with cardiovascular risk. Nucl Med Mol Imaging. 2018;52:279–86.
58. Malmberg C, Ripa RS, Johnbeck CB, et al. 64Cu-DOTATATE for noninvasive assessment of atherosclerosis in large arteries and its correlation with risk factors: head-to-head comparison with 68Ga-DOTATOC in 60 patients. J Nucl Med. 2015;56:1895–900.
59. Mateo J, Izquierdo-Garcia D, Badimon JJ, et al. Noninvasive assessment of hypoxia in rabbit advanced atherosclerosis using (1)(8)F-fluoromisonidazole positron emission tomographic imaging. Circ Cardiovasc Imaging. 2014;7:312–20.
60. Dai D, Chuang HH, Macapinlac HA, et al. Correlation of fluorine 18-labeled sodium fluoride uptake and arterial calcification on whole-body PET/CT in cancer patients. Nucl Med Commun. 2019;40:604–10.
61. Kitagawa T, Yamamoto H, Nakamoto Y, et al. Predictive value of (18)F-sodium fluoride positron emission tomography in detecting high-risk coronary artery disease in combination with computed tomography. J Am Heart Assoc. 2018;7:e010224.
62. Bellinge JW, Francis RJ, Majeed K, et al. In search of the vulnerable patient or the vulnerable plaque: (18)F-sodium fluoride positron emission tomography for cardiovascular risk stratification. J Nucl Cardiol. 2018;25:1774–83.
63. Kitagawa T, Yamamoto H, Toshimitsu S, et al. (18)F-sodium fluoride positron emission tomography for molecular imaging of coronary atherosclerosis based on computed tomography analysis. Atherosclerosis. 2017;263:385–92.
64. Hellberg S, Silvola JMU, Liljenback H, et al. Amyloid-targeting PET tracer [(18)F]Flutemetamol accumulates in atherosclerotic plaques. Molecules. 2019;24:1072.
65. McKenney-Drake ML, Moghbel MC, Paydary K, et al. (18)F-NaF and (18)F-FDG as molecular probes in the evaluation of atherosclerosis. Eur J Nucl Med Mol Imaging. 2018;45:2190–200.
66. Li X, Heber D, Cal-Gonzalez J, et al. Association between osteogenesis and inflammation during the progression of calcified plaque evaluated by (18)F-fluoride and (18)F-FDG. J Nucl Med. 2017;58:968–74.
67. Quirce R, Martinez-Rodriguez I, Banzo I, et al. New insight of functional molecular imaging into the atheroma biology: 18F-NaF and 18F-FDG in symptomatic and asymptomatic carotid plaques after recent CVA. Preliminary results. Clin Physiol Funct Imaging. 2016;36:499–503.
68. Ishiwata Y, Kaneta T, Nawata S, et al. Quantification of temporal changes in calcium score in active atherosclerotic plaque in major vessels by (18)F-sodium fluoride PET/CT. Eur J Nucl Med Mol Imaging. 2017;44:1529–37.
69. Irkle A, Vesey AT, Lewis DY, et al. Identifying active vascular microcalcification by (18)F-sodium fluoride positron emission tomography. Nat Commun. 2015;6:7495.
70. Alam MM, Lee J, Lee SY. Recent progress in the development of TSPO PET ligands for neuroinflammation imaging in neurological diseases. Nucl Med Mol Imaging. 2017;51(4):283–96.
71. Truillet C, et al. Longitudinal imaging of microglia-astrocyte activation in mouse mesial temporal lobe epilepsy with TSPO PET to identify the best therapeutic time windows. Médecine Nucléaire. 2018;42(3):179–80.
72. Maeda J, et al. In vivo positron emission tomographic imaging of glial responses to amyloid-beta and tau pathologies in mouse models of Alzheimer's disease and related disorders. J Neurosci. 2011;31(12):4720–30.
73. Dupont AC, et al. Translocator protein-18 kDa (TSPO) positron emission tomography (PET) imaging and its clinical impact in neurodegenerative diseases. Int J Mol Sci. 2017;18(4):E785.
74. Ji B, et al. Imaging of peripheral benzodiazepine receptor expression as biomarkers of detrimental versus beneficial glial responses in mouse models of Alzheimer's and other CNS pathologies. J Neurosci. 2008;28(47):12255–67.
75. Ji B, et al. Distinct binding of amyloid imaging ligands to unique amyloid-beta deposited in the presubiculum of Alzheimer's disease. J Neurochem. 2015;135(5):859–66.
76. Ishikawa A, et al. In vivo visualization of tau accumulation, microglial activation, and brain atrophy in a mouse model of tauopathy rTg4510. J Alzheimers Dis. 2018;61(3):1037–52.
77. Maeda J, et al. Longitudinal, quantitative assessment of amyloid, neuroinflammation, and anti-amyloid treatment in a living mouse model of Alzheimer's disease enabled by positron emission tomography. J Neurosci. 2007;27(41):10957–68.
78. Ni R, et al. Comparative in vitro and in vivo quantifications of pathologic tau deposits and their association with neurodegeneration in tauopathy mouse models. J Nucl Med. 2018;59(6):960–6.
79. Gargiulo S, et al. Imaging of brain TSPO expression in a mouse model of amyotrophic lateral sclerosis with (18) F-DPA-714 and micro-PET/CT. Eur J Nucl Med Mol Imaging. 2016;43(7):1348–59.
80. Walker MD, et al. [11C]PBR28 PET imaging is sensitive to neuroinflammation in the aged rat. J Cereb Blood Flow Metab. 2015;35(8):1331–8.
81. Gerhard A. TSPO imaging in parkinsonian disorders. Clin Transl Imaging. 2016;4:183–90.
82. Varnas K, et al. PET imaging of [(11)C]PBR28 in Parkinson's disease patients does not indicate increased binding to TSPO

despite reduced dopamine transporter binding. Eur J Nucl Med Mol Imaging. 2019;46(2):367–75.
83. Morrice JR, Gregory-Evans CY, Shaw CA. Animal models of amyotrophic lateral sclerosis: a comparison of model validity. Neural Regen Res. 2018;13(12):2050–4.
84. Jankowsky JL, Zheng H. Practical considerations for choosing a mouse model of Alzheimer's disease. Mol Neurodegener. 2017;12(1):89.
85. Owen DR, et al. An 18-kDa translocator protein (TSPO) polymorphism explains differences in binding affinity of the PET radioligand PBR28. J Cereb Blood Flow Metab. 2012;32(1):1–5.
86. Rizzo G, et al. Kinetic modeling without accounting for the vascular component impairs the quantification of [(11)C]PBR28 brain PET data. J Cereb Blood Flow Metab. 2014;34(6):1060–9.
87. Tomasi G, et al. Novel reference region model reveals increased microglial and reduced vascular binding of 11C-(R)-PK11195 in patients with Alzheimer's disease. J Nucl Med. 2008;49(8):1249–56.
88. Horti AG, et al. PET imaging of microglia by targeting macrophage colony-stimulating factor 1 receptor (CSF1R). Proc Natl Acad Sci U S A. 2019;116(5):1686–91.
89. Tanzey SS, et al. Synthesis and initial in vivo evaluation of [(11) C]AZ683—a novel PET radiotracer for colony stimulating factor 1 receptor (CSF1R). Pharmaceuticals (Basel). 2018;11(4):136.
90. Beaino W, et al. Purinergic receptors P2Y12R and P2X7R: potential targets for PET imaging of microglia phenotypes in multiple sclerosis. J Neuroinflammation. 2017;14(1):259.
91. Janssen B, et al. Identification of the allosteric P2X7 receptor antagonist [(11)C]SMW139 as a PET tracer of microglial activation. Sci Rep. 2018;8(1):6580.
92. Territo PR, et al. Characterization of (11)C-GSK1482160 for targeting the P2X7 receptor as a biomarker for neuroinflammation. J Nucl Med. 2017;58(3):458–65.
93. Berdyyeva T, et al. PET imaging of the P2X7 ion channel with a novel tracer [(18)F]JNJ-64413739 in a rat model of neuroinflammation. Mol Imaging Biol. 2019;21:871–8.
94. Kolb H, et al. Preclinical evaluation and non-human primate receptor occupancy study of (18)F-JNJ-64413739, a novel PET radioligand for P2X7 receptors. J Nucl Med. 2019;60:1154–9.
95. Koole M, et al. (18)F-JNJ-64413739, a novel PET ligand for the P2X7 ion channel: radiation dosimetry, kinetic modeling, test-retest variability and occupancy of the P2X7 antagonist JNJ-54175446. J Nucl Med. 2019;60:683–90.
96. Villa A, et al. Identification of new molecular targets for PET imaging of the microglial anti-inflammatory activation state. Theranostics. 2018;8(19):5400–18.
97. DiSabato DJ, Quan N, Godbout JP. Neuroinflammation: the devil is in the details. J Neurochem. 2016;139(Suppl 2):136–53.
98. Kawabori M, Yenari MA. Inflammatory responses in brain ischemia. Curr Med Chem. 2015;22(10):1258–77.
99. Hosomi S, Watabe T, Mori Y, et al. Inflammatory projections after focal brain injury trigger neuronal network disruption: an (18) F-DPA714 PET study in mice. Neuroimage Clin. 2018;20:946–54.
100. Chen WW, Zhang X, Huang WJ. Role of neuroinflammation in neurodegenerative diseases (review). Mol Med Rep. 2016;13(4):3391–6.
101. Prata J, Santos SG, Almeida MI, et al. Bridging autism spectrum disorders and schizophrenia through inflammation and biomarkers—pre-clinical and clinical investigations. J Neuroinflammation. 2017;14(1):179.
102. Vivash L, O'Brien TJ. Imaging microglial activation with TSPO PET: lighting up neurologic diseases? J Nucl Med. 2016;57(2):165–8.
103. Kreisl WC, Fujita M, Fujimura Y, et al. Comparison of [^{11}C]-(R)-PK 11195 and [^{11}C]PBR28, two radioligands for translocator protein (18 kDa) in human and monkey: implications for positron emission tomographic imaging of this inflammation biomarker. NeuroImage. 2010;49:2924–32.
104. Kobayashi M, Jiang T, Telu S, et al. ^{11}C-DPA-713 has much greater specific binding to translocator protein 18 kDa (TSPO) in human brain than ^{11}C-(R)-PK11195. J Cereb Blood Flow Metab. 2018;38:393–403.
105. Doorduin J, Klein HC, Dierckx RA, James M, Kassiou M, de Vries EF. [^{11}C]-DPA-713 and [^{18}F]-DPA-714 as new PET tracers for TSPO: a comparison with [^{11}C]-(R)-PK11195 in a rat model of herpes encephalitis. Mol Imaging Biol. 2009;11:386–98.
106. Owen DR, Yeo AJ, Gunn RN, et al. An 18-kDa translocator protein (TSPO) polymorphism explains differences in binding affinity of the PET radioligand PBR28. J Cereb Blood Flow Metab. 2012;32(1):1–5. https://doi.org/10.1038/jcbfm.2011.147.
107. Lavisse S, Guillermier M, Herard AS, et al. Reactive astrocytes overexpress TSPO and are detected by TSPO positron emission tomography imaging. J Neurosci. 2012;32:10809–18.
108. Watabe T, Kanai Y, Ikeda H, et al. Evaluation of recanalization of occluded middle cerebral artery and restored cerebral blood flow in rats with transient brain ischemia: a combination study of digital subtraction angiography and ^{15}O-water positron emission tomography. Cereb Blood Flow Metabolism. 2015;26(2):1–9.
109. Koizumi J, Yoshida Y, Nakazawa T, Oneda G. Experimental studies of ischemic brain edema. A new experimental model of cerebral embolism in rats in which recirculation can be introduced in the ischemia area. Jpn J Stroke. 1986;8:1–8.
110. Martin A, Boisgard R, Theze B, et al. Evaluation of the PBR/TSPO radioligand [(18)F]DPA-714 in a rat model of focal cerebral ischemia. J Cereb Blood Flow Metab. 2010;30(1):230–41.
111. Martin A, Boisgard R, Kassiou M, Dolle F, Tavitian B. Reduced PBR/TSPO expression after minocycline treatment in a rat model of focal cerebral ischemia: a PET study using [(18)F]DPA-714. Mol Imaging Biol. 2011;13(1):10–5.
112. Jin X, Ishii H, Bai Z, Itokazu T, Yamashita T. Temporal changes in cell marker expression and cellular infiltration in a controlled cortical impact model in adult male C57BL/6 mice. PLoS One. 2012;7(7):e41892.
113. Hosomi S, Koyama Y, Watabe T, Ohnishi M, Ogura H, Yamashita T, et al. Myeloid-derived suppressor cells infiltrate the brain and suppress neuroinflammation in a mouse model of focal traumatic brain injury. Neuroscience. 2019;406:457–66. https://doi.org/10.1016/j.neuroscience.2019.03.015.
114. Maeda J, Zhang MR, Okauchi T, Ji B, Ono M, Hattori S, et al. In vivo positron emission tomographic imaging of glial responses to amyloid-beta and tau pathologies in mouse models of Alzheimer's disease and related disorders. J Neurosci. 2011;31(12):4720–30.
115. Ji B, Maeda J, Sawada M, Ono M, Okauchi T, Inaji M, et al. Imaging of peripheral benzodiazepine receptor expression as biomarkers of detrimental versus beneficial glial responses in mouse models of Alzheimer's and other CNS pathologies. J Neurosci. 2008;28(47):12255–67.
116. Maier FC, Wehrl HF, Schmid AM, et al. Longitudinal PET-MRI reveals beta-amyloid deposition and rCBF dynamics and connects vascular amyloidosis to quantitative loss of perfusion. Nat Med. 2014;20(12):1485–92.
117. Shukuri M, Takashima-Hirano M, Tokuda K, Takashima T, Matsumura K, Inoue O, et al. In vivo expression of cyclooxygenase-1 in activated microglia and macrophages during neuroinflammation visualized by PET with 11C-ketoprofen methyl ester. J Nucl Med. 2011;52(7):1094–101.
118. Shukuri M, Mawatari A, Ohno M, Suzuki M, Doi H, Watanabe Y, et al. Detection of cyclooxygenase-1 in activated microglia during amyloid plaque progression: PET studies in Alzheimer's disease model mice. J Nucl Med. 2016;57(2):291–6.
119. Imamoto N, Momosaki S, Fujita M, Omachi S, Yamato H, Kimura M, et al. [11C]PK11195 PET imaging of spinal glial activation after nerve injury in rats. NeuroImage. 2013;79:121–8.
120. Belloli S, Zanotti L, Murtaj V, Mazzon C, Di Grigoli G, Monterisi C, et al. (18)F-VC701-PET and MRI in the in vivo neuroinflam-

mation assessment of a mouse model of multiple sclerosis. J Neuroinflammation. 2018;15(1):33.
121. Higuchi M, Ji B, Maeda J, et al. In vivo imaging of neuroinflammation in Alzheimer's disease. Clin Experiment Neuroimmunol. 2016;7:139–44.
122. Parvathenani LK, Tertyshnikova S, Greco CR, Roberts SB, Robertson B, Posmantur R. P2X7 mediates superoxide production in primary microglia and is up-regulated in a transgenic mouse model of Alzheimer's disease. J Biol Chem. 2003;278(15):13309–17.
123. Moore CS, Ase AR, Kinsara A, Rao VT, Michell-Robinson M, Leong SY, et al. P2Y12 expression and function in alternatively activated human microglia. Neurol Neuroimmunol Neuroinflamm. 2015;2(2):e80.
124. Kolb H, Barret O, Bhattacharya A, Chen G, Constantinescu C, Huang C, et al. Preclinical evaluation and non-human primate receptor occupancy study of (18)F-JNJ-64413739, a novel PET radioligand for P2X7 receptors. J Nucl Med. 2019;60:1154–9.
125. Koole M, Schmidt M, Hijzen A, Ravenstijn P, Vandermeulen C, Van Weehaeghe D, et al. (18)F-JNJ-64413739, a novel PET ligand for the P2X7 ion channel: radiation dosimetry, kinetic modeling, test-retest variability and occupancy of the P2X7 antagonist JNJ-54175446. J Nucl Med. 2019;60:683–90.
126. Fu Z, Lin Q, Hu B, Zhang Y, Chen W, Zhu J, et al. P2X7 radioligand (18)F-PTTP for the differentiation of lung tumor and inflammation. J Nucl Med. 2019; https://doi.org/10.2967/jnumed.118.222547.
127. Narayanaswami V, Dahl K, Bernard-Gauthier V, Josephson L, Cumming P, Vasdev N. Emerging PET radiotracers and targets for imaging of neuroinflammation in neurodegenerative diseases: outlook beyond TSPO. Mol Imaging. 2018;17:1536012118792317. https://doi.org/10.1177/1536012118792317.
128. Papadopoulos V, Baraldi M, Guilarte TR, et al. Translocator protein (18 kDa): new nomenclature for the peripheral-type benzodiazepine receptor based on its structure and molecular function. Trends Pharmacol Sci. 2006;27:402–9.
129. Zhang MR, Kida T, Noguchi J, Furutsuka K, Maeda J, Suhara T, Suzuki K. [^{11}C]DAA1106: radiosynthesis and in vivo binding to peripheral benzodiazepine receptors in mouse brain. Nucl Med Biol. 2003;30:513–9.
130. Maeda J, Suhara T, Zhang MR, et al. Novel peripheral benzodiazepine receptor ligand [^{11}C]DAA1106 for PET: an imaging tool for glial cells in the brain. Synapse. 2004;52:283–91.
131. Ikoma Y, Yasuno F, Ito H, et al. Quantitative analysis for estimating binding potential of the peripheral benzodiazepine receptor with [^{11}C]DAA1106. J Cereb Blood Flow Metab. 2007;27:173–84.
132. Zhang MR, Maeda J, Furutsuka K, et al. [^{18}F]FMDAA1106 and [^{18}F]FEDAA1106: two positron-emitter labeled ligands for peripheral benzodiazepine receptor (PBR). Bioorg Med Chem Lett. 2003;13:201–4.
133. Zhang MR, Maeda J, Ogawa M, et al. Development of a new radioligand, N-(5-fluoro-2-phenoxyphenyl)-N-(2-[^{18}F]fluoroethyl-5-methoxybenzyl)acetamide, for pet imaging of peripheral benzodiazepine receptor in primate brain. J Med Chem. 2004;47:2228–35.
134. Fujimura Y, Ikoma Y, Yasuno F, et al. Quantitative analyses of ^{18}F-FEDAA1106 binding to peripheral benzodiazepine receptors in living human brain. J Nucl Med. 2006;47:43–50.
135. Zhang MR, Kumata K, Maeda J, et al. ^{11}C-AC-5216: a novel PET ligand for peripheral benzodiazepine receptors in the primate brain. J Nucl Med. 2007;48:1853–61.
136. Miyoshi M, Ito H, Arakawa R, et al. Quantitative analysis of peripheral benzodiazepine receptor in the human brain using PET with ^{11}C-AC-5216. J Nucl Med. 2009;50:1095–101.
137. Yanamoto K, Kumata K, Yamasaki T, et al. [^{18}F]FEAC and [^{18}F]FEDAC: two novel positron emission tomography ligands for peripheral-type benzodiazepine receptor in the brain. Bioorg Med Chem Lett. 2009;19:1707–10.
138. Yui J, Maeda J, Kumata K, et al. ^{18}F-FEAC and ^{18}F-FEDAC: PET of the monkey brain and imaging of translocator protein (18 kDa) in the infarcted rat brain. J Nucl Med. 2010;51:1301–9.
139. Kawamura K, Kumata K, Takei M, et al. Efficient radiosynthesis and non-clinical safety tests of the TSPO radioprobe [^{18}F]FEDAC: prerequisites for clinical application. Nucl Med Biol. 2016;43:445–53.
140. Yanamoto K, Kumata K, Fujinaga M, et al. In vivo imaging and quantitative analysis of TSPO in rat peripheral tissues using small-animal PET with [^{18}F]FEDAC. Nucl Med Biol. 2010;37:853–60.
141. Hatori A, Yui J, Yamasaki T, et al. PET imaging of lung inflammation with [^{18}F]FEDAC, a radioligand for translocator protein (18 kDa). PLoS One. 2012;7:e45065.
142. Xie L, Yui J, Hatori A, et al. Translocator protein (18 kDa), a potential molecular imaging biomarker for non-invasively distinguishing non-alcoholic fatty liver disease. J Hepatol. 2012;57:1076–82.
143. Hatori A, Yui J, Xie L, et al. Visualization of acute liver damage induced by cycloheximide in rats using PET with [^{18}F]FEDAC, a radiotracer for translocator protein (18 kDa). PLoS One. 2014;9:e86625.
144. Hatori A, Yui J, Xie L, et al. Utility of translocator protein (18 kDa) as a molecular imaging biomarker to monitor the progression of liver fibrosis. Sci Rep. 2015;5:17327.
145. Xie L, Yamasaki T, Ichimaru N, et al. [^{11}C]DAC-PET for noninvasively monitoring neuroinflammation and immunosuppressive therapy efficacy in rat experimental autoimmune encephalomyelitis model. J Neuroimmune Pharmacol. 2012;7:231–42.
146. Chung SJ, Yoon HJ, Youn H, et al. ^{18}F-FEDAC as a targeting agent for activated macrophages in DBA/1 mice with collagen-induced arthritis: comparison with ^{18}F-FDG. J Nucl Med. 2018;59:839–45.
147. Chung SJ, Youn H, Jeong EJ, et al. In vivo imaging of activated macrophages by ^{18}F-FEDAC, a TSPO targeting PET ligand, in the use of biologic disease-modifying anti-rheumatic drugs (bDMARDs). Biochem Biophys Res Commun. 2018;506:216–22.
148. Cunningham C. Microglia and neurodegeneration: the role of systemic inflammation. Glia. 2013;61:71–90.
149. Rezaie P, Patel K, Male DK. Microglia in the human fetal spinal cord; patterns of distribution, morphology and phenotype. Dev Brain Res. 1999;115:71–8.
150. Ren L, Lubrich B, Biber K, Gebicke-Haerter PJ. Mol Brain Res. 1999;65:198–205.
151. Suzumura A, Sawada M, Takayanagi T. Production of interleukin-12 and expression of its receptors by murine microglia. Brain Res. 1998;787:139–42.
152. Katoh Y, Niimi M, Yamamoto Y, Kawamura T, Morimoto-Ishizuka T, Sawada M, Takemori H, Yamatodani A. Histamine production by cultured microglial cells of the mouse. Neurosci Lett. 2001;305:181–4.
153. Okada M, Irie S, Sawada M, Urae R, Urae A, Iwata N, Ozaki N, Akazawa K, Nakanishi H. Pepstatin a induces extracellular acidification distinct from aspartic protease inhibition in microglial cell lines. Glia. 2003;43:167–74.
154. Shimizu E, Kawahara K, Kajizono M, Sawada M, Nakayama H. Interleukin-4-induced selective clearance of oligomeric beta-amyloid peptide1-42 by rat primary type-2 microglia. J Immunol. 2008;181:6503–13.
155. Ling EA, Wong WC. The origin and nature of ramified and amoeboid microglia: a historical review and current concepts. Glia. 1993;7:9–18.
156. Sawada M, Suzumura A, Yamamoto H, Marunouchi T. Activation and proliferation of the isolated microglia by colony stimulating factor-1 and possible involvement of protein kinase C. Brain Res. 1990;509:119–24.
157. Witmer-Pack MD, Hughes DA, Schuler G, Lawson L, McWilliam A, Inaba K, Steinman RM, Gordon S. Identification of macro-

phages and dendritic cells in the osteopetrotic (*op/op*) mouse. J Cell Sci. 1993;104:1021–9.
158. Wiktor JW, Bartocci A, Ferrante AJ, Ahmed AA, Sell KW, Pollard JW, Stanley ER. Total absence of colony-stimulating factor 1 in the macrophage-deficient osteopetrotic (*op/op*) mouse. Proc Natl Acad Sci U S A. 1990;87:4828–32.
159. Yoshida H, Hayashi S, Kunisada T, Ogawa M, Nishikawa S, Okamura H, Sudo T, Shultz LD, Nishikawa S. The murine mutation osteopetrosis is in the coding region of the macrophage colony stimulating factor gene. Nature. 1990;345:442–4.
160. Gehrmann J, Matsumoto Y, Kreutzberg GW. Microglia: intrinsic immuneffector cell of the brain. Brain Res Brain Res Rev. 1995;20:269–87.
161. Ziegler-Heitbrock HWL, Ulevitch RJ. CD14: cell surface receptor and differentiation marker. Immunol Today. 1993;14:121–5.
162. Freeman MW. Macrophage scavenger receptors. Curr Opin Lipidol. 1994;5:143–8.
163. Suzumura A, Marunouchi T, Yamamoto H. Morphological transformation of microglia in vitro. Brain Res. 1991;545:301–6.
164. Sawada M, Suzumura A, Itoh Y, Marunouchi T. Production of interleukin-5 by mouse astrocytes and microglia in culture. Neurosci Lett. 1993;155:175–8.
165. Sawada M, Suzumura A, Marunouchi T. Induction of functional interleukin-2 receptor in mouse microglia. J Neurochem. 1995;64:1973–9.
166. Kovacs E, Brock B, Varesio L, Young H. IL-2 induction of IL-1 beta mRNA expression in monocytes. J Immunol. 1989;143:3532–7.
167. Wahl S, McCartney-Francis N, Hunt D, Smith P, Wahl L, Katona I. Monocyte interleukin-2-receptor gene expression and interleukin-2 augmentation of microbicidal activity. J Immunol. 1987;139:1342–7.
168. Sawada M, Suzumura A, Marunouchi T. Down regulation of CD4 expression in cultured microglia by immunosuppressants and lipopolysaccharide. Biochem Biophys Res Commun. 1992;189:869–76.
169. Lassmann H, Schmied M, Vass K, Hickey WF. Bone marrow derived elements and resident microglia in brain inflammation. Glia. 1993;7:19–24.
170. Matsumoto Y, Fujiwara M. Absence of donor-type major histocompatibility complex class I antigen- bearing microglia in the rat central nervous system of radiation bone marrow chimeras. J Neuroimmunol. 1987;17:71–82.
171. MatsumotoY, HaraN, TanakaR, FujiwaraM. Immunohistochemical analysis of the rat central nervous system during experimental allergic encephalomyelitis, with special reference to Ia-positive cells with dendritic morphology. J Immunol. 1986;136:3668–76.
172. Rocha B, von BH, Guy GD. Selection of intraepithelial lymphocytes with CD8 alpha/alpha co-receptors by self-antigen in the murine gut. Proc Natl Acad Sci U S A. 1992;89:5336–40.
173. Nakata K, Akagawa KS, Fukayama M, Hayashi Y, Kadokura M, Tokunaga T. Granulocyte-macrophage colony-stimulating factor promotes the proliferation of human alveolar macrophages in vitro. J Immunol. 1991;147:1266–72.
174. Dexter DT, Nanayakkara I, Goss-Sampson MA, Muller DP, Harding AE, Marsden CD, et al. Nigral dopaminergic cell loss in vitamin E deficient rats. Neuroreport. 1994;5:1773–6.
175. Nagatsu T, Sawada M. Cellular and molecular mechanisms of Parkinson's disease: neurotoxins, causative genes, and inflammatory cytokines. Cell Mol Neurobiol. 2006;26:781–802.
176. Sawada M, Imamura K, Nagatsu T. Role of cytokines in inflammatory process in Parkinson's disease. J Neural Transm Suppl. 2006;70:373–81.
177. Imamura K, Hishikawa N, Sawada M, Nagatsu T, Yoshida M, Hashizume Y. Distribution of major histocompatibility complex class II-positive microglia and cytokine profile of Parkinson's disease brains. Acta Neuropathol. 2003;106:518–26.
178. Wu DC, Jackson-Lewis V, Vila M, Tieu K, Teismann P, Vadseth C, et al. Blockade of microglial activation is neuroprotective in the 1methyl-4-phenyl-1,2,3,6-tetrahydropyridine mouse model of Parkinson disease. J Neurosci. 2002;22:1763–71.
179. Wu DC, Teismann P, Tieu K, Vila M, Jackson-Lewis V, Ischiropoulos H, et al. NADPH oxidase mediates oxidative stress in the 1-methyl4-phenyl-1,2,3,6-tetrahydropyridine model of Parkinson disease. Proc Natl Acad Sci U S A. 2003;100:6145–50.
180. Ito S, Sawada M, Haneda M, Ishida Y, Isobe K. Amyloid-beta peptides induce several chemokine mRNA expressions in the primary microglia and Ra2 cell line via PI3K/Akt and/or ERK pathway. Neurosci Res. 2006;56:294–9.
181. Sawada H, Hashida R, Hirata Y, Ono K, Suzuki H, Muramatsu SI, et al. Activated microglia affect the nigro-striatal dopamine neurons differently in neonatal and aged mice treated with 1-methyl-4-phenyl 1,2,3,6-tetra-hydropyridine. J Neurosci Res. 2007;85:1752–61.
182. Imai F, Suzuki H, Oda J, Ninomiya T, Ono K, Sano H, et al. Neuroprotective effect of exogenous microglia in global brain ischemia. J Cereb Blood Flow Metab. 2007;27:488–500.
183. Vilhardt F, Plastre O, Sawada M, Suzuki K, Wiznerowicz M, Kiyokawa E, et al. The HIV-1 Nef protein and phagocyte NADPH oxidase activation. J Biol Chem. 2002;277:42136–43.
184. Sawada M, Suzumura A, Marunouchi T. Cytokine network in the central nervous system and its roles in growth and differentiation of glial and neuronal cells. Int J Dev Neurosci. 1995;13:253–64.
185. Alderman TS, Frothingham R, Sempowski GD. Validation of an animal isolation imaging chamber for use in animal biosafety level-3 containment. Appl Biosaf. 2010;15:62–6.
186. Lei XY, Liu MM, Yu XJ. Severe fever with thrombocytopenia syndrome and its pathogen SFTSV. Microbes Infect. 2015;17:149–54.
187. Hayasaka D, Nishi K, Fuchigami T, et al. 18F-FDG PET imaging for identifying the dynamics of intestinal disease caused by SFTSV infection in a mouse model. Oncotarget. 2016;7:140–7.
188. Fuchigami T, Ono H, Oyadomari K, et al. Development of a (68) Ge/(68)Ga generator system using polysaccharide polymers and its application in PET imaging of tropical infectious diseases. *ACS*. Omega. 2017;2:1400–7.
189. Sauerbrunn BJ, Andrews GA, Hubner KF. Ga-67 citrate imaging in tumors of the genito-urinary tract: report of cooperative study. J Nucl Med. 1978;19:470–5.
190. Rossleigh MA, Murray IP, Mackey DW, Bargwanna KA, Nayanar VV. Pediatric solid tumors: evaluation by gallium-67 SPECT studies. J Nucl Med. 1990;31:168–72.
191. Tsan MF. Mechanism of gallium-67 accumulation in inflammatory lesions. J Nucl Med. 1985;26:88–92.
192. Mougneau E, Bihl F, Glaichenhaus N. Cell biology and immunology of Leishmania. Immunol Rev. 2011;240:286–96.

2 FDG-PET/CT in Patients with Inflammation or Fever of Unknown Origin (IUO and FUO)

Kazuo Kubota, Motoki Takeuchi, Qian Wang, and Yuji Nakamoto

2.1 Role of FDG-PET/CT in the Diagnosis of Fever or Inflammation of Unknown Origin (FUO/IUO)

Kazuo Kubota

Abstract Fever of unknown origin (FUO) is a syndrome of fever without obvious cause, and it is regarded as a difficult diagnostic challenge. Inflammation of unknown origin (IUO) is similar to FUO, except that it is not associated with elevated body temperature. FDG-PET/CT may cover the diagnosis of a wide spectrum of diseases causing FUO/IUO, namely tumors and inflammation, under the conditions that the disease is active (consuming a lot of glucose), and the lesion is focal and of a size that is sufficiently larger than the limit of detectability. Promising results of FDGPET/CT for the diagnosis of FUO/IUO have been reported from many institutions. FDGPET/CT is very helpful for recognizing and excluding diseases, directing further diagnostic decisions, and avoiding unnecessary invasive examinations. If confirmed by further studies, FDG-PET/CT may become established as an initial, noninvasive diagnostic tool in the evaluation of FUO/IUO.

K. Kubota (✉)
Department of Radiology, Southern TOHOKU General Hospital, Koriyama, Fukushima, Japan
e-mail: kkubota@cpost.plala.or.jp

M. Takeuchi
Department of Emergency and General Internal Medicine, Fujita Health University School of Medicine, Toyoake, Aichi, Japan

Department of General Internal Medicine, Japanese Red Cross Nagoya Daini Hospital, Nagoya, Aichi, Japan
e-mail: mtakeuchi7117@gmail.com

Q. Wang
Department of Nuclear Medicine, Peking University People's Hospital, Beijing, China
e-mail: wangqian20135@163.com

Y. Nakamoto
Kyoto University Hospital, Kyoto, Japan
e-mail: ynakamo1@kuhp.kyoto-u.ac.jp

Keywords: Fever of unknown origin (FUO), Inflammation of unknown origin (IUO), Disease prevalence, Markers of inflammation, FDGPET/CT

2.1.1 What Is FUO?

Fever of unknown origin (FUO) is a syndrome of fever, the cause of which is not obvious. It was named and defined to facilitate the search for causative diseases and other medical considerations. FUO was first defined by Petersdorf and Beeson, in 1961, as an (a) illness of more than 3 weeks duration, (b) fever higher than 101 °F (38.3 °C) on several occasions, (c) diagnosis remaining uncertain even after 1 week of investigations at a hospital. The period of 3 weeks in the definition was set to eliminate acute-limited infectious diseases, and fever higher than 38.3 °C was set to eliminate the entity of habitual hyperthermia (higher body temperature due to the normal variations or various physiological causes). A prospective study conducted in 100 patients of FUO revealed the following distribution of causative diseases: infection 36, neoplastic disease 19, collagen disease 13, pulmonary embolism, etc. 3, pericarditis 2, sarcoidosis 2, hypersensitivity status 4, cranial arteritis 2, periodic diseases 5, miscellaneous diseases 4, factitious fever 3, and indeterminate diagnosis 7. These results serve to emphasize that most patients with FUO do not suffer from unusual diseases, but instead exhibit atypical manifestations of common illnesses [1].

Thirty years later, Durack DT and Street AC modified and subdivided the standard definition of FUO [2]. They modified the definition from "1-week of investigation at the hospital" to "at least three outpatient visits or at least 3 days at a hospital," in response to the medical trend of shorter hospitalization with the accelerated pace of investigations. They proposed four definitions as follows: (a) classical FUO, (b) nosocomial FUO, (c) neutropenic FUO, and (d) HIV-associated FUO (Table 2.1). This modification was proposed because the spectrum of underlying diseases, especially in the latter three categories, is different. Also, for patients with

H. Toyama et al. (eds.), *PET/CT for Inflammatory Diseases*, https://doi.org/10.1007/978-981-15-0810-3_2

Table 2.1 New definition and classification of fever of unknown origin (FUO)[a]

Classical FUO
• Fever 38.3 °C (101 °F) or higher on several occasions
• Fever of more than 3 weeks duration
• Diagnosis uncertain despite appropriate investigations, after at least three outpatient visits or at least 3 days at the hospital
Nosocomial FUO
• Fever 38.3 °C (101 °F) or higher on several occasions in a hospitalized patient receiving acute care
• Infection not present or incubating at hospital admission
• Diagnosis still uncertain after 3 days despite appropriate investigation, including at least 2 days of incubation of microbiologic culture
Neutropenic FUO
• Fever 38.3 °C (101 °F) or higher on several occasions
• Peripheral blood neutrophil count less than 500/mm^3 or expected to fall below 500/mm^3 within 1–2 days
• Diagnosis still uncertain after 3 days despite appropriate investigation days, including at least 2 days incubation of microbiologic culture
HIV-associated FUO
• Fever 38.3 °C (101 °F) or higher on several occasions
• Confirmed positive serology for HIV infection
• Fever of more than 4 weeks duration for outpatients, or more than 3 days at the hospital
• Diagnosis uncertain after 3 days despite appropriate investigation, including at least 2 days incubation of microbiologic culture

[a]Modified from ref. [2]

immune dysfunction, early empirical antimicrobial therapy may be required rather than the standard diagnostic approach.

2.1.2 What Is IUO?

FUO is regarded as a difficult diagnostic challenge. Since the original and revised definitions have been laid out, a search for the causes of FUO has been accelerated, and another revision has been proposed. Petersdorf introduced the cutoff value of the body temperature of 38.3 °C, to exclude cases with habitual hyperthermia, a very common entity in the 1950s. Knockaert et al. proposed inclusion of patients with either an oral temperature of over 38.3 °C or a low-grade fever, on the condition that signs of inflammation (increased erythrocyte sedimentation rate (ESR) or increased serum C-reactive protein level (CRP)) are present. An oral temperature of >37.2 °C (morning) or >37.8 °C (any time) as the sole criterion resulted in inclusion of a large number of patients with chronic fatigue syndrome and fibromyalgia [3]. Perrin et al. reported a retrospective study of 47 patients (pts) with inflammation that remained undiagnosed during hospital admission. Their inclusion threshold was a serum CRP level of 15 mg/L. Diagnosis was established in 14 pts (30%) during follow-up and was most frequently polymyalgia rheumatica or giant cell arteritis [4]. Vanderscheuren et al. conducted a matched study of 57 pts with inflammation of unknown origin (IUO) and 57 pts with FUO of the same gender and mean age. Diagnosis was established in 35 pts with IUO (61%) and in 33 pts with FUO (58%). Noninfectious inflammatory diseases were the largest diagnostic category in the IUO group (16 pts), while the FUO group included similar numbers of malignancy (10 pts), infections (9 pts), and noninfectious inflammatory diseases (9 pts). FDG-PET contributed comparably to the diagnosis in both groups (36% pts in the IUO and 40.33% pts in the FUO group). In both groups, 7 pts died during the average follow-up period of 1 year. They concluded that the diagnostic yield, case-mix, contribution of FDG-PET to the diagnosis and the prognosis were similar in the two groups with IUO and FUO. The findings suggest that the threshold of 38.3 °C may be arbitrary and that the diagnostic approaches used for FUO can also be applied for IUO [5]. Their definition of IUO was (3 weeks duration, serum CRP >30 mg/L, and/or ESR >age/2 in men or (age+10)/2 in women on >3 occasions, undiagnosed after three outpatient visits or 3 days at a hospital).

2.1.3 Why FDG-PET/CT for FUO/IUO?

FDG-PET/CT enables not only detection of malignancy but also detection of active inflammatory processes, including infections and noninfectious inflammatory lesions. In other words, FDG-PET/CT may cover the diagnosis of a wide spectrum of causative diseases of FUO/IUO, provided that the disease is active (consuming a lot of glucose) and the lesion is focal and of a size that is sufficiently larger than the limit of detectability of PET/CT (around 1 cm). Using FDG-PET/CT, we can search for active lesions through real whole-body scanning, with a high rate of detectability. Figure 2.1 shows our proposed protocol for the usage of FDG-PET/CT in the evaluation of FUO/IUO. If an active lesion is detected on FDG-PET, biopsy for histopathological examination or aspiration for bacteriology may lead to the specific diagnosis and therapy. If no active lesion is detected, the possibility of a systemic disease without focal lesions would be considered, such as drug fever, viral infection, some form of micro-vessel vasculitis etc., and further evaluation along these lines would be performed. No active lesion on FDG-PET/CT may also mean no active disease in the patient, and lead to the adoption of a wait-and-watch policy or palliative therapy.

2.1.4 Results of FDG-PET/CT for FUO/IUO

Muto et al. studied 124 elderly pts hospitalized for IUO (definition: over 50 years old, fever of 38.3 °C or over on three occasions, serum CRP over 2.5 mg/dL, more than 3 weeks

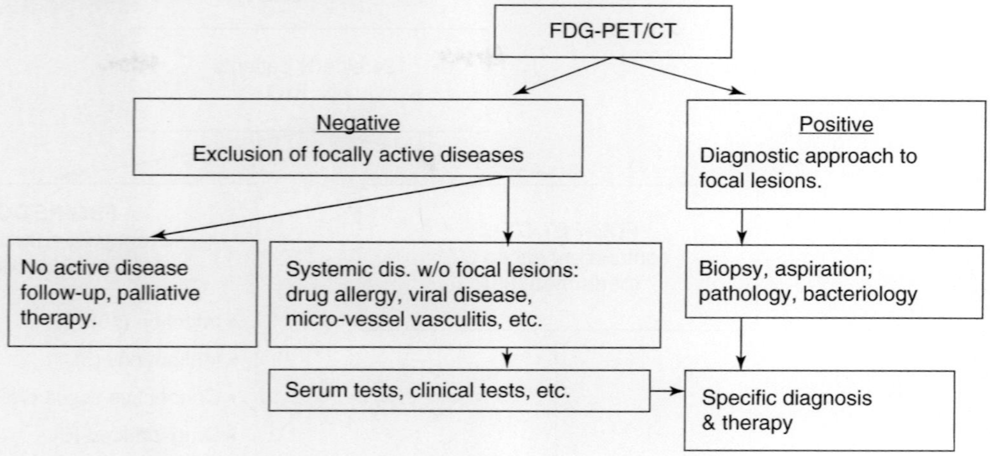

Fig. 2.1 Merits of FDG-PET/CT in the evaluation of FUO/IUO

duration, undiagnosed after three visits or 3 days in hospital). Of the 124 pts, 88 were examined by FDG-PET/CT, which yielded the diagnosis of large-vessel vasculitis (LVV) in 13 pts (13/124; 10.5%); LVV was diagnosed only in the FDG-PET/CT group. The predominant causative diseases in the elderly IUO pts were connective tissue diseases (48/124; 38.7%, not including LVV), infection (31 pts, 25%), and malignancy (18 pts, 14.5%) (Fig. 2.2). LVV, only detected by FDG-PET/CT, is an important cause of IUO with nonspecific symptoms in the elderly. They also performed evaluation of therapy for LVV and concluded that FDG-PET/CT is useful for early diagnosis and treatment evaluation of LVV, allowing amelioration of reversible aortic wall thickening [6].

Kubota et al. reported a multicenter retrospective study of FDG-PET for the evaluation of FUO in Japan [7]. FUO was defined as the presence of a recurrent or persistent fever of 38 °C or higher lasting for 2 weeks or longer and remaining undiagnosed after appropriate inpatient or outpatient evaluation. (Note that the Celsius unit is used nationwide in Japan and a threshold of 38.3 °C (101 °F) is not practical.). A total of 96 pts from six institutions were enrolled over a period of 18 months, and 81 were effectively entered in the analysis (Fig. 2.3). A final diagnosis was obtained in 61 pts (61/81; 75.3%), including infection in 29 pts (HIV infection 4, aortic graft infection 4, tuberculosis 2, etc.), noninfectious inflammatory disease in 26 pts (Takayasu arteritis 5, rheumatoid arthritis 2, adult onset of Still's disease 2, polymyalgia rheumatica 2, IgG4-related disease 2, histiocytic necrotizing lymphadenitis 2, etc.), malignancy in 3 pts, other disease in 3 pts. The diagnostic yield in the 76 pts who were entered in the final analysis was as follows: sensitivity 81% (42/52), specificity 75% (18/24), positive predictive value 87.5% (42/48), and contribution rate 55.3% (true positive/total pts: 42/76). As compared to other studies, the diagnostic performance was quite high, but the population with malignancy was small; this was speculated as cases of lymphoma, etc., which can be diagnosed early by CT and staged by FDG-PET, were excluded from this study.

2.1.5 Factors Affecting the Results

2.1.5.1 Disease Prevalence and Positivity

Figure 2.4 shows the diagnostic yield analyzed by the disease category of the final diagnosis reported by Kubota et al. Higher FDG uptake scores, a higher sensitivity of PET CT, more additional information from the test, and a higher clinical impact of the imaging examination were observed in patients with infection or tumor/granuloma than in those with arthritis/vasculitis/collagen diseases and other diseases/indeterminate diagnosis. Differences in the study population, prevalence of the causative diseases, especially of infectious diseases, such as tuberculosis, in the population may be expected to affect these results. Hospitals treating a large number of pts with infections and acute-phase diseases may see a higher diagnostic yield of FDGPET/CT in pts with FUO, while tertiary-care hospitals and those offering advanced medical consulting, which may see a larger number of cases of noninfectious inflammatory diseases, miscellaneous diseases, or unknown diseases, may not achieve high diagnostic yields of FDG-PET/CT in pts with FUO. Such bias depending on the prevalence pattern of diseases can be corrected by conducting a multicenter study or by using appropriate patient inclusion criteria.

2.1.5.2 Markers of Inflammation

Balink et al. [7] showed, from a retrospective study of 331 pts with FUO or IUO, that elevated serum CRP more often predicted a true-positive FDGPET/CT outcome than elevated ESR. Garcia-Vincent et al. [8] reported from their retrospective study of 67 pts of FUO, that pts with positive inflammation markers and elevated serum CRP or positive pathologic protein analysis were more likely to show true-positive PET/CT results. Schönau et al. [9] analyzed a prospective cohort of 240 pts with FUO or IUO or exFUO/IUO examined by FDG-PET/CT. Predictors of positive diagnostic findings on

a

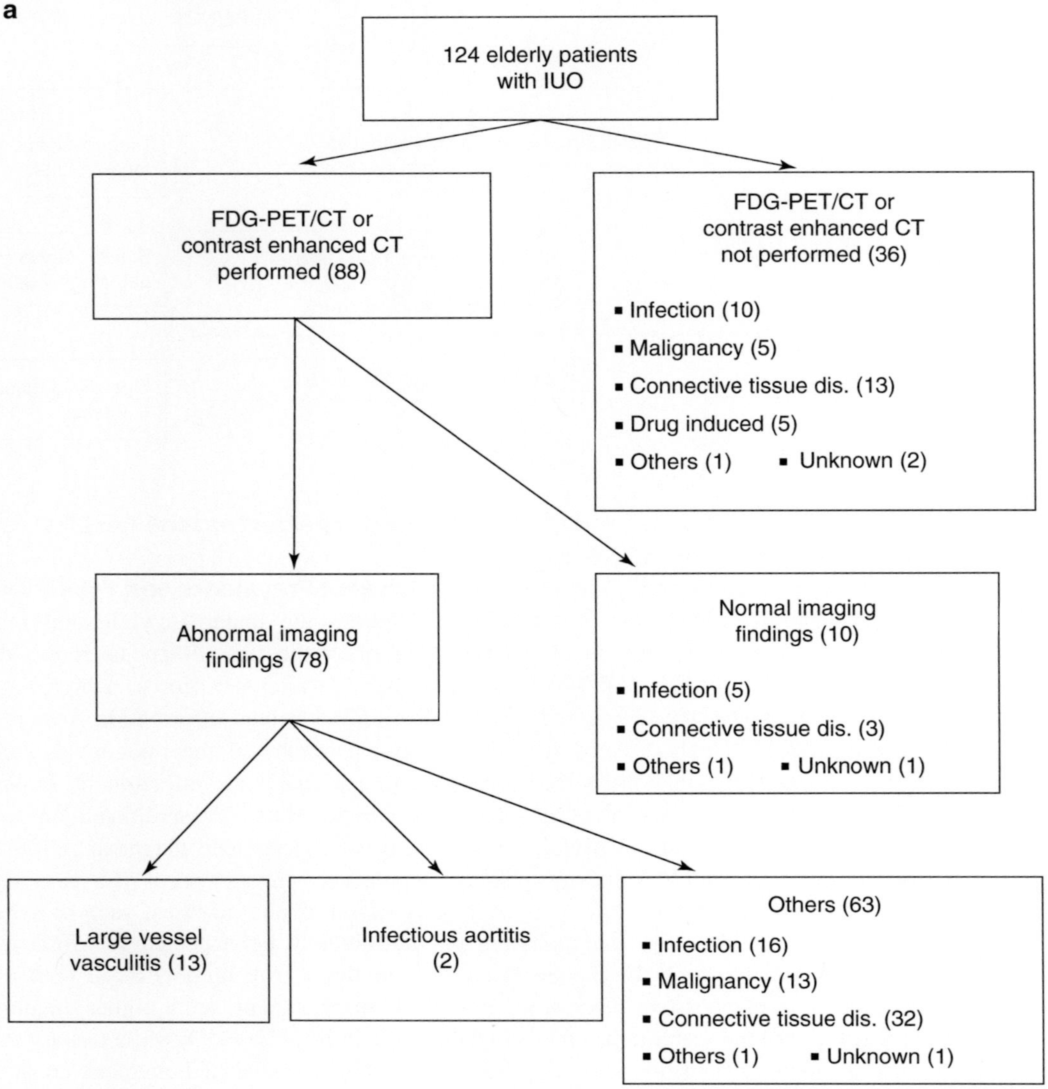

b

Final diagnosis(All; 124pts)		
FDGPET/CT study group (88)		
Connective tissue disease	35	48
Infection	21	31
Malignancy	13	18
Large vessel vasculitis	13	13
Infectious aortitis	2	2
Drug-induced	0	5
Others	2	3
Unknown	2	4

Fig. 2.2 (**a**) Flow chart of a retrospective study of IUO (modified from ref. [6]). (**b**) Causative diseases of IUO, all pts and the pts examined by FDG-ET/CT (modified from ref. [6])

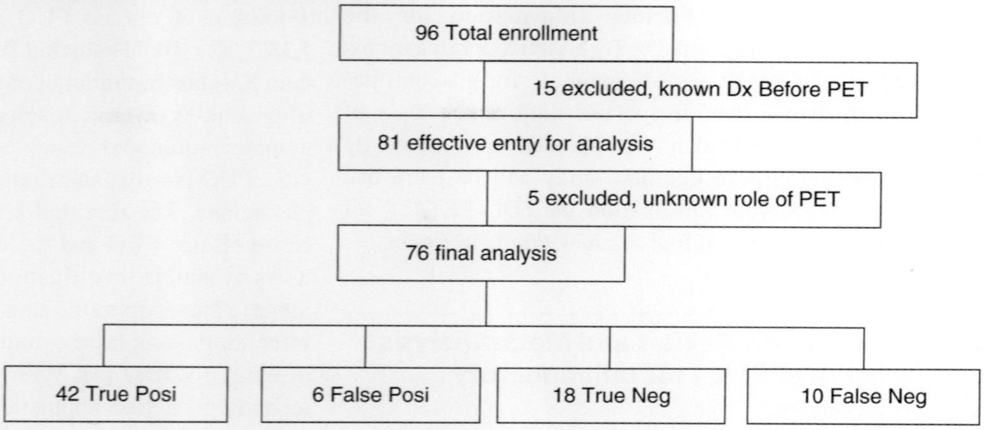

Fig. 2.3 Diagnostic yield of FDG-PET for FUO in a multicenter study (modified from ref. [16]). Sensitivity 81% (42/52), specificity 75% (18/24), positive predictive value 87.5% (42/48). Contribution 55.3% (true positive/total pts = 42/76)

Fig. 2.4 Results by disease category of the final diagnosis (modified from ref. [16])

Disease categories	**Infection**	**Tumor/ Granuloma**	Arthritis/Vasculitis/ Collagen dis.	Others/ Unknown
No.Patients	29	8	21	23
FDG score	**2.5**	**2.6**	1.7	1.3
Sensitivity%	**89**(24/27)	**100**(7/7)	65(11/17)	0(0/1)
Specificity%	0(0/2)	100(1/1)	50(1/2)	**84**(16/19)
Additional Info.%	**76**(22/29)	**75**(6/8)	43(9/21)	23(5/22)
Clinical Impact(Ave.)	**2.1**	**2.3**	1.4	1.2

FDG-PET/CT were age over 50 years (p = 0.019), serum C-reactive protein (CRP) level over 30 mg/L (p = 0.002), and absence of fever (p = 0.001). Based on these reports, the elevated serum CRP level may be one of the most important predictors of a true-positive result of FDGPET/CT in pts with FUO/IUO.

2.1.5.3 Structured Evaluation FUO/IUO

Workup of FUO/IUO pts begins with thorough history-taking, physical examination, and laboratory tests. Imaging examinations like ultrasound, chest X-ray, or even CT would be the next step. FDGPET/CT had until now been considered only in the late stage of investigation of FUO because of its limited availability, high cost, and high radiation exposure. In their multicenter study of FUO, Bleeker-Rovers et al. [10] used FDG-PET as a part of their structured diagnostic protocol for FUO. They prospectively recruited FUO patients from five community/university hospitals. If there were no potentially diagnostic clues, FDG-PET was performed within 1–2 weeks. They concluded that FDG-PET is a valuable imaging technique that must be included in the diagnostic protocol for FUO patients in the general population with a raised ESR or serum CRP. It is important to determine the optimal timing for the test and to assess the impact of the test on the management and outcomes in pts with FUO [11]. Abnormal PET findings are associated with substantial increase in the final diagnostic rate in pts with FUO. Therefore, FDG-PET could be considered for inclusion in the first-line diagnostic workup for FUO [12]. Takeuchi et al. suggested that undiagnosed classic FUO patients with negative PET/CT findings had a high likelihood of spontaneous remission after a series of unsuccessful investigations [13]. FDGPET/CT is very helpful for recognizing and excluding diseases, directing further diagnostic decisions and avoiding unnecessary invasive examinations. Recently, it has been suggested that FDG-PET/CT should be considered as one of the first-line diagnostic tools for patients with FUO/IUO [14, 15].

2.1.6 Conclusion

In addition to our experiences described above, recent reviews and meta-analyses have also shown a promising role of FDGPET/CT in the diagnostic evaluation for FUO/IUO. If confirmed by further studies, FDG-PET/CT may become established as an initial, noninvasive diagnostic tool in the evaluation of FUO/IUO.

Acknowledgments and Further Information for the Reader I would like to thank Dr. Toshiyuki Saginoya for his kind support, and Dr. Ryogo Minamimoto for his contribution to complete our new prospective multicenter study of FDG-PET/CT for FUO that was planned and started by Kazuo Kubota. I believe this new study will be published soon providing definite information on FDG-PET/CT for FUO. Hope the reader will find our new article in future.

2.2 Systematic Review and Meta-Analysis in FDG-PET/CT for Inflammatory Diseases

Motoki Takeuchi

Abstract Fever of unknown origin (FUO) is a common clinical dilemma encountered in general medical practice. With the advances in diagnostic technology, identifying the source of fever in cases of undiagnosed classic FUO that could not be diagnosed with these sophisticated imaging tests has become difficult in contemporary clinical practice. FDG-PET and FDG-PET/CT are functional imaging tests for identifying focal inflammatory or malignant lesions that cannot be detected by anatomical imaging. Although several studies have evaluated their diagnostic value for patients with classic FUO, the clinical role and impact of these modalities remain unclear because of small sample sizes and heterogeneous study designs. We, therefore, performed a systematic review and meta-analysis to quantitatively evaluate the current evidence. Our first study reported test performance and diagnostic yield of FDG-PET/CT and FDG-PET for diagnosing FUO. The summary sensitivity and specificity of FDG-PET/CT were 0.86 (95% CI, 0.81–0.90) and 0.52 (95% CI, 0.36–0.67), respectively. In the second study, we reported the association of FDG-PET/CT with spontaneous remission of FUO for evaluating the predictive ability of negative FDG-PET/CT. Patients with negative FDG-PET/CT results were significantly more likely to experience spontaneous regression than those with positive results (summary RR = 5.6, 95% CI: 3.4–9.2, $P < 0.001$, $I^2 = 0\%$).

Keywords: Fever of unknown origin, Systematic review, Meta-analysis, Diagnostic accuracy, Diagnostic yield, Spontaneous remission

2.2.1 Introduction; Nuclear Imaging Tests and Classic Fever of Unknown Origin

Classic fever of unknown origin (FUO) was defined by Petersdorf and Besson in 1961 [17]. The most recent definition of classic FUO is community-acquired fever ≥38.3 °C (101 °F) lasting for a period equal to or greater than 3 weeks in immunocompetent individuals and explicitly excludes fever in hospitalized patients or patients with human immunodeficiency virus infection or neutropenia [18]. FUO is a diagnostic and clinical challenge for several physicians. The fact that several diseases can potentially cause classic FUO and the difficulty in arriving at a diagnosis by simple investigations alone contribute to the challenge. The common causes of classic FUO include infections, neoplasms, and noninfectious inflammatory diseases (NIIDs) [3]. With recent advances in diagnostic technologies, like sophisticated imaging tests, improved culture techniques, and molecular diagnostics, infections, and neoplasms have become less common causes of FUO and undiagnosed cases have become more challenging to investigate [19, 20].

When the temporal changes of the diagnostic disease rate of classic FUO are considered, the combined proportion of infections and neoplasms have been gradually decreasing, and the rate of undiagnosed cases has been increasing [20]. Familiar imaging tests such as US, CT, and MRI often provide important diagnostic information for FUO. In addition to these tests, nuclear imaging has been used for patients with FUO which has been difficult to diagnose.

^{67}Ga scintigraphy is used as a staging modality in oncology [21]. Since gallium accumulates in both malignant tumors and inflammation, gallium scintigraphy is used as a part of workup strategies for patients with classic FUO [3, 22]. For the identification of the site of infectious disease, scintigraphy using autologous white blood cells labeled with ^{111}In or ^{99m}Tc was also used in some facilities [3, 12, 22]. FDG-PET emerged in the 1990s. Clinical studies reporting diagnostic accuracy of FDG-PET/CT for FUO have increased in recent years, and PET/CT is a popular examination option in developed countries, when there is no diagnostic clue for FUO [19].

In this article, we review the relationship between FDG-PET/CT and FUO, focusing on data from the two systematic reviews and meta-analyses we previously reported.

2.2.2 Our Systematic Review and Meta-Analysis for Nuclear Imaging Tests and Classic Fever of Unknown Origin

Our first study which reported test performance and diagnostic yield of nuclear imaging tests including FDG-PET/CT for diagnosing FUO was published in 2016 [14]. In 2018, we reported the association of FDG-PET/CT with spontaneous remission of FUO for evaluating the predictive ability of negative FDG-PET/CT [23].

2.2.3 Test Performance and Diagnostic Yieldof 18F-FDG-PET and PET/CT for Classic FUO

In our first systematic review and meta-analysis, we searched Pubmed and Scopus from their inception till October 31, 2015, without language restrictions. We included studies that evaluated diagnostic accuracy of FDG-PET/CT, FDG-PET, gallium scintigraphy, and leukocyte scintigraphy for adults with classic FUO.

Although previous systematic reviews evaluating similar studies have been published [24–27], our review attempted to address new challenges by evaluating current evidence. First, we adopted the diagnostic yield (the proportion of patients in whom the imaging results were reported to contribute to the diagnosis of FUO causes) as a parameter of diagnostic accuracy. Second, our review attempted analyses to compare the utility of each nuclear imaging tests.

A total of 43 unique publications met our eligibility criteria. Twenty-two studies (1137 patients) evaluated FDG-PET/CT and 12 (522 patients) evaluated FDG-PET. Studies of FDG-PET were conducted between 1996 and 2003, while those on FDG-PET/CT were conducted between 2008 and 2015.

From data synthesis of these studies revealed summary sensitivity and specificity of FDG-PET/CT to be 0.86 (95% CI, 0.81–0.90) and 0.52 (95% CI, 0.36–0.67). For FDG-PET, summary sensitivity and specificity were 0.76 (95% CI, 0.66–0.83) and 0.50 (95% CI, 0.30–0.70), respectively. The summary diagnostic yield of FDG-PET/CT and FDG-PET were 0.58 (95% CI, 0.51–0.64) and 0.44 (95% CI, 0.31–0.58), respectively.

Our findings regarding the test performance of FDG-PET and FDG-PET/CT are in general agreement with previous systematic reviews [24–27]. As mentioned above, advances in diagnostic techniques make it easier to diagnose infections and neoplasms.

In meta-regression under the hypothesis that FDG-PET/CT is useful to diagnose those disease groups, studies reporting a higher proportion of neoplasms and infections as the cause of FUO also reported a higher diagnostic yield (Spearman's $\rho = 0.44$, $P = 0.038$). A similar tendency was observed also with FDG-PET (Spearman's $\rho = 0.66$, $P = 0.020$).

We divided the causes of FUO into infections, neoplasms, and NIID and calculated the failure rate which FDG-PET/CT (18 studies) and FDG-PET (12 studies) indicate positive scan results for each eligible study. In the neoplasm group, 13 out of 18 FDG-PET/CT studies (72%) and 10 out of 12 FDG-PET studies (83%) had 100% positive scan results. In the infection group, 9 out of 18 FDG-PET/CT studies (50%) and 6 out of 12 FDG-PET studies (50%) had failure rates below 20%. In contrast, in the NIID group, 7 out of 18 FDG-PET/CT studies (39%) and 2 out of 12 FDG-PET studies (17%) had failure rates below 20%. Thus, it was inferred that the detection of findings to diagnose NIID was difficult. Adult-onset Still's disease, tuberculosis, and polymyalgia rheumatica were the three causes which most often showed no pathologic uptake, making diagnosis possible. Although these results have not been reported in earlier systematic reviews, it may be concluded that FDG-PET/CT and FDG-PET are less useful when causes other than infection and malignancy are unlikely.

2.2.4 Comparisons of Test Performance and Diagnostic Yield Among Nuclear Imaging Tests

We considered the importance of the comparison with other nuclear imaging modalities to the utility of FDG-PET/CT. We ought to have evaluated data from studies that directly compare test performance between some test modalities. However, we did not perform meta-analysis of comparative studies because very few studies were available for each direct comparison. Therefore, we compared test performance indirectly for each test modality.

We estimated relative diagnostic odds ratios (rDORs) as the measure of comparative accuracy between two alternative imaging tests. Evidence from indirect comparisons of test performance suggested that FDG-PET/CT outperformed standalone FDG-PET (rDOR = 3.10, CrI: 1.00–9.53), gallium scintigraphy (rDOR = 5.07, CrI: 1.13–23.57), and leukocyte scintigraphy (rDOR = 11.18, CrI: 1.67–90.47). Regarding diagnostic yield, evidence from indirect comparisons suggested that FDG-PET/CT was the most helpful imaging modality in localizing the anatomical locations of the source of FUO among the four tests. Although these results were calculated from indirect comparisons, they are indicative of the reason for the shift to PET/CT from other imaging modalities for the diagnosis of FUO.

2.2.5 Association of Negative ^{18}F-FDG-PET, PET/CT Results, and Spontaneous Remission

While identifying the source of fever in cases of undiagnosed classic FUO in contemporary clinical practice has become more difficult, spontaneous remissions during clinical follow-up have been reported in up to 75% of these diagnostically challenging cases [28]. Therefore, we considered that revealing predictors of spontaneous remission would improve management strategies, which can potentially reduce unnecessary invasive investigations, such as tissue biopsy or empirical treatments with antibiotics or steroids. Moreover, it may allow us to keep stable patients merely under watchful waiting without treatment.

Our clinical hypothesis was that the absence of abnormal FDG uptakes in FDG-PET/CT or FDG-PET is a good predictor of spontaneous remission. We performed systematic review and meta-analysis for evaluating the associations between negative FDG-PET/CT or FDG-PET results and spontaneous remission in diagnostically challenging cases of classic FUO.

We searched Pubmed and Scopus from their inception till June 30, 2018, in the same manner as our systematic review for diagnostic accuracy. The eligible studies evaluated at least one patient with spontaneous remission of fever and had to have followed up the patients for ≥3 months after PET or PET/CT scans. We defined a patient with spontaneous remission as a patient in whom FUO symptoms were reported to have regressed spontaneously without any therapeutic intervention, before reaching a diagnosis during the clinical follow-up.

A total of 13 publications met our eligibility criteria, including 4 studies (128 patients) on FDG-PET results and 9 studies (418 patients) evaluating FDG-PET/CT results. Only 4 studies (2 for FDG-PET and 2 for FDG-PET/CT) had a prospective design.

The minimum follow-up duration after FDG-PET or FDG-PET/CT assessment for undiagnosed FUO ranged from 3 to 16 months.

The average spontaneous remission rate in the eligible studies was 20% (minimum–maximum: 6–45%). The cumulative incidence of spontaneous remission ranged from 20% to 78% in patients with negative FDG-PET/CT results and from 0% to 48% in those with positive results. Overall, patients with a negative FDG-PET/CT result had a significantly higher incidence of spontaneous regression compared with those with a positive scan. The summary risk ratio (RR) for a negative scan was 5.6 (95% CI: 3.4–9.2, $p < 0.001$, $I^2 = 0\%$). In contrast, there was no evidence that either a positive or a negative PET scan had a higher incidence of spontaneous remission. The summary RR for a negative scan was 0.83 (favoring a positive scan; 95% CI: 0.14–5.0, $p = 0.77$, $I^2 = 32\%$). Our meta-analysis found that patients with a negative PET/CT result had an approximately five times higher chance of spontaneous remission than those with a negative PET/CT result.

We surmise that careful watchful waiting may be a reasonable approach for stable patients with negative FDG-PET/CT in clinical settings where the incidence of spontaneous remission is reasonably high, based on these results. However, during follow-up special attention should be given to NIIDs that are difficult to diagnose with FDG-PET/CT.

2.3 FDG-PET/CT in Fever of Unknown Origin and Inflammation of Unknown Origin: a Chinese Multicenter Study

Qian Wang

Abstract A multicenter study of 376 patients from 12 hospitals in China was conducted to evaluate the clinical value of FDG-PET/CT for the diagnosis of inflammation or fever of unknown origin (IUO and FUO). In this study, the infectious diseases accounted for 33.0% of patients, rheumatologic diseases for 32.4%, malignancies for 19.1%, miscellaneous causes for 6.6%, and cause unknown for 8.8%. The etiological distribution among hospitals was varied. On FDG-PET/CT examinations, 358 (95.2%) of the patients had a positive finding. Within them, local high uptake lesion was found in 219 cases, and nonspecific abnormal uptake was found in 187 cases. FDG uptake in malignant diseases was significantly higher than in other category diseases. Based on a clinical questionnaire survey, PET/CT provided additional diagnostic information for 77.4% of patients, and 89.6% of patients benefited from PET/CT examination. This study proves FDG-PET/CT is a valuable tool for clinical diagnosis of IUO & FUO.

Keywords: Fever of unknown origin (FUO), Inflammation of unknown origin (IUO), Positron emission tomography (PET), Fluorodeoxyglucose (FDG)

2.3.1 Introduction of the Multi-Center Study

In the search for an explanation of FUO or IUO, patients may undergo extensive and expensive investigations and medical treatment. Some of these may be invalid and unnecessarily risky. In contrast to the conventional diagnostic workup, diagnosis of underlying disease may be improved by FDG-PET/CT [5, 10, 29]. In 2018, a multicenter study was conducted by Chinese Society of Nuclear Medicine to evaluate the clinical value of FDG-PET/CT for the diagnosis of inflammation or fever of unknown origin (IUO and FUO). A total of 376 patients from 12 hospitals were included in the study, who met the criteria of FUO or IUO and underwent FDG-PET/CT examinations [3, 5]. PET/CT scans were performed with a standard technique, based on the guidelines issued by Chinese Society of Nuclear Medicine [30]. Data analysis included the etiological distribution in the study population, image characteristics in different category of diseases, and clinical significance of PET/CT. The significance of PET/CT in diagnosis of FUO/IUO was evaluated through a questionnaire survey to the clinicians [16].

2.3.2 Major Data and Point of View of the Multi-Center Study

In the 376 patients, there were 195 males and 181 females; their age ranged from 4 to 91 years, with a mean age of 51.6 ± 20.1 years. Among them, 346 met the FUO standard and 30 met the IUO standard. Final clinical diagnosis and etiological classification for the 376 patients are listed in Table 2.2. It was demonstrated that infection and rheumatologic disease are the most common causes for FUO/IUO. Compared to the previous Chinese survey [31], the proportion of rheumatologic diseases (32.4% vs. 20.1%) in Chinese FUO patients is on the rise over time. The study also revealed a difference in the etiological distribution among hospitals due to the different medical characteristics of each hospital (Table 2.3).

On PET/CT examinations, 358 (95.2%) patients had a positive finding. Within these patients, local high uptake lesion was found in 219 cases, including 74 of infectious diseases, 63 of rheumatologic diseases, 67 of malignancies, 10 of miscellaneous causes, and 5 of cause unknown. And nonspecific abnormal uptake (NAU) was found in 187 patients, which manifested as spleen and bone marrow diffuse high uptake and multiple reactive hyperplasia lymph nodes with high uptake and symmetrical distribution. NAU more commonly occurred in the rheumatologic disease, followed by cause unknown and miscellaneous causes (Table 2.4). In 74.3% (139/187) of these patients, NAU was the only positive finding on PET/CT. In patients with NAU, multiple high uptake lymph nodes were found in 84.5% (158/187) of cases, and histopathologic evidence of nonspecific reactive hyperplasia was obtained in 82.7% (105/127) of these patients. Many previous studies defined the focal FDG uptake as a positive PET/CT, and NAU was not given much discussion. In some literatures [29, 32, 33], NAU has been considered as false-positive or noncontributing to diagnosis. However, in our study, about half of patients showed NAU on PET/CT. We regard NAU as the positive finding for PET/CT, and the results not only have a high positive rate but also have a positive impact for the clinical diagnosis and management, especially for those patients with rheumatologic disease. NAU was more commonly occurred in the rheumatologic diseases, such as adult-onset Still's disease, it might reflect the activation of the immune system and the secretion of cytokines in the procedure of inflammation.

Table 2.2 Clinical diagnosis and etiological classification in 376 patients with FUO & IUO

Etiology classification	Case number	Proportion	Clinical diagnosis
Infection	124	33.0%	***Pathogen:*** Tubercle bacillus (19), Epstein-Barr virus (14), Bacterium burgeri (8), *Burkholderia cepacia* (2), *Salmonella gallinarum* (1), Spirochaeta (1), *Penicillium marneffei* (1), *Escherichia coli* (1), Klebsiella pneumonia (1), Mycoplasma pneumonia (1), uncertain (75)
			Infection site: Lung (31), urinary tract (11), periprosthesis (7), lymph node (4), peritoneum (3), bone (2), intestinal tract (2), ovary or uterus (2), pericardiac (1), liver (1), muscle (1), spleen (1), kidney (1), meninges (1), epididymis (1), multiple sites (17), uncertain (38)
Rheumatologic disease	122	32.4%	Adult-onset Still's disease (39), undifferentiated connective tissue disease (19), systemic vasculitis (16), idiopathic inflammatory myopathy (10), systemic lupus erythematosus (9), polymyalgia rheumatic (7), relapsing polychondritis (4), rheumatoid arthritis (3), Sjogren syndrome (3), panniculitis (3), juvenile idiopathic arthritis (3), IgG4-related disease (2), reactive arthritis (2), ankylosing spondylitis (1), antiphospholipid syndrome (1)
Malignancy	72	19.1%	Lymphoma (56), leukemia (9), lung cancer (2), myelodysplastic syndrome (2), colon cancer (1), gastric cancer (1), hepatic cellular cancer (1)
Miscellaneous	25	6.6%	Drug allergy (11), histiocytic necrotizing lymphadenitis (4), Castleman disease (3), primary hemophagocytic syndrome (2), inflammatory bowel disease (2), Rosai-Dorfman disease (1), limbic encephalitis (1), hyperthyroidism (1)
Unknown	33	8.8%	Uncertain (33)

Table 2.3 Distribution of etiological diseases in different hospitals

	Cases provided	Infection	Rheumatologic disease	Malignancy	Miscellaneous	Unknown
Peking University People's Hospital	170	47 (27.6%)	78 (45.9%)	22 (12.9%)	14 (8.2%)	9 (5.3%)
Huashan Hospital	38	17 (44.7%)	12 (31.6%)	4 (10.5%)	3 (7.9%)	2 (5.3%)
Nanfang Hospital	38	9 (23.7%)	10 (26.3%)	14 (36.8%)	4 (10.5%)	1 (2.6%)
Beijing Anzhen Hospital	25	23 (92.0%)	0 (0.0%)	1 (4.0%)	0 (0.0%)	1 (4.0%)
The First Hospital of China Medical University	20	5 (25.0%)	6 (30.0%)	4 (20.0%)	1 (5.0%)	4 (20.0%)
Other hospitals	85	23 (27.1%)	16 (18.8%)	27 (31.8%)	3 (3.5%)	16 (18.8%)
Total	376	124	122	72	25	33

Table 2.4 Nonspecific abnormal uptake in different category diseases

	Infection	Rheumatologic disease	Malignancy	Miscellaneous	Unknown	Total
Case number	41	99	5	17	25	187
Proportion	33.1%	81.1%	6.9%	68.0%	75.8%	49.7%

Table 2.5 FDG uptake in different etiological diseases

FDG uptake		Infection	Rheumatologic disease	Malignancy	Miscellaneous	Unknown
SUV_{max}	Mean ± SD	5.4 ± 3.6	4.5 ± 3.0	9.4 ± 7.0	5.0 ± 3.3	4.3 ± 2.6
	Range	0.5–18.9	1.3–27.1	2.8–47.3	1.3–13.0	1.2–11.2
Visual score	Mean ± SD	2.3 ± 0.7	2.3 ± 0.5	2.8 ± 0.4	2.4 ± 0.8	2.1 ± 0.7
	Range	0–3	0–3	1–3	0–3	0–3

Table 2.5 shows FDG uptake in different category diseases. The FDG uptake in malignant diseases was significantly higher than in other category of diseases both on SUV_{max} and on visual scores (t value ranges from 4.098 to 5.612, all P value <0.001). Although there were some overlaps between different types of disease. The lesion uptake of FDG combined with the structural information provided by CT may be helpful in differential diagnosis.

Histopathologic examinations were obtained in 372 of the patients (98.9%), including lymph node (217 cases), bone marrow (169 cases), and other tissues (105 cases). Among these patients, 165 underwent histopathologic examination before the PET/CT, though none obtained direct diagnostic clues. However, 105/242 of patients (43.4%) achieved etiological diagnosis through histopathologic examination performed after PET/CT, including 21 infections, 6 rheumatologic diseases, 65 malignancies, and 13 miscellaneous diseases. The pathological examination results of the patients in this group show that, during the diagnostic process of FUO, pathological diagnosis has significant value for the detection of malignant lesions, but the value is limited in nonneoplastic diseases, which highlights the significance of PET/CT. Since FDG-PET/CT has multiple functions in the diagnostic procedure, especially in nonneoplastic diseases, its diagnostic value in FUO/IUO cannot be fully demonstrated by simply evaluating its role in detecting malignant tumors or infectious lesions.

In order to avoid nonobjective judgment caused by the lack of understanding of the clinical situation by radiologists, in this study we evaluated the significance of PET/CT in FUO/IUO by using a questionnaire to the clinician according to Kubota's method [16]. Based on the clinical questionnaire survey, PET/CT provided additional diagnostic information for 291 patients (77.4%). If G2 and G3 were considered as helpful, 89.6% of patients in the study benefited from the PET/CT examination. PET/CT examination tended to provide more help in the diagnostic process for rheumatic disease and malignancies.

For FUO/IUO patients, establishing an etiologic diagnosis is often difficult when simply relying on clinical manifestation, laboratory examination, conventional imaging, and sometimes even invasive histopathological examination. Comprehensive judgment of various information is important. In this process, the role of PET/CT can be quite complex. It can help to detect or exclude malignant tumors in the early stage, which will contribute to the etiological diagnosis or the decision of experimental treatment [34]; for certain diseases, PET/CT can also reveal the characteristic manifestations of the disease through observing lesion site and distribution, which probably may lead to final clinical diagnosis. In conclusion, FDG-PET/CT is a valuable tool for diagnosing FUO/IUO. From the current study results obtained in FUO or IUO patients, it is suggested that it is of great importance to further investigate the usefulness of PET/CT in nonneoplastic diseases.

2.4 Inflammation of Unknown Origin

Yuji Nakamoto

Abstract A 67-year-old diabetic woman underwent FDG-PET/CT for fever of unknown origin. She had a history of aortic valve replacement and had been treated with steroids for systemic lupus erythematosus. FDG-PET revealed moderate uptake in the mediastinum, especially around the ascending aorta, which was surrounded by a soft tissue density mass. Contrast-enhanced CT demonstrated a contrast material leak, indicating pseudoaneurysm of the aorta. The patient was treated with emergency operation.

Keywords: Fever, Diabetes, Aortic valve, Rupture, Pseudoaneurysm

2.4.1 Clinical Presentation

A 67-year-old diabetic woman, who had a history of aortic valve replacement and had been treated with steroids for systemic lupus erythematosus, complained of a fever lasting 2 weeks despite treatment with antibiotics. Chest and abdominal CT revealed no abnormal findings for inflammation. For this reason, FDG-PET/CT was performed to detect occult malignancies or an active inflammatory focus.

2.4.2 Key Images

PET/CT with 18F-FDG (Fig. 2.5a–d) was performed to detect an occult malignancy or active inflammatory foci.

2.4.3 Technique

- The patient fasted for at least 4 h before administration of the radiopharmaceutical.
- 191 MBq of 18f-FDG was administered intravenously.

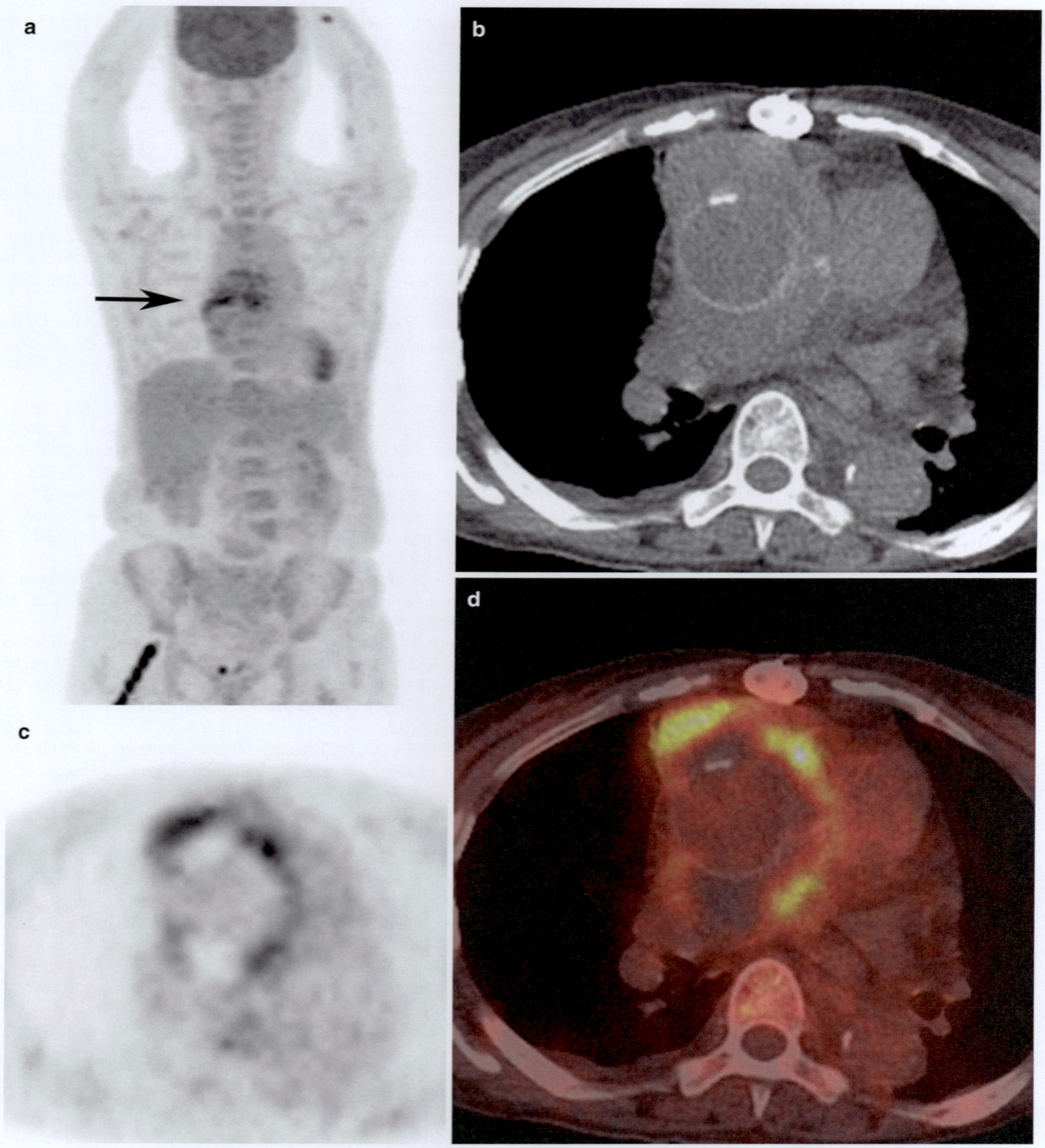

Fig. 2.5 A maximum intensity projection image (**a**), axial images of CT (**b**), PET (**c**), and fusion (**d**) demonstrate increased tracer uptake in the mediastinum (**a**, arrow), especially around the ascending aorta, where a soft tissue density mass is also noted. Because CT images obtained 2 weeks before demonstrated no soft tissue density mass around the ascending aorta, it is speculated that infection around the area caused a rupture, resulting in pseudoaneurysm of the aorta and hematoma. Because of the patient's high plasma glucose level, physiological uptake in the brain is low. In addition, the kidneys and bladder are not depicted because of chronic renal failure

- The imaging device was a whole-body PET/CT camera (GE Discovery STE) with a resolution of 5.0 mm FWHM.
- The patient's plasma glucose level was 214 mg/dL at FDG injection due to her diabetes.

2.4.4 Differential Diagnosis

- Pseudoaneurysm.

2.4.5 Diagnosis and Clinical Follow-Ups

After saline infusion, a contrast-enhanced CT scan was performed, and leakage of the contrast material was observed around the ascending aorta (arrowhead), indicating pseudoaneurysm of the aorta. An emergency operation was performed, and a stent graft was placed in the aorta.

2.4.6 Discussion

The advantage of 18F-FDG-PET/CT for fever of unknown origin is in detecting active inflammatory foci for a whole body. In this case, an inflammatory focus causing pseudoaneurysm of the aorta was identified and properly treated. It is generally believed that FDG-PET scans should be postponed or canceled when a patient's plasma glucose level is more than 150–200 mg/dL because of decreased accumulation of FDG into lesion; however, even in such a case, FDG-PET studies under hyperglycosemia can often provide useful information for developing therapeutic strategies.

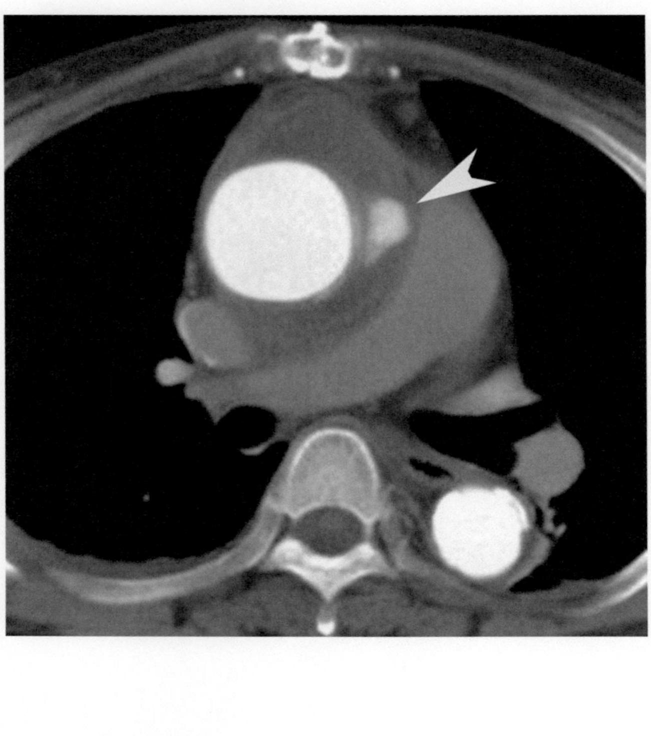

References

1. Petersdorf RG, Beeson PB. Fever of unexplained origin: report on 100 cases. Medicine. 1961;40:1–30.
2. Durack DT, Street AC. Fever of unknown origin-reexamined. Curr Clin Top Infect Dis. 1991;11:35–51.
3. Knockaert DC, Vanderschueren S, Blockmans D. Fever of unknown origin in adults: 40 years on. J Intern Med. 2003;253:263–75.
4. Perrin AE, Goichot B, Andès E, et al. [Development and long-term prognosis of unexplained persistent inflammatory biologic syndromes] in French. Rev Med Interne. 2002;23(8):683–9.
5. Vanderschueren S, Biondo ED, Ruttens D, et al. Inflammation of unknown origin versus fever of unknown origin: two of a kind. Eur J Intern Med. 2009;20:415–8.
6. Muto G, Yamashita H, Takahashi Y, et al. Large vessel vasculitis in elderly patients: early diagnosis and steroid-response evaluation with FDG-PET/CT and contrast-enhanced CT. Rheumatol Int. 2014;34(11):1545–54.
7. Balink H, Veeger NJ, Bennink RJ, et al. The predictive value of C-reactive protein and erythrocyte sedimentation rate for 18F-FDG PET/CT outcome in patients with fever and inflammation of unknown origin. Nucl Med Commun. 2015;36:604–9.
8. Garcia-Vincent AM, Tello-Galán MJ, Amo-Salas M, et al. Do clinical and laboratory variables have any impact on the diagnostic performance of 18F-FDGPET/CT in patients with fever of unknown origin? Ann Nucl Med. 2018;32:123–31.
9. Schönau V, Vogel K, Englbrecht M, et al. The value of 18F-FDGPET/CT in identifying the cause of fever of unknown origin (FUO) and inflammation of unknown origin (IUO): data from a prospective study. Ann Rheum Dis. 2018;77:70–7.
10. Bleeker-Rovers CP, Vos FJ, Mudde AH, et al. A prospective multicentre study of the value of FDG-PET as part of a structured diagnostic protocol in patients with fever of unknown origin. Eur J Nucl Med Mol Imaging. 2007;34:694–703.
11. Takeuchi M, Dahabreh IJ, Nihashi T, et al. Nuclear imaging for classic fever of unknown origin: meta-analysis. J Nucl Med. 2016;57:1913–9.
12. Besson FL, Chaumet-Riffaud P, Playe M, et al. Contribution of 18F-FDG PET in the diagnostic assessment of fever of unknown origin (FUO): a stratification-based meta-analysis. Eur J Nucl Med Mol Imaging. 2016;43:1887–95.
13. Takeuchi M, Nihashi T, Gafter-Gvili A, et al. Association of 18F-FDG PET or PET/CT results with spontaneous remission in classic fever of unknown origin; a systematic review and meta-analysis. Medicine. 2018;97(43):e12909.
14. Palestro CJ, Love C. Nuclear medicine imaging in fever of unknown origin: the new paradigm. Curr Pharm Des. 2017; https://doi.org/10.2174/1381612824666171129194507.
15. Kan Y, Wang W, Liu J, et al. Contribution of 18F-FDGPET/CT in a case-mix of fever of unknow origin and inflammation of unknown origin: a meta-analysis. Acta Radiol. 2019;60:716–25. https://doi.org/10.1177/0284185118799512.
16. Kubota K, Nakamoto Y, Tamaki N, et al. FDG-PET for the diagnosis of fever of unknown origin: a Japanese multi-center study. Ann Nucl Med. 2011;25:355–64.
17. Petersdorf RG, Beeson PB. Fever of unexplained origin: report on 100 cases. Medicine (Baltimore). 1961;40:1–30.
18. Bleeker-Rovers CP, van der Meer JWM. Fever of unknown origin. In: Fauci A, Hauser S, Longo D, Jameson J, Loscalzo J, Kasper D, editors. Harrison's principles of internal medicine. 19th ed. New York: McGraw Hill; 2015. p. 135–42.
19. Varghese GM, Trowbridge P, Doherty T. Investigating and managing pyrexia of unknown origin in adults. BMJ. 2010;341:C5470.
20. Horowitz HW. Fever of unknown origin or fever of too many origins? N Engl J Med. 2013;368(3):197–9.
21. Hicks RJ, Hofman MS. Is there still a role for SPECT–CT in oncology in the PET–CT era? Nat Rev Clin Oncol. 2012;9(12):712–20.

22. Rennen HJM, Bleeker-Rovers C, Oyen WG. Imaging infection and inflammation. In: Baert AL, Sartor K, Schiepers C, editors. Diagnostic nuclear medicine. Berlin Heidelberg: Springer; 2006. p. 113–26.
23. Takeuchi M, Nihashi T, Gafter-Gvili A, García-Gómez FJ, Andres E, Blockmans D, et al. Association of 18F-FDG PET or PET/CT results with spontaneous remission in classic fever of unknown origin. Medicine. 2018;97(43):e12909.
24. Dong MJ, Zhao K, Liu ZF, Wang GL, Yang SY, Zhou GJ. A meta-analysis of the value of fluorodeoxyglucose-PET/PET-CT in the evaluation of fever of unknown origin. Eur J Radiol. 2011;80(3):834–44.
25. Hao R, Yuan L, Kan Y, Li C, Yang J. Diagnostic performance of 18F-FDG PET/CT in patients with fever of unknown origin: a meta-analysis. Nucl Med Commun. 2013;34(7):682–8.
26. van der Ende EL, Punwasia RVG, van Daeleb PLA, Schurinkc KAM. Diagnostic value of FDG-PET/CT in fever of unknown origin. Erasmus J Med. 2013;3:32–7.
27. Sioka C, Assimakopoulos A, Fotopoulos A. The diagnostic role of18F fluorodeoxyglucose positron emission tomography in patients with fever of unknown origin. Eur J Clin Investig. 2015;45(6):601–8.
28. Mulders-Manders C, Simon A, Bleeker-Rovers C. Fever of unknown origin. Clin Med (Lond). 2015;15(3):280–4.
29. Schönau V, Vogel K, Englbrecht M, et al. The value of 18F-FDG-PET/CT in identifying the cause of fever of unknown origin (FUO) and inflammation of unknown origin (IUO): data from a prospective study. Ann Rheum Dis. 2018;77:70–7.
30. Chinese Society of Nuclear Medicine. Basic requirements of clinical quality control and quality assurance on SPECT (/CT) and PET/CT (2014 edition). Chin J Nucl Med Mol Imaging. 2014:343–448.
31. Tan XY, He QY. Chinese literature review of etiology distribution of adult patients with fever of unknown origin from1979 to 2012. Chin J Intern Med. 2013;52:1013–7.
32. Keidar Z, Gurman-Balbir A, Gaitini D, et al. Fever of unknown origin: the role of 18F-FDG PET/CT. J Nucl Med. 2008;49:1980–5.
33. Ergül N, Halac M, Cermik TF, et al. The diagnostic role of FDG PET/CT in patients with fever of unknown origin. Mol Imaging Radionucl Ther. 2011;20:19–25.
34. Mulders-Manders CM, Simon A, Bleeker-Rovers CP. Rheumatologic diseases as the cause of fever of unknown origin. Best Pract Res Clin Rheumatol. 2016;30:789–801.

3 FDG-PET/CT for a Variety of Infectious Diseases

Hiroshi Toyama, Koji Satoh, Taroh Okui, Chao Cheng, Kimiteru Ito, Jingping Zhang, Miyako Morooka, Motoyuki Takaki, Kentaro Inoue, Yoshinori Tsuchiya, Nobuyuki Honma, and Yuji Nakamoto

3.1 Anti-Resorptive Agents-Related Osteonecrosis of the Jaw (ARONJ)

Koji Satoh and Taroh Okui

Abstract A 70-year-old man presented with right mandibular pain and history of right mandibular third molar extraction 20 months back. Examination revealed purulence, exposed bone, and mental nerve hypoesthesia. He was previously prescribed zoledronate to treat bone metastases from pulmonary adenocarcinoma. PET/CT images taken 5 months before the first visit demonstrated increased mandibular FDG uptake. The inflammation remained symptomatic despite zoledronate discontinuation and antibiotic administration, with left mandibular bone exposure. SPECT/CT images demonstrated increased MDP uptake and bilateral mandibular bone destruction. Mandibular resection and pathological investigation revealed a sequestrum, indicating chronic osteomyelitis, leading to diagnosis of ARONJ (stages III and I).

Keywords: Anti-resorptive agents-related osteonecrosis of the jaw (ARONJ), bisphosphonate, FDG-PET/CT, SPECT/CT

3.1.1 Clinical Presentation

A 70-year-old man present with right mandibular pain and history of right lower third molar extraction performed 20 months ago. Examination revealed purulence, exposed bone, and mental nerve hypoesthesia (Fig. 3.1). For 5 years, the patient was administered 4 mg of zoledronate intravenously to treat bone metastases of pulmonary adenocarcinoma (T1aN1M1b).

H. Toyama (✉)
Department of Radiology, Fujita Health University, Toyoake, Aichi, Japan
e-mail: htoyama@fujita-hu.ac.jp

K. Satoh · T. Okui
Department of Dentistry and Oral-Maxillofacial Surgery, School of Medicine, Fujita Health University, Toyoake, Aichi, Japan
e-mail: kjsato@fujita-hu.ac.jp; taro1003@fujita-hu.ac.jp

C. Cheng
Shanghai Changhai Hospital, Shanghai, China
e-mail: chao_cheng_1999@163.com

K. Ito
Department of Diagnostic Radiology, National Cancer Center Hospital, Tokyo, Japan
e-mail: kimito@ncc.go.jp

J. Zhang
The First Hospital of China Medical University, Shenyang, China
e-mail: zjp809302@163.com

M. Morooka
Toho University Omori Medical Center, Tokyo, Japan
e-mail: miyako.morooka@med.toho-u.ac.jp

M. Takaki
Fukushima Medical University/Southern TOHOKU General Hospital, Koriyama, Fukushima, Japan
e-mail: riverplate@me.com

K. Inoue
Department of Radiology, Sendai Kousei Hospital, Sendai, Japan
e-mail: kentaro_inoue@sendai-kousei-hospital.jp

Y. Tsuchiya
Department of Nephrology, Japan Community Health Care Organization (JCHO) Sendai Hospital, Sendai, Japan
e-mail: yossitsutti@gmail.com

N. Honma
Department of Surgery, Japan Community Health Care Organization (JCHO) Sendai Hospital, Sendai, Japan

Y. Nakamoto
Kyoto University Hospital, Kyoto, Japan
e-mail: ynakamo1@kuhp.kyoto-u.ac.jp

H. Toyama et al. (eds.), *PET/CT for Inflammatory Diseases*, https://doi.org/10.1007/978-981-15-0810-3_3

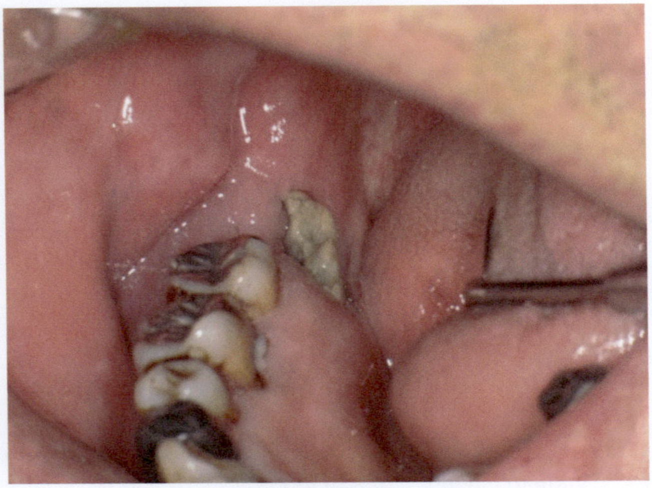

Fig. 3.1 Intraoral image

3.1.2 Key Images

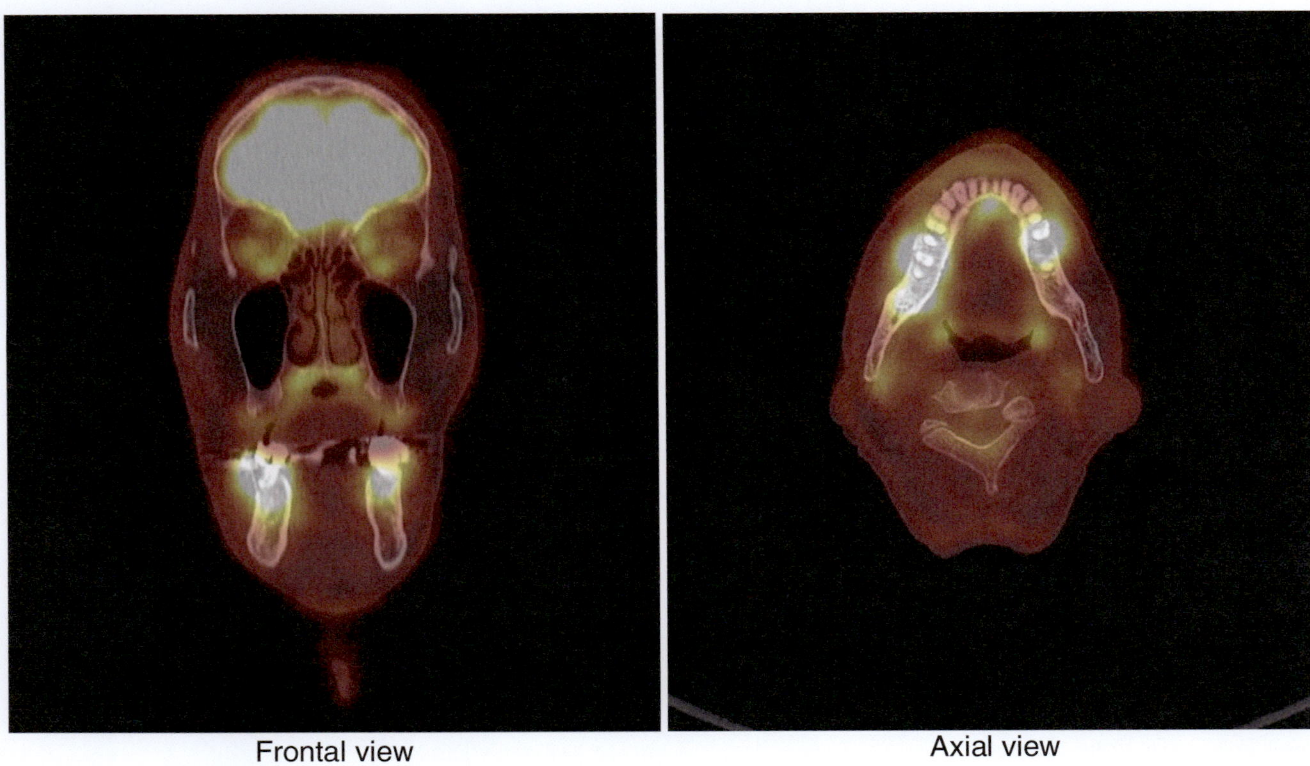

Fig. 3.2 FDG-PET/CT. Frontal view (left) and axial view (right)

3.1.3 Technique

- Patient preparation: patient did not consume anything by mouth for 6 h before the administration of the radiopharmaceutical.
- PET images were acquired 60 min after intravenous injection of FDG (4 MBq/kg).
- Imaging device: whole-body PET/CT camera (Biograph mCT with 3D/OSEM+TOF+PSF, Siemens Japan, Tokyo) was used.
- Attenuation correction: emission scanning was carried out for 1.5 min per bed following the CT image acquisition.

3.1.4 Image Interpretation

PET/CT images (Fig. 3.2) taken 5 months before the first visit demonstrated increased FDG uptake, seen bilaterally in the mandible. H-MDP bone SPECT/CT images (Fig. 3.3)

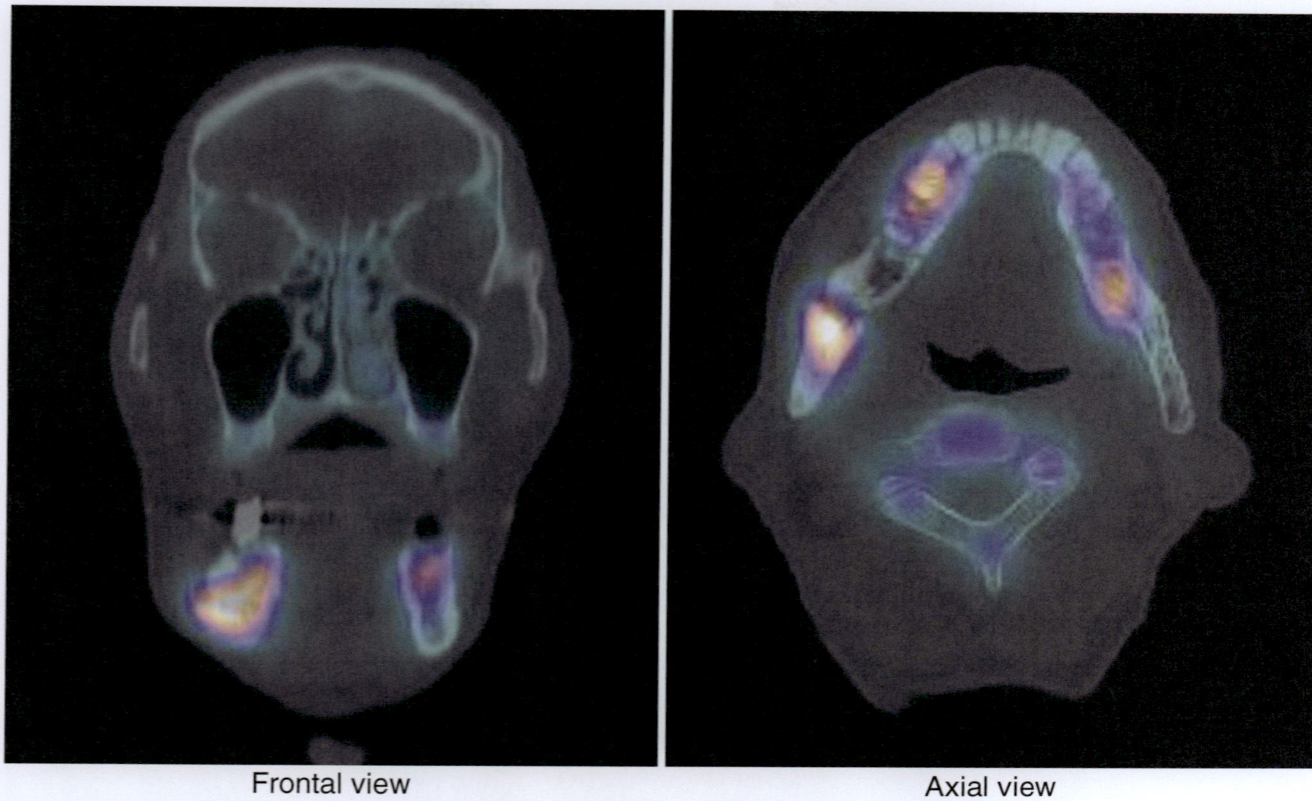

Fig. 3.3 SPECT/CT. Frontal view (left) and axial view (right)

taken 2 years later, preoperatively, demonstrated cold areas in the bone destruction areas along with increased uptake in the surrounding mandible bilaterally.

3.1.5 Differential Diagnosis

- ARONJ
- Radiation osteonecrosis
- Bone metastases

3.1.6 Diagnosis and Clinical Follow-Ups

The patient had not undergone radiation therapy of the jaws. Segment resection and marginal resection were performed on the right and left sides, respectively (Fig. 3.4). Pathological investigation revealed a sequestrum that indicated chronic osteomyelitis. Diagnosis of ARONJ (stages III and I) was made, with no signs of recurrence in follow-ups.

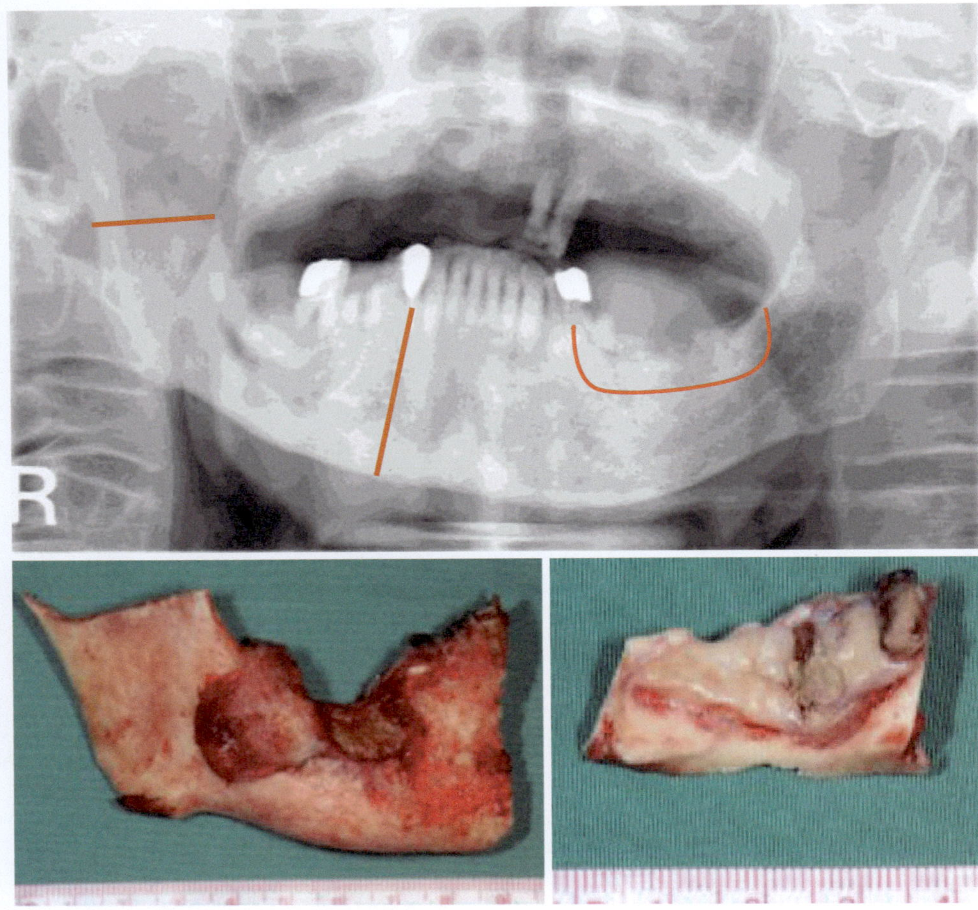

Fig. 3.4 Panoramic X-ray image and resected lesions

3.1.7 Discussion

Surgical management of ARONJ requires sufficient resection to prevent recurrence. Hybrid FDG-PET/CT and SPECT/CT systems (combining RI tomographic scanning and low-dose CT) could significantly increase the certainty of anatomical localization, and facilitate diagnosis and treatment planning by identifying functional changes, visualizing chronic osteomyelitis, and identifying bone metabolism preceding bone destruction [1, 2].

3.2 Tuberculosis 1

Chao Cheng

Abstract Tuberculosis is a chronic infectious disease caused by *Mycobacterium tuberculosis*. It can invade multiple organs, among which pulmonary infection is the most common. Tuberculosis is caused by low-grade fever (significant afternoon), night sweat, feeble, bone pain, and other clinical features. This disease often attacks the lung, the intestinal tract, the spine, and the kidney. The imaging manifestations of tuberculosis invading the spine must be differentiated from spinal tumor and degenerative osteoarthropathy. The main MR criteria for spine tuberculosis are hypointensity on T1-weighted sequences and hyperintensity sequences; sometimes empty hole, dead bone, and a cold abscess can be seen. F-18 FDG PET/CT scan can provide additional information on early change, metabolism, and spread of the disease, compared to MRI.

Keywords: Tuberculosis, FDG, PET/CT

3.2.1 Clinical Presentation

A 34-year-old man known with neck mass appeared 4 months ago, about 2 cm × 2 cm, with a fever up to 39.5°. Laboratory examination: leukocyte count 5.2 × 10^9/L, neutrophils 73.9 × 10^9/L, monocyte 9.0 × 10^9/L; blood platelet 309 × 10^9/L; plasma D-diploid 0.84 μg/mL; hepatitis B surface antibody anti-HBs(+); hepatitis B surface antibody, anti-HBc(+) (Figs. 3.5 and 3.6).

3.2.2 Key Images

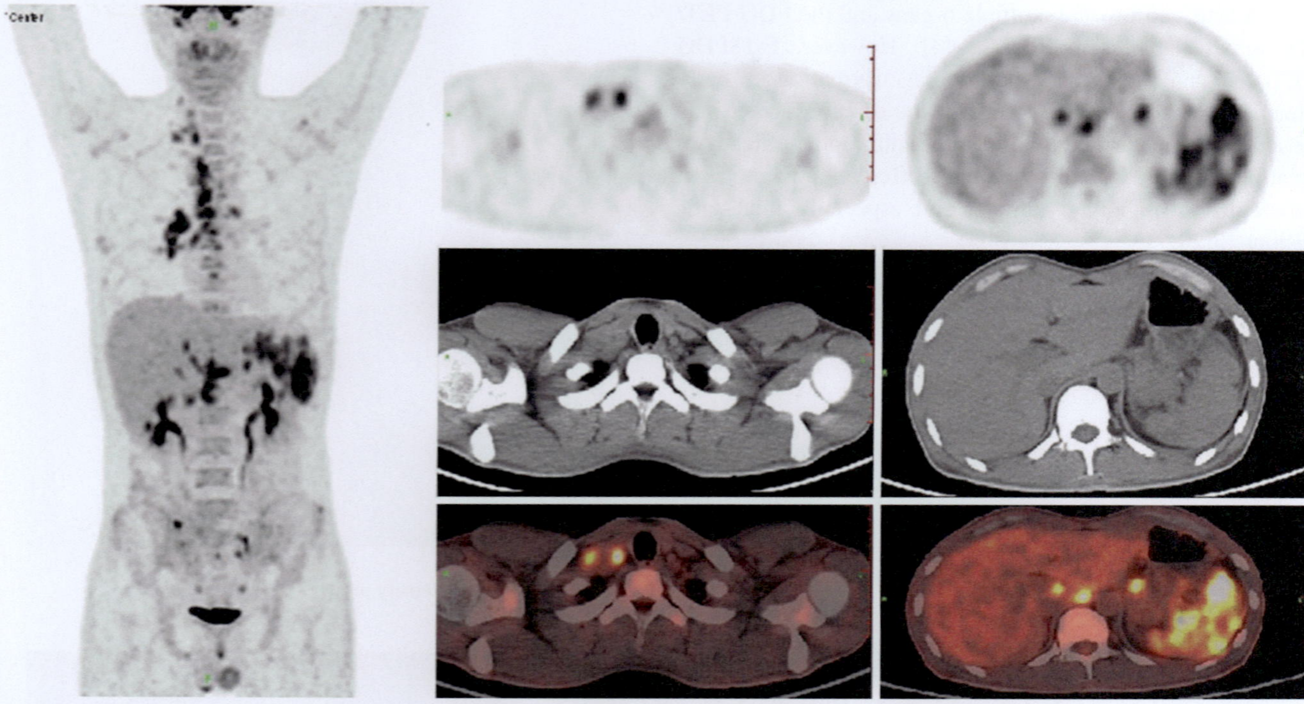

Fig. 3.5 Demonstrates multiple nodules in the upper right lung without increased metabolism, and short articles in the lower left lung. Enlargement and abnormal uptake of lymph nodes can be seen in the mediastinum, right hilum, and right septal angle of the heart. High metabolism nodules can be seen in the right lobe, SUV_{max} = 5.8. Increased radioactive uptake could be seen in the leading edge of the right 3 and 4 ribs. Color ultrasound showed right cervical lymph node enlargement

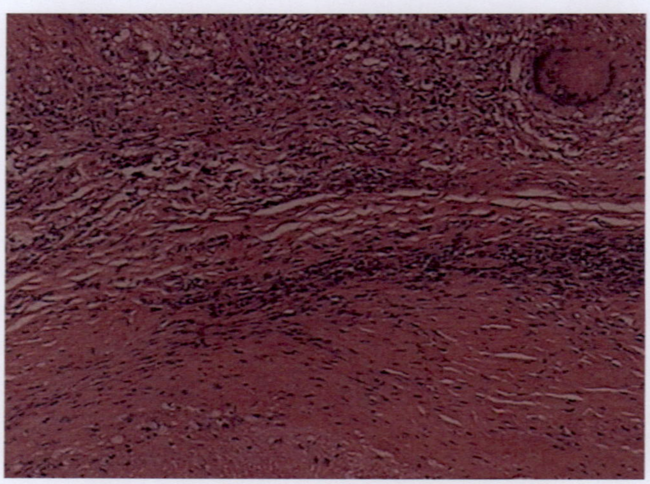

Fig. 3.6 Shows neck lymph nodes biopsy result, epithelioid granuloma, and caseous necrosis

3.2.3 Technique

- Patient preparation: patient should not take anything by mouth for 6 h before administration of radiopharmaceutical.
- 281.2 MBq of 18FDG administered intravenously (body weight = 49 kg)
- Imaging device: whole-body PET/CT camera (Siemens biograph 64) with resolution of 4.0 mm FWHM.

3.2.4 Differential Diagnosis

- Lymphoma
- Metastatic tumor

3.2.5 Diagnosis and Clinical Follow-Ups

The patient received a cervical lymph node biopsy and diagnosed as tuberculosis. Patients were referred to other hospital for TB specialist treatment.

3.2.6 Discussion

Tuberculosis is a chronic infectious disease caused by *Mycobacterium tuberculosis*. The top three extrapulmonary tuberculosis are lymph node tuberculosis, bone and joint tuberculosis, and urogenital tuberculosis [3]. Extrapulmonary tuberculosis can involve multiple organs and the FDG PET/CT manifestations are diverse [4]. However, F-18FDG PET/CT scan can provide additional information on early change, metabolism, and spread of the disease, and it may be a complementary method for determining the efficacy of treatment. FDG PET/CT scan helps differential diagnosis of tuberculosis, malignant tumors, and especially metastatic lesions [5, 6].

3.3 Tuberculosis 2

Kimiteru Ito

Abstract In 2016, 10.4 million new cases of active tuberculosis and 1.7 million deaths due to tuberculosis were reported worldwide, and >60% of these patients were located in Africa and Asia. Malignancies indicating high-uptake lesions can be detected using ^{18}F-FDG PET. Active tuberculosis lesions commonly result in high ^{18}F-FDG uptake because tuberculous granulomas comprise activated macrophages and lymphocytes that have a high avidity to glucose. Therefore, in endemic countries, positive ^{18}F-FDG PET should be interpreted with caution to avoid misdiagnosis. Notably, all radiologists must be familiar with the clinical features and ^{18}F-FDG PET of tuberculosis.

Keywords: Tuberculosis, ^{18}F-FDG, PET, Granuloma, Tuberculoma

3.3.1 Clinical Presentation

A 57-year-old man was incidentally diagnosed with a pulmonary nodule at the left upper lobe using computed tomography (CT). The nodule was resected as lung cancer.

3.3.2 Key Images

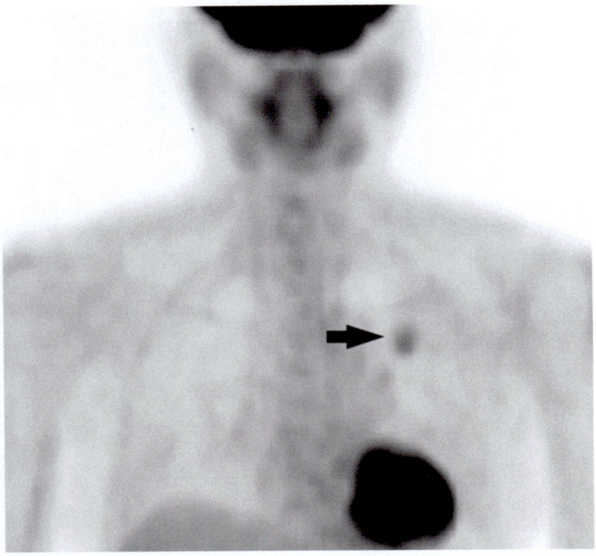

Fig. 3.7 Maximum intensity projection

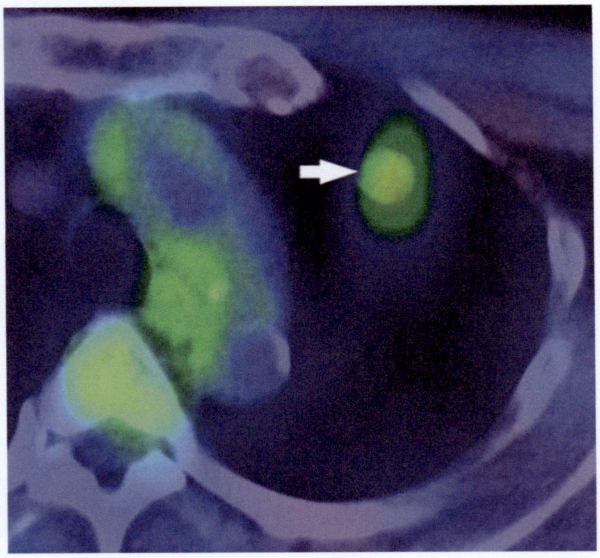

Fig. 3.8 Fusion image of PET/CT

3.3.3 Technique

- Patient preparation: The patient should not take anything orally up to 4 h before the administration of ^{18}F-FDG.
- 4–6 MBq/kg of ^{18}F-FDG was intravenously administered.
- Imaging device: Whole-body PET/CT camera (Siemens biograph 16) with a resolution of 3.75 mm FWHM was used.

3.3.4 Image Interpretation

An MIP of ^{18}F-FDG PET/CT (Fig. 3.7) showed mild ^{18}F-FDG uptake in the upper lobe in the left lung (black arrow); however, no other lesions were detected in both lungs. Axial fused PET/CT image (Fig. 3.8) showed increased ^{18}F-FDG uptake in the nodular lesion [white arrow; maximum standardized uptake value (SUV_{max}), 2.7].

3.3.5 Differential Diagnosis

- Nontuberculous mycobacteria
- Various malignancies (for example, lung cancer and lymphoma)
- Sarcoidosis
- Collagen diseases
- Inflammatory diseases

3.3.6 Diagnosis and Clinical Follow-Ups

CT (Fig. 3.9) showed calcified part as a faint high density (white arrow). In a sectioned macroscopic specimen of the nodule, ivory white cut surfaces were observed (Fig. 3.10). Histological slice at the center of the nodule revealed a tuberculous granuloma with caseous necrosis (Fig. 3.11).

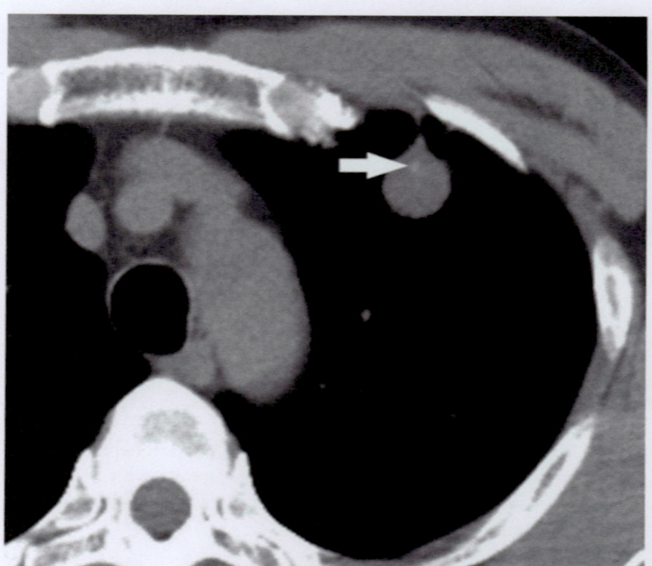

Fig. 3.9 CT image

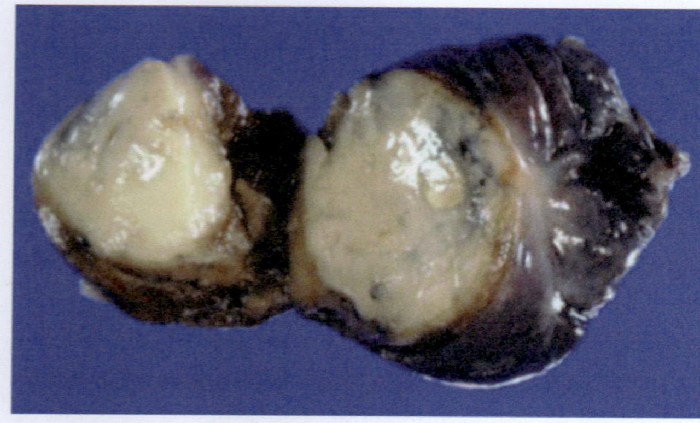

Fig. 3.10 Macroscopic finding

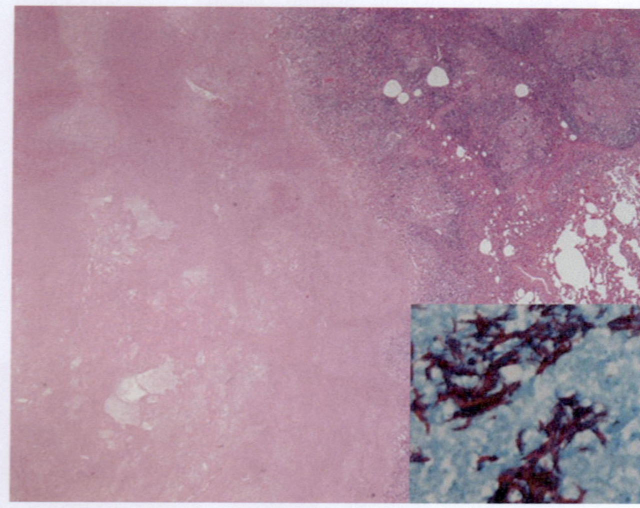

Fig. 3.11 Microscopic finding

3.3.7 Discussion

Features of ^{18}F-FDG PET/CT in tuberculosis frequently mimic those in many malignancies [7–9]. Moreover, tuberculosis must be suspected in high-risk populations in Asia and Africa [10] when PET/CT imaging detected high FDG uptake lesions with calcification. Notably, all radiologists must be familiar with these findings to accurately interpret ^{18}F-FDG PET/CT of tuberculosis.

3.4 Fungal Granuloma

Chao Cheng

Abstract Systemic disseminated fungal infections were mostly found in patients with extensive application of anti-tumor drugs and immunosuppressive agents, patients with abuse of broad-spectrum antibiotics, and patients with dialysis, intubation, organ transplantation, bone marrow transplantation, diabetes, and AIDS. The common pathogenic bacteria are *Candida albicans*, followed by pathogens such as aspergillus and cryptococcus. Systemic disseminated fungal infection is prone to misdiagnosis due to its lack of specificity clinical symptoms.

Keywords: Fungal granuloma, FDG, PET/CT

3.4.1 Clinical Presentation

A 32-year-old man was presented with lumbar pain for more than a month after fever, and was treated with anti-infective therapy in the local hospital. The temperature could be recovered to normal, but the temperature rose again after the treatment was stopped. Specialized examination suggested oral mucosa leukoplastic plaque, gastroscopy suggested mycotic esophagitis, and abdominal CT suggested the possibility of retroperitoneal tumor and abdominal aortic dissection aneurysm. C-reactive protein, 95.2 mg/L; white blood cell count 12.2×10^9/L–14.31×10^9/L (Fig. 3.12).

3.4.2 Key Images

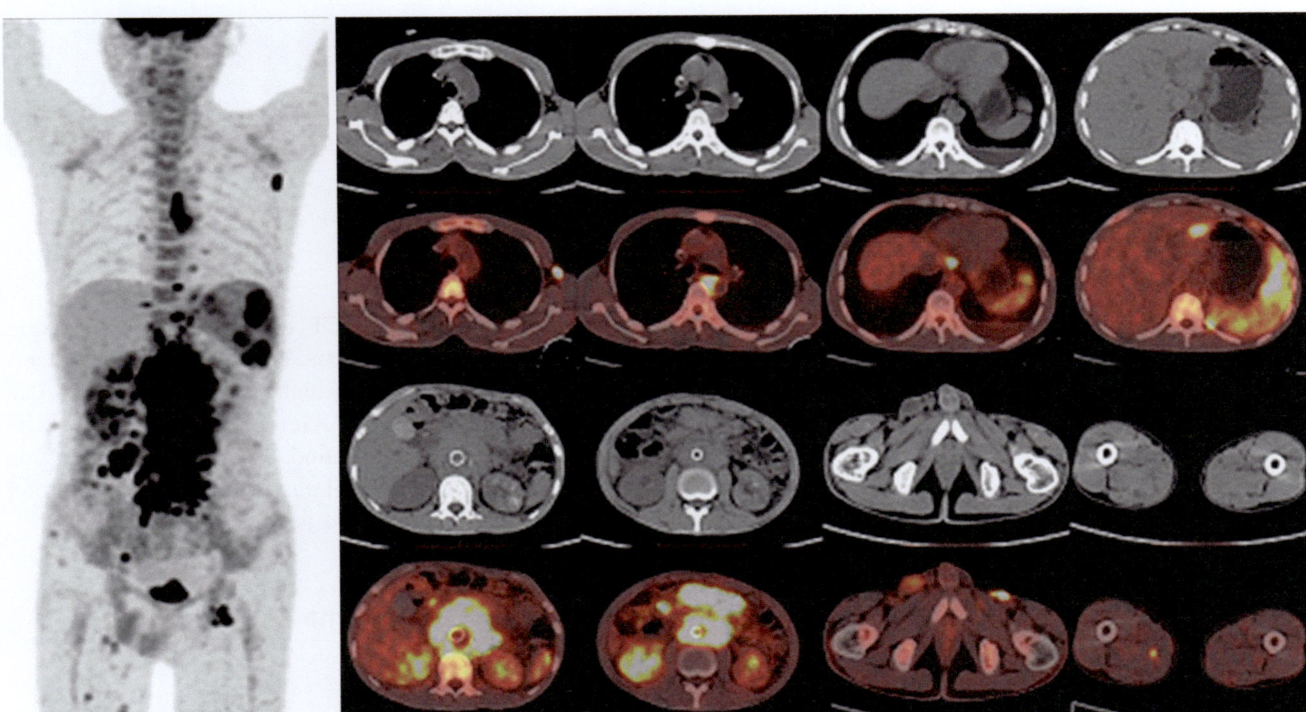

Fig. 3.12 PET/CT showed multiple enlarged lymph nodes in the left axillary, mediastinum, right hilar, left internal mammary, diaphragm, hepatic portal, small omental bursa, retroperitoneal, mesenteric area, the right fossa, basin on the right side, on both sides of the inguinal region and right leg muscle clearance, and showed intense FDG uptake with SUV_{max} of 21.8, two side pleural effusion, the left hepatic lobe in the ventral subcapsular showed intense FDG uptake with SUV_{max} of 4.7; spleen volume increased with different sizes nodules with intense FDG uptake with SUV_{max} of 8.8

3.4.3 Technique

- Patient preparation: patient should not take anything by mouth for 6 h before administration of radiopharmaceutical.
- 325 MBq of 18FDG administered intravenously (body weight = 42 kg).
- Imaging device: whole-body PET/CT camera (Siemens biograph 64) with resolution of 4.0 mm FWHM (Fig. 3.13).

3.4.4 Differential Diagnosis

- Lymphoma
- Tuberculosis of lymph nodes
- Sarcoidosis

3.4.5 Diagnosis and Clinical Follow-Ups

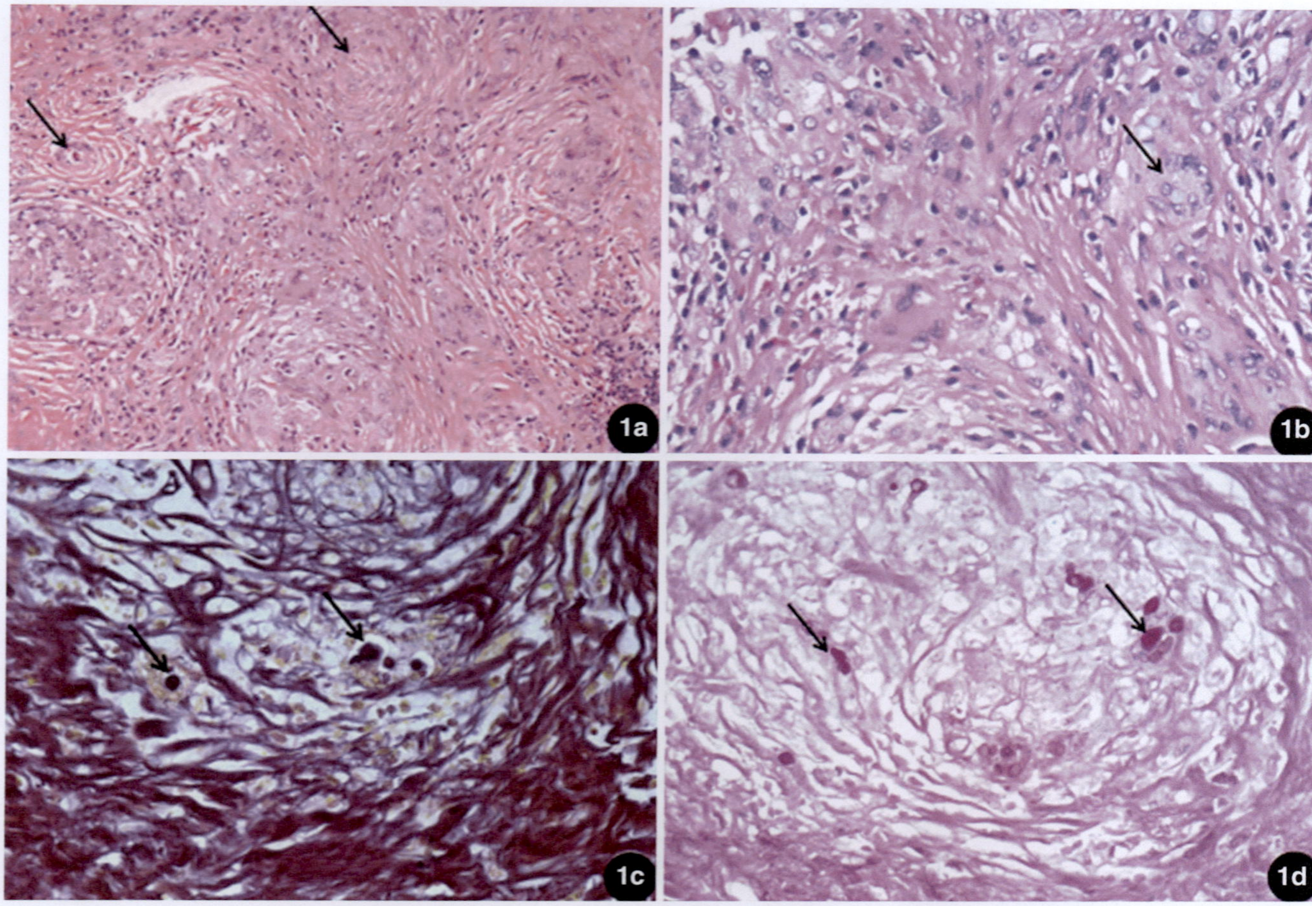

Fig. 3.13 Pathology and special staining of retroperitoneal masses: (**a**) Granulomatous lesions (HE×200). (**b**) Granulomatous lesions (HE×400). (**c**) Positive silver staining (×400). (**d**) PAS positive staining (×400). The pathology HE of retroperitoneal mass (**a**, **b**) showed that diffuse granulomatous lesions were formed in the retroperitoneal mesenteric tissue and surrounding lymph nodes, epithelioid cells, and polynuclear giant cells; lymphocyte hyperplasia and infiltration were observed in granuloma; and small circular fungal spore deposition was observed in granuloma. Both silver staining (**c**) and PAS staining (**d**) were positive, and the final diagnosis was fungal granuloma

3.4.6 Discussion

Systemic disseminated fungal infection mainly presented systemic multiple lymph node enlargements was very rare, and it was difficult to distinguish from lymphoma by FDG PET/CT. Although PET/CT has a high diagnostic value for lymphoma, it may be misdiagnosed in this case only depending on PET/CT imaging. PET/CT diagnosis should be based on a variety of comprehensive imaging, clinical presentation, and laboratory tests. Therefore, in this case, we should also attach great importance to the mycotic esophagitis revealed by Gastroscopy, a white spot of the oral mucosa, fungi D-glucan testing positive for clinical data, only fully combined the clinical and imaging, is likely to make close to the accurate diagnosis of disseminated fungal infection [11–14].

3.5 Infective Endocarditis 1

Chao Cheng

Abstract Infective endocarditis (IE) is an infectious disease due to the pathogens that infect and destroy the cardiac valves or endocardium, which often involves unhealthy valves (such as caused by rheumatic valvular disease) or hearts with congenital heart diseases. The implantation of a valvular prosthesis or pacemaker is also a risk factor for IE. The patients of IE may suffer fever, fatigue, joints pain, or other atypical symptoms related to infection, while some may have the Osler nodes or other symptoms due to infarction of organs. Currently, practice guidelines use modified Duke criteria for the diagnosis of IE, and transesophageal echocardiography (TEE) and CT angiography (CTA) are the first-line imaging choices for the diagnosis. F-18 FDG PET/CT scan can detect a metabolic change of valves and endocardium that may provide more information for developing IE diagnosis.

Keywords: Infective endocarditis, FDG, PET/CT

3.5.1 Clinical Presentation

A 43-year-old woman with aortic stenosis for over 20 years and suffered repeated fever for 1 month. The maximum body temperature was 39.0 °C. Laboratory examinations showed that ESR and CRP was 71 mm/h and 19.3 mg/L, respectively. The heart echocardiography manifested severe aortic stenosis with the formation of valvular vegetation and abscess (Fig. 3.14).

3.5.2 Key Images

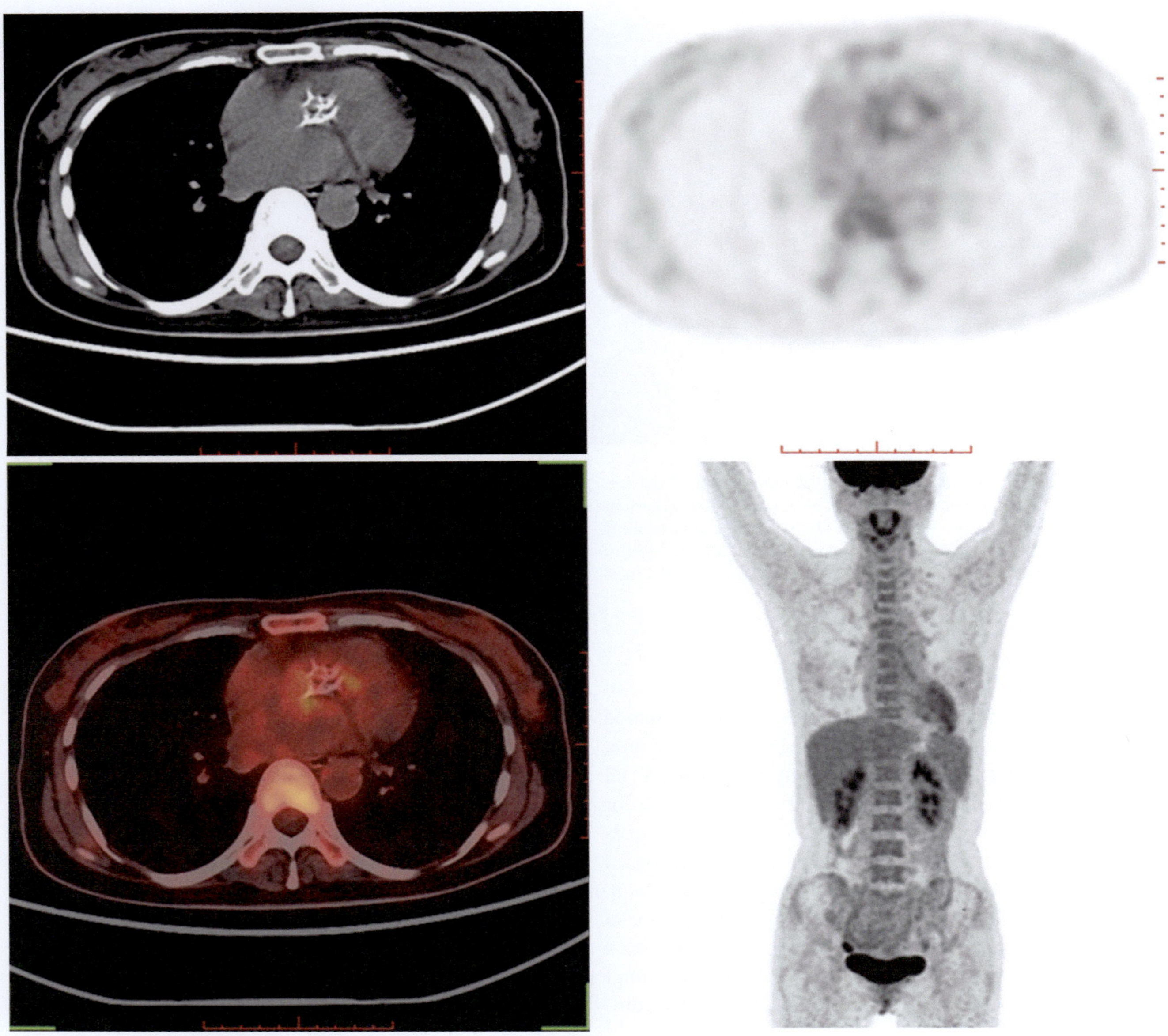

Fig. 3.14 Images demonstrate notable calcification of aortic valve on CT and mild increased FDG uptake of soft tissue around the calcified foci on the fusion image ($SUV_{max} = 3.1$)

3.5.3 Technique

- Patient preparation: patient should not take anything by mouth for 6 h before administration of radiopharmaceutical.
- 350 MBq of F-18 FDG administered intravenously (body weight = 46 kg).
- Imaging device: whole-body PET/CT camera (Siemens biograph 64) with resolution of 4.0 mm FWHM,

3.5.4 Differential Diagnosis

- Rheumatic valvular disease
- Elderly degenerative heart valve disease

3.5.5 Diagnosis and Clinical Follow-Ups

This patient was received antibiotic treatment using penicillin and vancomycin and then underwent surgical aortic valve replacement after exclusion of surgical contraindications. The patient recovered well after surgery and discharged 17 days later.

3.5.6 Discussion

Infective endocarditis is a dangerous fatal disease caused by virus, bacterias, or fungus [15]. TEE and CTA are the baseline imaging methods that provide information about structural and hemodynamic abnormalities. According to F18-FDG PET/CT images, IE may be characterized as mild to the high uptake of FDG along the endocardium or around cardiac valves, especially the ones with baseline valvular diseases or congenital heart diseases. FDG PET/CT may provide information related to infection, evaluate infective embolism and primary extra-cardiac infection source, and reflect the changes of conditions, particularly in patients with suspected prosthetic valve endocarditis [16–19].

3.6 Infective Endocarditis 2

Chao Cheng

Abstract Infective endocarditis (IE) is an infectious disease due to the pathogens that infect and destroy the cardiac valves or endocardium, which often involves unhealthy valves (such as caused by rheumatic valvular disease) or hearts with congenital heart diseases. The implantation of a valvular prosthesis or pacemaker is also a risk factor for IE. The patients of IE may suffer fever, fatigue, joints pain, or other atypical symptoms related to infection, while some may have the Osler nodes or other symptoms due to infarction of organs. Currently, practice guidelines use modified Duke criteria for the diagnosis of IE, and transesophageal echocardiography (TEE) and CT angiography (CTA) are the first-line imaging choices for the diagnosis. F-18 FDG PET/CT scan can detect a metabolic change of valves and endocardium that may provide more information for developing IE diagnosis.

Keywords: Infective endocarditis, FDG, PET/CT

3.6.1 Clinical Presentation

A 63-year-old woman with ventricular septal defect (VSD) for over 30 years who suffered fever with anorexia and weight loss for 3 months. The fever could be controlled by antibiotics, but relapsed after cessation. The white blood cell counts were 6.52×10^9/L, and ESR was 93 mm/h. The heart echocardiography showed VSD with IE, tricuspid valvular insufficiency with vegetation formation (Figs. 3.15 and 3.16).

3.6.2 Key Images

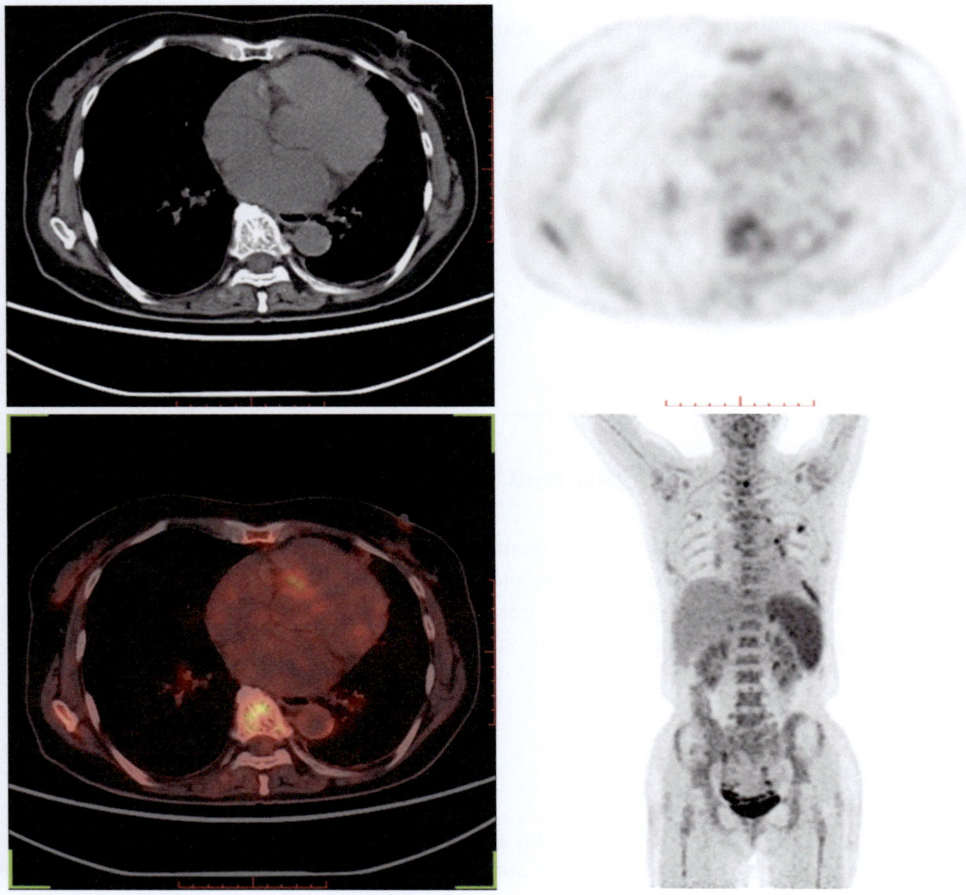

Fig. 3.15 The transverse image demonstrates mild increased FDG uptake of soft tissue around the tricuspid valve on the fusion image ($SUV_{max} = 2.9$)

Fig. 3.16 . Multiple pulmonary lesions with avid FDG uptake implied infection on lung window CT image and MIP image. MIP map shows enlarged spleen with diffuse high FDG uptake (SUV_{max} = 4.9)

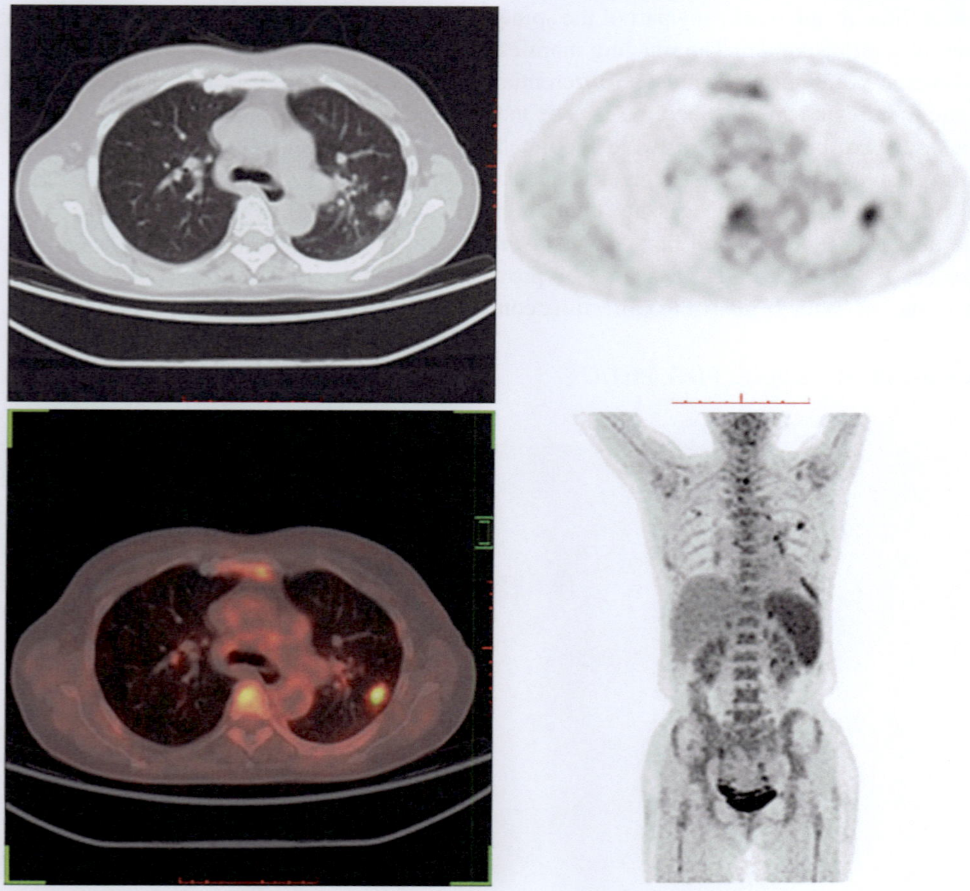

3.6.3 Technique

- Patient preparation: patient should not take anything by mouth for 6 h before administration of radiopharmaceutical.
- 333 MBq of F-18 FDG administered intravenously (body weight = 58 kg).
- Imaging device: whole-body PET/CT camera (Siemens biograph 64) with resolution of 4.0 mm FWHM.

3.6.4 Differential Diagnosis

- Rheumatic valvular disease
- Elderly degenerative heart valve disease

3.6.5 Diagnosis and Clinical Follow-Ups

This patient was received antibiotic treatment using penicillin and teicoplanin, and then underwent surgical repair of VSD and tricuspid valve replacement after exclusion of surgical contraindications. The patient discharged 18 days after the surgery and kept on antibiotic treatment in a community hospital.

3.6.6 Discussion

Infective endocarditis is a dangerous fatal disease caused by virus, bacterias, or fungus [15]. TEE and CTA are the baseline imaging methods that provide information about structural and hemodynamic abnormalities. According to F18-FDG PET/CT images, IE may be characterized as mild to the high uptake of FDG along the endocardium or around cardiac valves, especially the ones with baseline valvular diseases or congenital heart diseases. FDG PET/CT may provide information related to infection, evaluate infective embolism and primary extra-cardiac infection source, and reflect the changes of conditions, particularly in patients with suspected prosthetic valve endocarditis [16–19].

3.7 Brucella melitensis

Chao Cheng

Abstract Brucellosis is a systemic infectious and allergic disease caused by Brucella, which is caused by fever, sweating, joint pain, hepatosplenomegaly, and other clinical features. This disease often attacks the spine and causes spondylitis; it can invade any part of the spine; most patients present with back pain. The imaging manifestations of brucellosis invading the spine must be differentiated from metastatic tumors and spinal tuberculosis. The main MR criteria for suspected spondylodiskitis were hypointensity of the disc and vertebral bodies on T1-weighted sequences, hyperintensity on T2-weighted sequences, and contrast enhancement of the disc, adjacent vertebral bodies and involved paraspinal tissues. F-18 FDG PET/CT scan can provide additional information on the spread of the infection, compared to MRI.

Keywords: Brucellosis, FDG, PET/CT

3.7.1 Clinical Presentation

A 57-year-old man known with low fever in the afternoon for more than 1 month without obvious incentives. The body temperature fluctuated at 38 °C, with obvious head, neck, and shoulder pain. Shoulder movements on both sides were slightly restricted. Laboratory examination found: ESR, 86 mm/H; CRP, 120 mg/L; OT test (negative). The levels of tumor markers were normal (Fig. 3.17).

3.7.2 Key Images

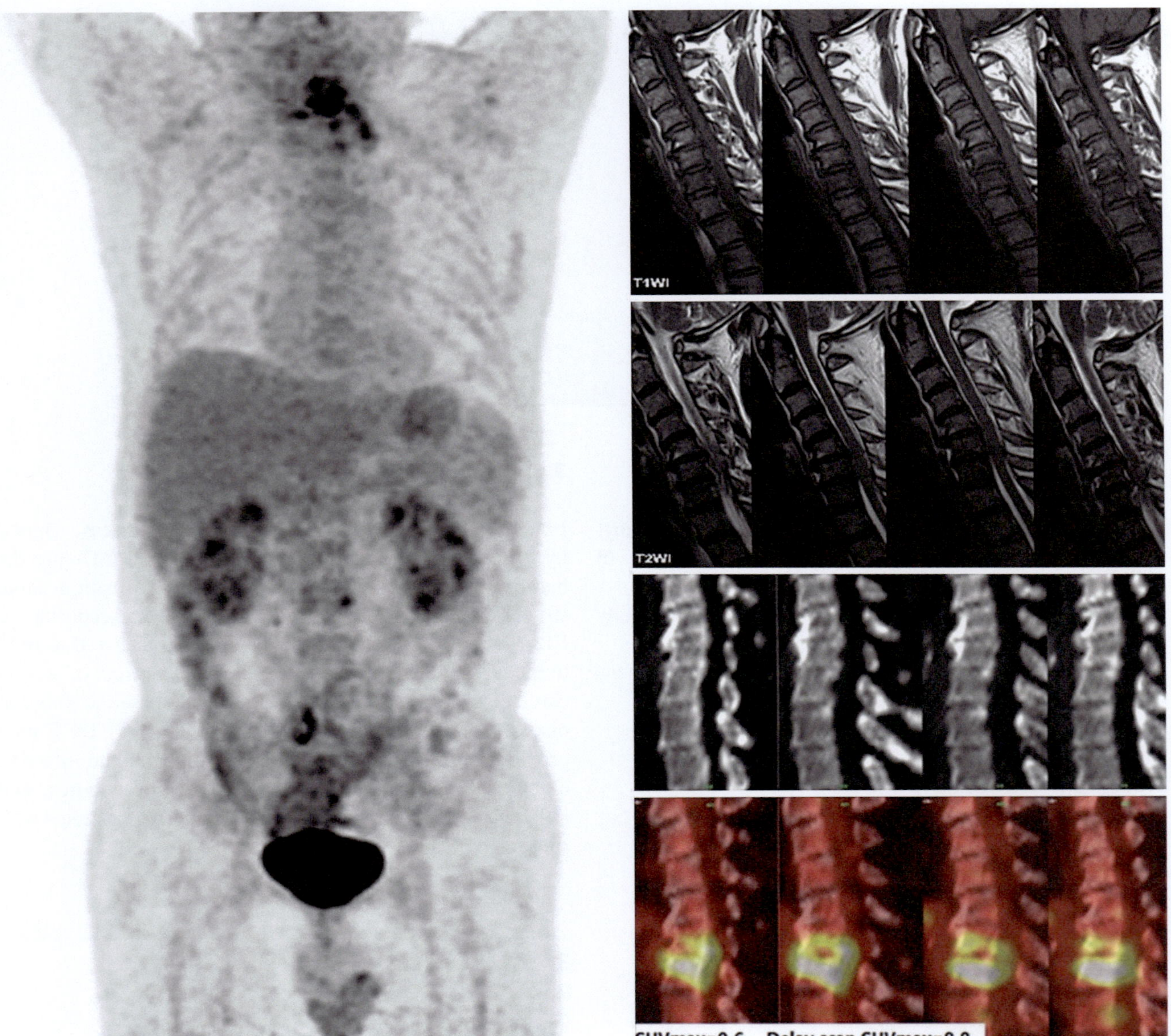

Fig. 3.17 Images demonstrate increased FDG uptake for PET/CT images in the cervical vertebrae ($SUV_{max} = 9.6$), and the bone density of C6 and C7 vertebral bodies was uneven. MRI showed low T1WI unevenness, uneven T2WI, and slightly higher signal changes, which indicated an increase in FDG uptake in PET/CT images

3.7.3 Technique

- Patient preparation: patient should not take anything by mouth for 6 h before administration of radiopharmaceutical.
- 380 MBq of 18FDG administered intravenously (body weight = 72 kg).
- Imaging device: whole-body PET/CT camera (Siemens biograph 64) with resolution of 4.0 mm FWHM.

3.7.4 Differential Diagnosis

- Spinal tuberculosis
- Spinal metastatic tumor

3.7.5 Diagnosis and Clinical Follow-Ups

This patient was living in a town close to Inner Mongolia Autonomous Region of China, where the brucellosis incidence rate is markedly higher compared with other areas. Blood culture found brucella maltese. The patient received anti-Brucella therapy (rifampicin, minocycline, streptomycin, and Moxifloxacin hydrochloride) and recovered promptly.

3.7.6 Discussion

Brucellosis is a widespread zoonotic disease caused by facultative intracellular bacteria. An MRI scan is the best imaging modality for the diagnosis of spondylodiskitis. However, F18-FDG PET/CT scan can provide additional information on the spread of brucellae spondylitis, and it may be a complementary method for determining the efficacy of treatment. The possibility of Brucella infection should be considered in interpreting FDG PET/CT images, especially in brucellosis epidemic regions [20–23].

3.8 Splenic Amoeba

Chao Cheng

Abstract Amoeba disease is caused by lytic tissue amoeba infection, which is often parasitic in the colon, presenting abdominal pain and diarrhea; occasionally, it could invade intestinal mucosa and can spread to other organs, such as causing liver damage, leading to amoeba hepatitis, and amoeba liver abscess. In addition, amoeba lung abscess and amoeba brain abscess are rare clinically. The clinical manifestations were mainly related to the lesion site and size. Simple splenic amoebas infection is rare in the clinic.

Keywords: Splenic, Amebomas, FDG PET/CT

3.8.1 Clinical Presentation

A 38-year-old man with severe pneumonia due to inhalation of swimming pool water 18 months ago complained of night sweat, tiredness, and anorexia for 1 month. Laboratory tests revealed decreased white and red blood cells and increased percentage of eosinophils. Erythrocyte sedimentation rate and C-reactive protein were elevated. Abdominal ultrasound showed multiple nodules in the spleen (Figs. 3.18 and 3.19).

3.8.2 Key Images

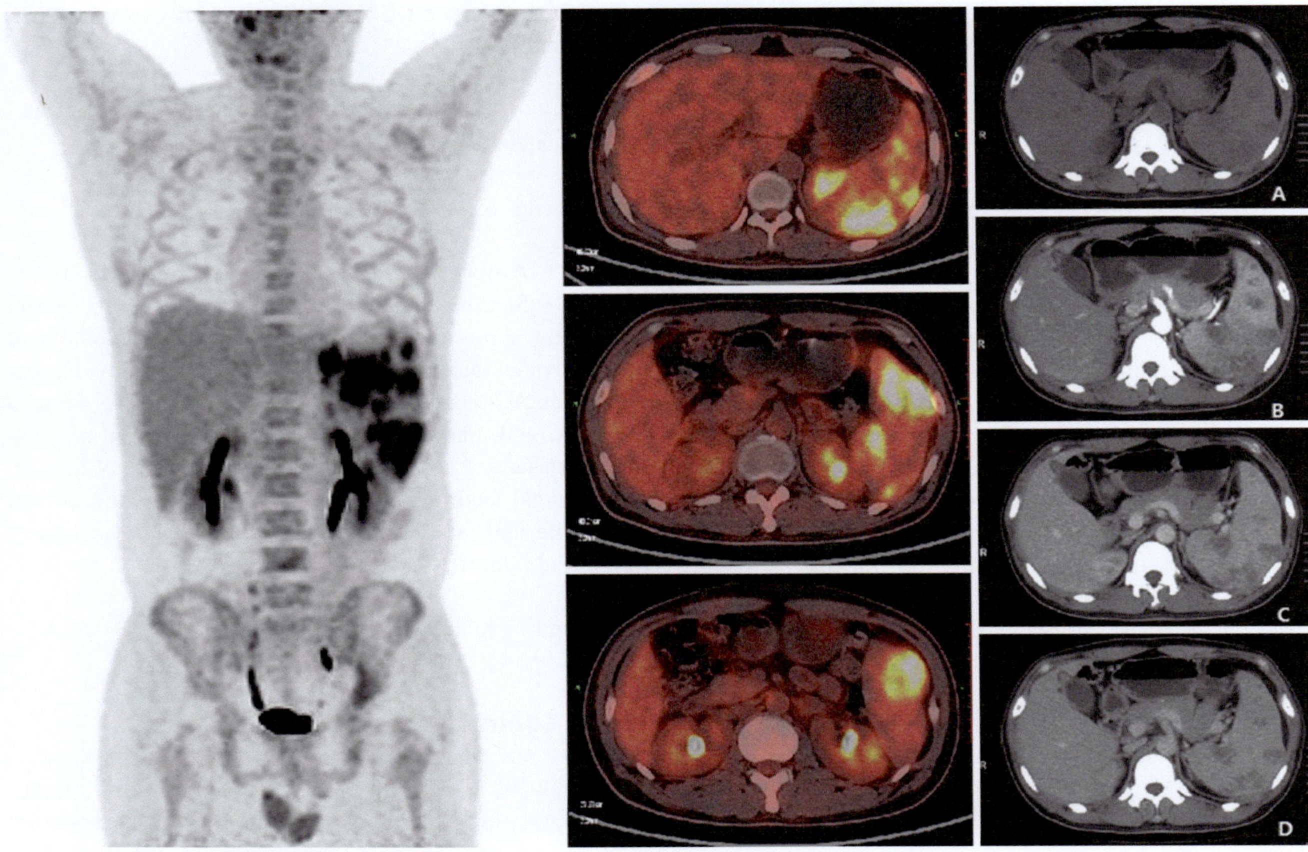

Fig. 3.18 FDG PET/CT images showed intense FDG uptake of the splenic lesions with SUV_{max} of 10.3. Unenhanced CT images (**a**) showed multiple hypodense nodules with different sizes in the spleen. Corresponding enhanced CT images in the arterial phase (**b**), portal phase (**c**), and venous phase (**d**) showed slight enhancement of the nodules. Malignancy was suspected

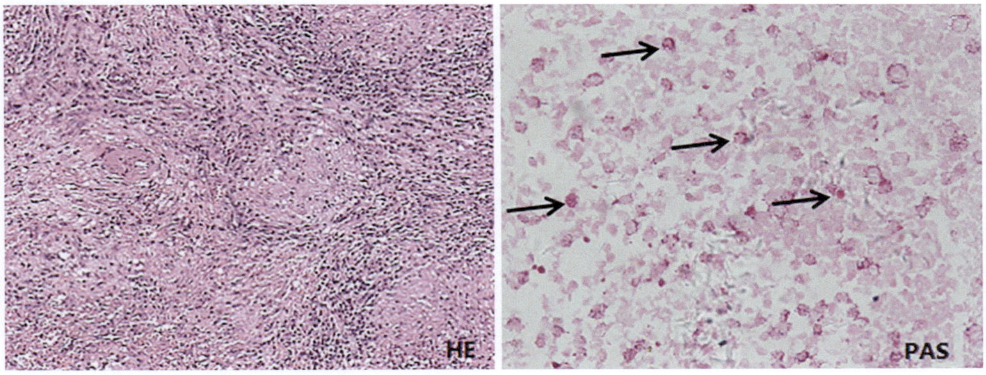

Fig. 3.19 Pathological results after spleen resection showed that multiple splenic amebomas were confirmed by pathology (HE stain). Periodic acid-Schiff staining (original magnification×600) showed numerous amebic trophozoites (arrows)

3.8.3 Technique

- Patient preparation: patient should not take anything by mouth for 6 h before administration of radiopharmaceutical.
- 400 MBq of 18FDG administered intravenously (body weight = 67 kg).
- Imaging device: whole-body PET/CT camera (Siemens biograph 64) with resolution of 4.0 mm FWHM.

3.8.4 Differential Diagnosis

- Lymphoma.
- Metastasis
- Angiosarcoma

3.8.5 Diagnosis and Clinical Follow-Ups

Patient received a Laparoscopic splenectomy. Extensive multifocal granulomatous lesions are seen in spleen specimens. Free-living amoebae were also detected in samples of pleural effusion and blood. The diagnosis was protozoosis, amoeba infection.

3.8.6 Discussion

Splenic amoebas infection is very rare and its clinical manifestations are nonspecific. PET/CT images are easily misdiagnosed as lymphoma and metastatic tumor. Diagnosis is based on the demonstration of Entamoeba in the stool or the colonic mucosa of the patients, and serologic exams can also be performed. It is difficult to diagnose spleen amoeba infection by imaging. The primary goal of the PET/CT diagnosis is to exclude other tumor diseases and combine with clinical examination data to guide further clinical examination [24–28].

3.9 Liver Abscess

Jingping Zhang

Abstract A 63-year-old man had chest and back pain and stomach upset for 1 month. Abdominal CT showed space-occupying lesion in the right lobe of the liver with multiple enlarged lymph nodes, considering liver cancer, low-density point lesion in the delayed stage in the left lobe of the liver. Laboratory examination: AFP: 23.43 (0–5.8) CEA: 10.12 (0–3.4). PET showed abnormal FDG uptake in the right posterior lobe of the liver. He had history of cirrhosis. After treatment the lesion was disappeared. The diagnosis was hepatic abscess.

Keywords: ^{18}F-FDG PET/CT, Liver cancer, Abscess

3.9.1 Clinical Presentation

A 63-year-old man presented with chest and back pain for 1 month and stomach upset. No fever, loss of weight, had constipation. CT showed space-occupying lesion in the right lobe of the liver with multiple enlarged lymph nodes, considering liver cancer. However, after treatment, the lesion was disappeared. The diagnosis was hepatic abscess (Figs. 3.20 and 3.21).

3.9.2 Key Images

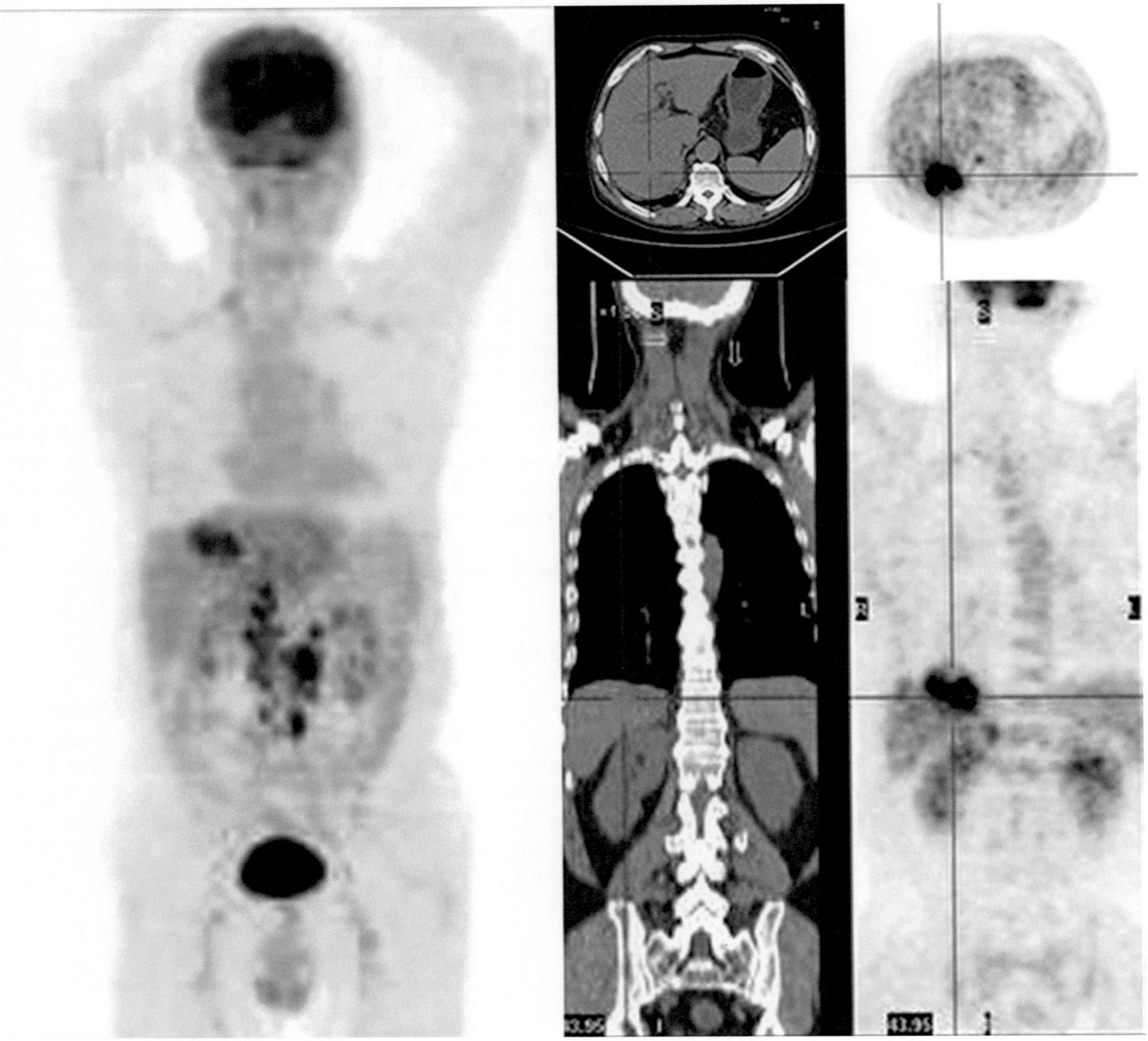

Fig. 3.20 PET/CT—The density of the right posterior lobe of the liver decreased slightly, metabolism increased, which maybe malignant lesions

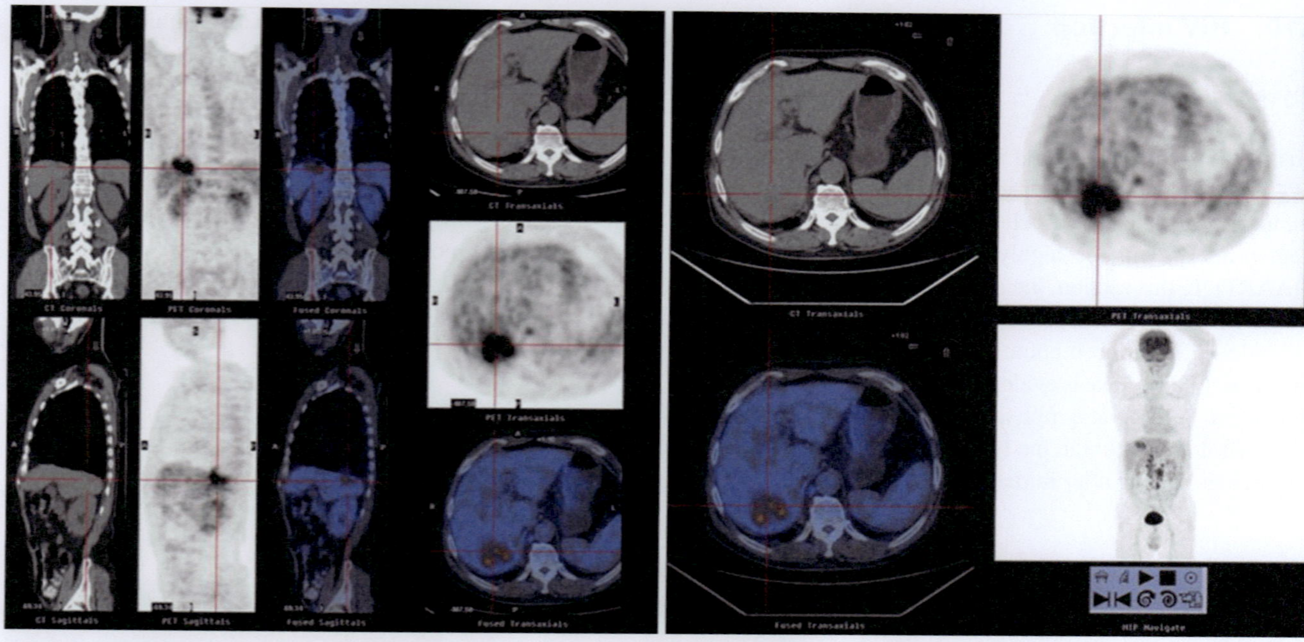

Fig. 3.20 (continued)

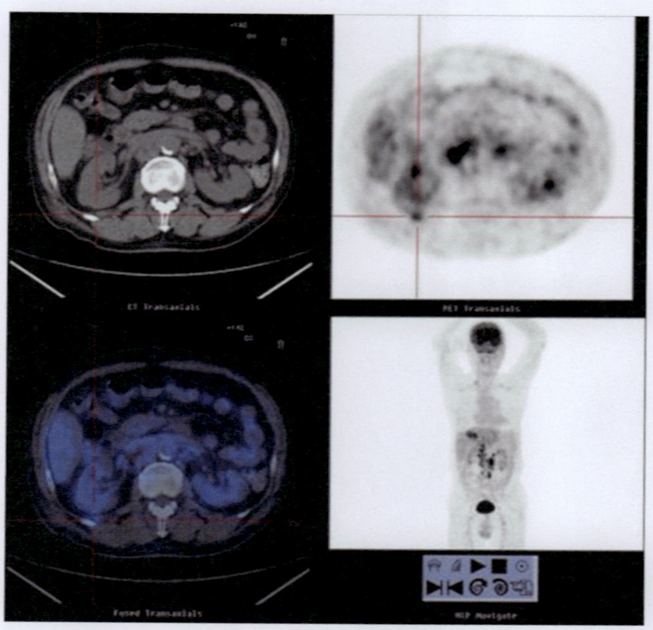

Fig. 3.21 PET/CT—Nodule shadow of right posterior abdominal wall, metabolism increased, malignant lesions metastasis is not excluded

3.9.3 Technique

- Patient preparation: patient should not take anything by mouth for 6 h before administration of radiopharmaceutical.
- 185 MBq of ^{18}F-FDG administered intravenously.
- Imaging device: Whole-body PET/CT scanning was performed using Siemens biograph mCT scanner with resolution of 5.0 mm FWHM.

3.9.4 Differential Diagnosis

- Subphrenic abscess
- Liver cancer

3.9.5 Diagnosis and Clinical Follow-Ups

CT showed space-occupying lesion in the right lobe of the liver with multiple enlarged lymph nodes.

PET/CT demonstrated abnormal FDG uptake in the right posterior lobe of the liver. The patient recovered after antibiotic therapy, and the lesion was disappeared. The diagnosis was hepatic abscess.

3.9.6 Discussion

The advantage of 18FDG PET/CT scan of hepatic lesion is safety, and it can comprehensively detect the lesions, accurately locate and judge the benign and malignant lesions, so it can detect the lesions early, quickly, accurately, and comprehensively.

3.10 HIV Infection

Miyako Morooka

Abstract To understand and interpret FDG PET imaging in HIV infection, some clinical data on infection status are useful, including the CD4+ T cell count, viral load, and management with or without highly active antiretroviral therapy (HAART). In this section, the author presents a representative image of immunovirological status before starting HAART, with a low CD4+ T cell count (<500 cells/μL) and high HIV viral load. FDG uptake is evident in the cervical, axillary, hilar, abdominal, and pelvic lymph nodes bilaterally. These findings reflect viral replication in the lymph nodes. Most importantly, the findings change after initiation of HAART.

Keywords: HIV, lymphadenopathy, CD4, viral load, highly active antiretroviral therapy (HAART)

3.10.1 Clinical Presentation

A 27-year-old man presented with cervical lymphadenopathy. He was HIV-positive and had a CD4+ T cell count of 234/μL and a viral load of 7.2 × 105 copies/mL. CT showed systemic lymphadenopathy, but no specific abnormal lesions in other areas.

3.10.2 Key Images

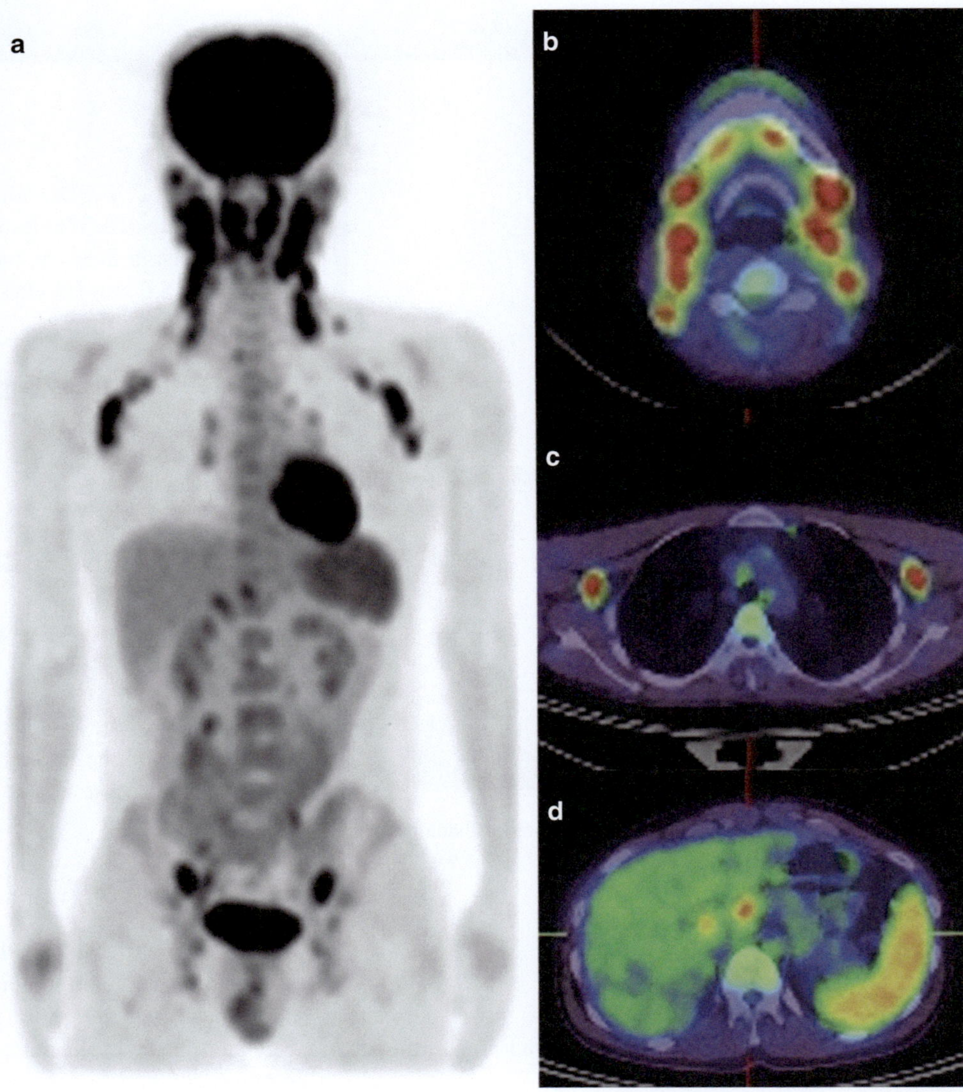

Fig. 3.22 The systemic lymphadenopathy with high FDG uptake. (**a**) A maximum intensity projection (MIP) image showing abnormal FDG uptake in the bilateral cervical, axially, hilar, abdominal, and pelvic lymph nodes. (**b**) An axial FDG PET/CT image showing increased FDG uptake in cervical lymph nodes bilaterally. (**c**) In axially lymph nodes bilaterally. (**d**) In the abdominal (portal) lymph node and diffuse increased uptake in the spleen

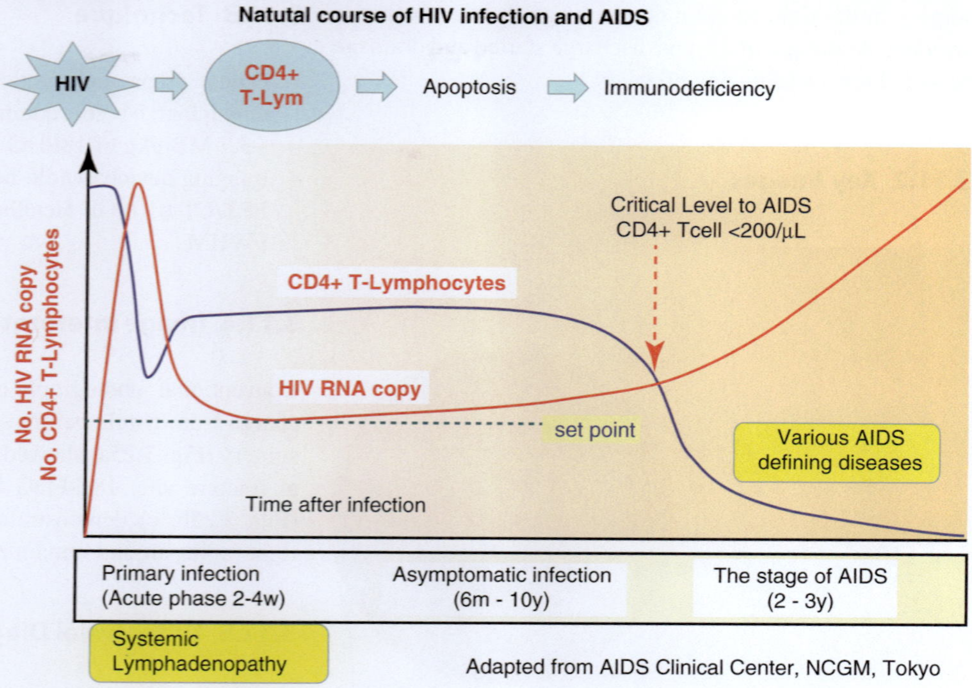

Fig. 3.23 The natural course of HIV infection and AIDS-related diseases

3.10.3 Technique

– Patient preparation: *Nil* per os for 5 h before administration of radiopharmaceutical.
– 250 MBq of 18FDG administered intravenously
– Imaging device: Whole-body PET/CT camera (Siemens Biograph) with resolution of 5.0 mm FWHM.

3.10.4 Image Interpretation

Figure 3.22 shows increased uptake in the cervical, axillary, hilar, abdominal, and pelvic lymph nodes bilaterally. Uptake in the spleen is also increased. These findings are typical of the immunovirological status before starting HAART, namely a lower CD4+ T cell count and a higher HIV RNA copy number.

3.10.5 Differential Diagnosis

– Lymphoma
– Tuberculosis

3.10.6 Diagnosis and Clinical Follow-Up

Figure 3.23 shows the natural course of HIV infection and AIDS-related diseases. Systemic lymphadenopathy is seen in the primary infection (acute phase, 2–4 weeks). The present patient had representative FDG images in this phase. After diagnosis, HAART therapy was started, and his viral load and lymphadenopathy subsequently decreased.

3.10.7 Discussion

The advantage of FDG whole-body PET/CT in HIV infection is the ability to detect and differentiate the immunovirological status associated with HIV infection from that of AIDS-related diseases [29–31]. Increased uptake is sometimes seen only in the lymph nodes of the upper torso, and never only in the lower torso [32].

3.11 Traumatic Osteomyelitis

Motoyuki Takaki

Abstract The post-traumatic osteomyelitis is one of the most severe complication of the fractures. The treatment can be difficult often because there is no method for detecting accurate location of the infection focus. Effectiveness of 18F-FDG PET/CT in detecting osteomyelitis has been reported recently. The present case explains the treatment strategies followed for a post-traumatic osteomyelitis of the right forearm. We decided the extent of surgical debridement following presurgical 18F-FDG PET/CT results. The present patient underwent surgical debridement with long-term antibiotic therapy. He has remained symptom-free at 3 years.

Keywords: FDG-PET/CT, Osteomyelitis, Post trauma

3.11.1 Clinical Presentation

A 75-year-old man presenting high fever and redness of his right forearm with pus discharge. He had undergone a surgery in the right forearm 60 years ago due to a worker's accident. At the age of 45, pus discharge started and drainage persisted for the following 30 years.

3.11.2 Key Images

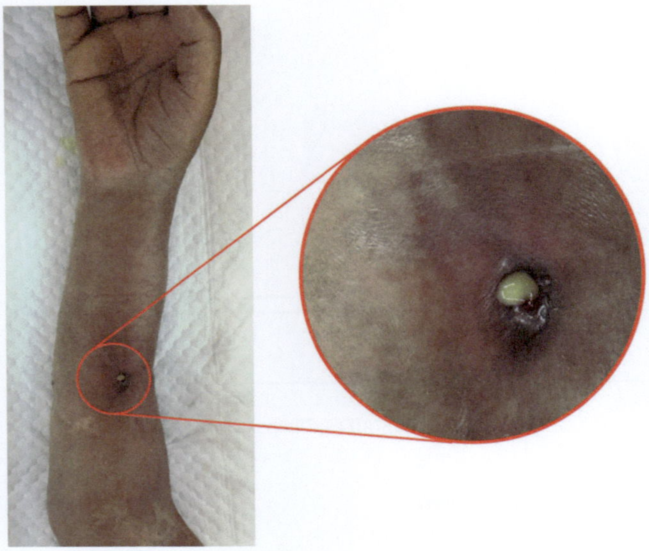

Fig. 3.24 Conventional photograph from the initial diagnosis. A fistula can be confirmed at the right forearm. The skin around the fistula showed redness and discharge

3.11.3 Technique

- Patient preparation: patient should not take anything by mouth for 6 h before administration of radiopharmaceutical.
- −3.7 MBq/kg of 18FDG administered intravenously.
- Imaging device: whole-body PET/CT camera (Discovery PET/CT 610; GE Healthcare) with resolution of 3.3 mm FWHM.

3.11.4 Image Interpretation

Conventional photograph of right forearm with pus discharge from fistula before surgery (Fig. 3.24). X-ray before surgery (Fig. 3.25a) showed remaining intramedullary sonde at fracture site. 18F-FDG PET/CT images before surgery (Fig. 3.25b, c) demonstrate increased tracer uptake in the right radius around remaining intramedullary sonde.

3.11.5 Differential Diagnosis

- Osteomyelitis of the right radius
- Subcutaneal abscess of the right forearm

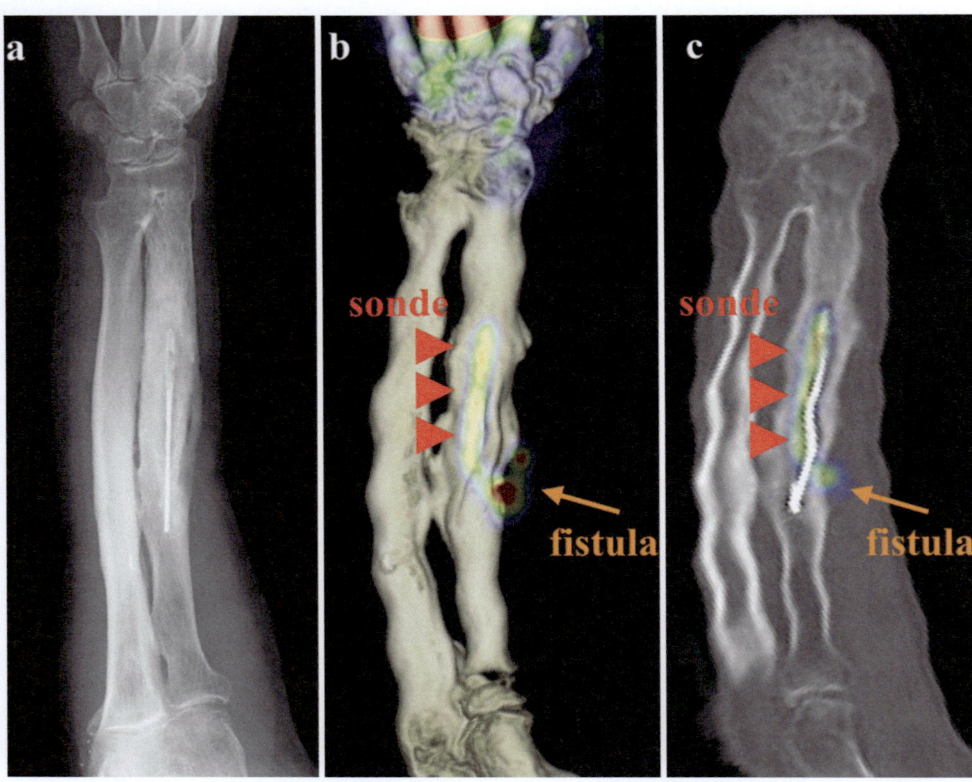

Fig. 3.25 (**a**) X-rays from the initial diagnosis showed osteosclerotic change around the intramedullary sonde. (**b**, **c**) FDG-PET/CT of the right forearm. A high degree of FDG accumulation was seen around the intramedullary sonde (red arrows) and the fistula (orange arrow)

3.11.6 Diagnosis and Clinical Follow-Ups

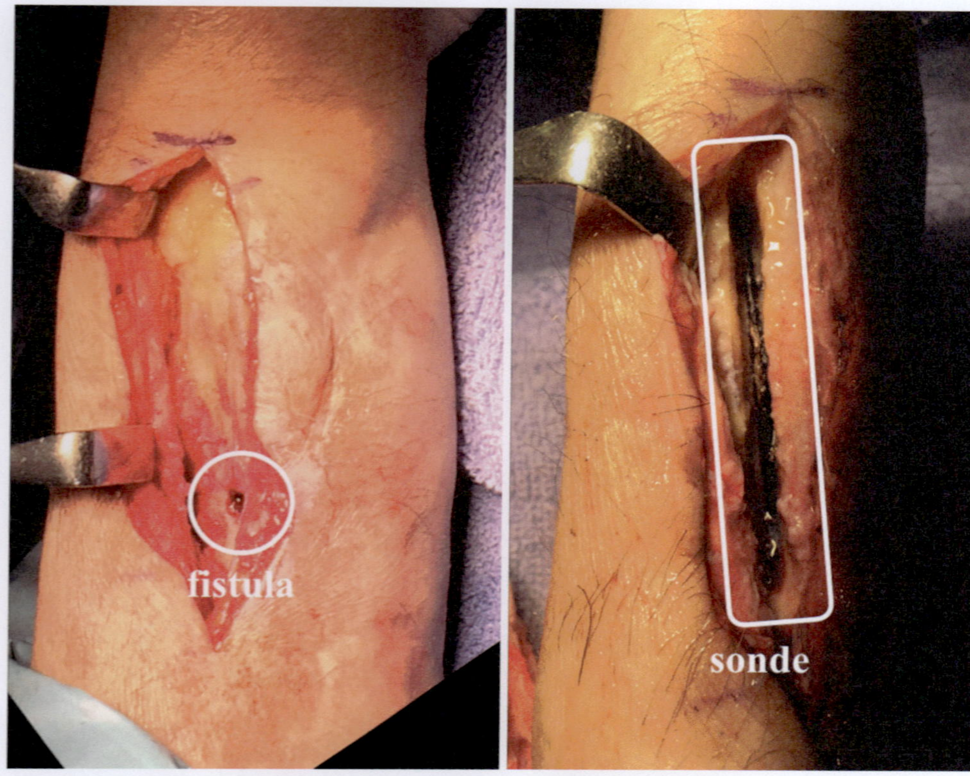

Fig. 3.26 Conventional photograph at surgery. There was fistula at the proximal third of the right radius. The sonde was seen through the entire length after cortical bone fenestration

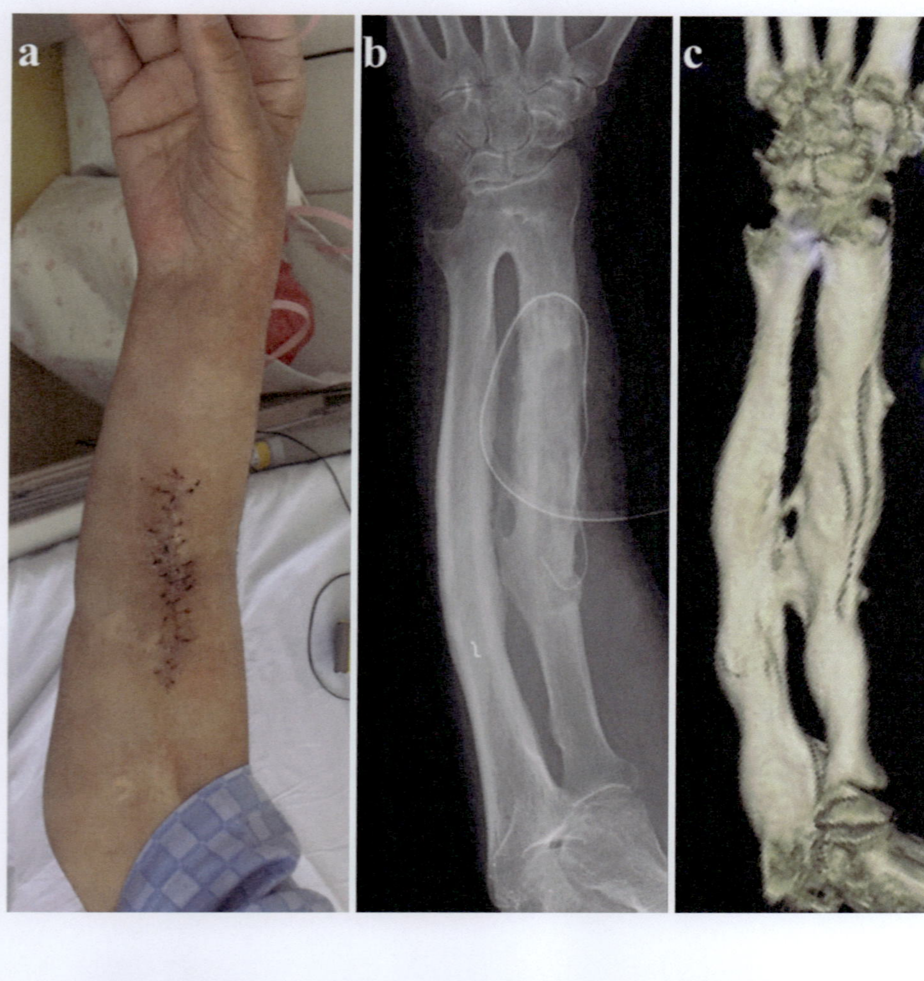

Fig. 3.27 (**a**) Conventional photograph after surgery. (**b**) Postoperative X-ray of the right forearm showing removal of the sonde. (**c**) FDG-PET/CT of the right forearm after surgery showing vanishing tracer uptake

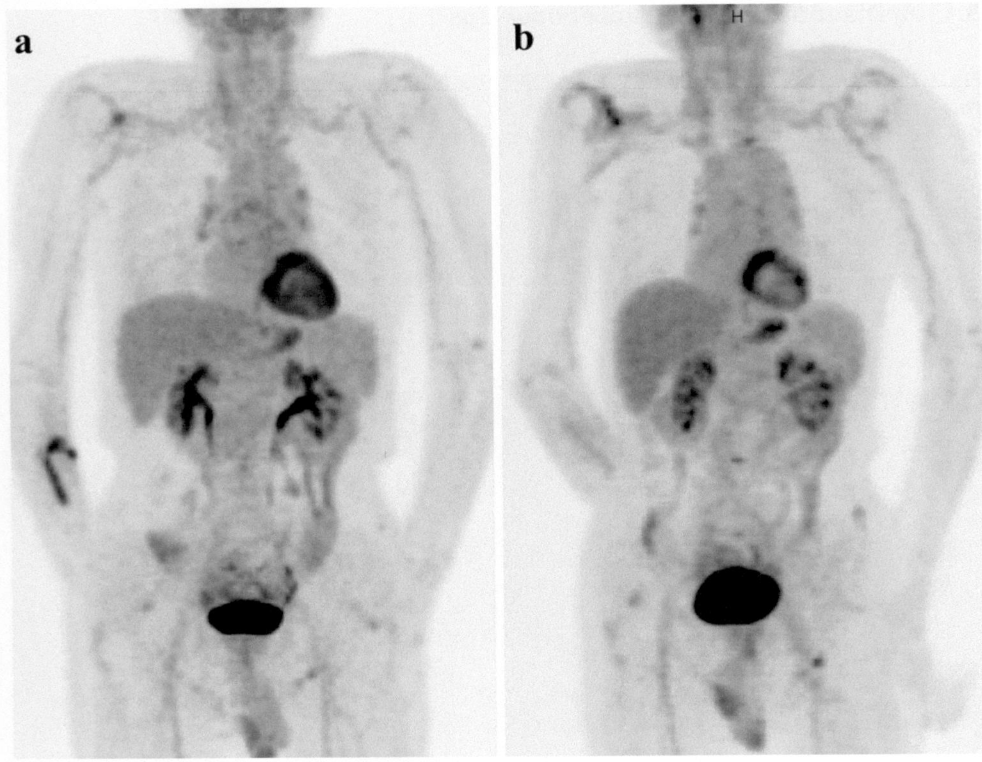

Fig. 3.28 FDG PET colonal MIP image before (**a**) and after (**b**) surgery showed successful treatment

The surgery was done to remove the remaining sonde (Fig. 3.26) and debridement. Cultures from the surgical specimen grew MRSA (methicillin-resistant *Staphylococcus aureus*). Histopathological examination showed formation of abscesses. Surgical wound was healed promptly (Fig. 3.27a), and 18F-FDG PET/CT images after surgery demonstrate vanishing tracer uptake (Fig. 3.27c). FDG PET colonal MIP image before (Fig. 3.28a) and after (Fig. 3.28b) surgery showed successful treatment.

3.11.7 Discussion

Treatment of osteomyelitis requires the through excision of the infection focus. But, there are currently no methods for accurately localizing the infection focus of osteomyelitis [33]. Effectiveness of 18F-FDG PET/CT in detecting osteomyelitis has been reported recently [34, 35]. 18F-FDG PET/CT scan is helpful for detecting the infecting lesion and deciding the extent of surgical resection and evaluating treatment effect.

3.12 Hepatic Cyst Infection in Polycystic Kidney Disease

Kentaro Inoue, Yoshinori Tsuchiya, and Nobuyuki Honma

Abstract Autosomal dominant polycystic kidney disease (ADPKD) is the most common hereditary kidney disease, characterized by multiple renal cysts leading to end-stage renal disease. Hepatic cysts are also common. Cyst infection is a common complication that frequently leads to hospitalization and often requires invasive treatment. Diagnosis of infection of cysts within multiple renal and hepatic cysts is often difficult with conventional radiologic modalities, such as ultrasonography, computed tomography (CT), magnetic resonance imaging (MRI), especially in patients with renal failure. This case illustrates that FDG-PET/CT can be helpful for the identification of infected cysts in patients with ADPKD.

Keywords: Autosomal dominant polycystic kidney disease, ADPKD, Cyst infection

3.12.1 Clinical Presentation

A 62-year-old woman with a medical history of ADPKD and hemodialysis had a prolonged hospitalization with a suspicion of cyst infection. Treatment with antibiotics did not improve her clinical condition. Conventional imaging studies failed to identify an infected cyst, so an FDG-PET/CT scan was ordered.

3.12.2 Key Images

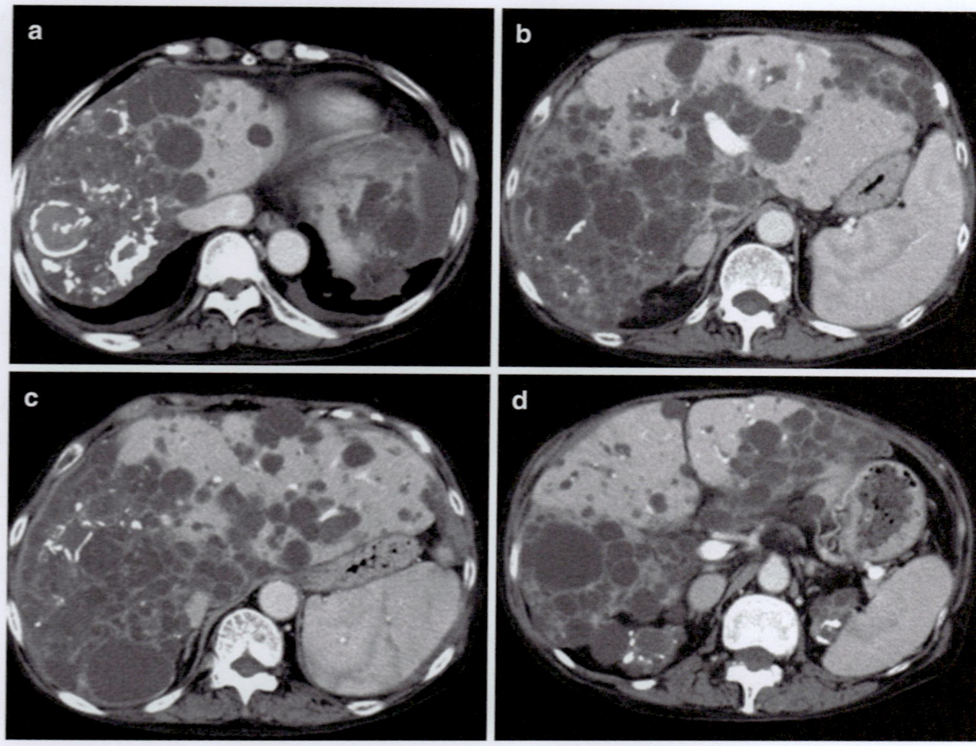

Fig. 3.29 Axial contrast-enhanced CT images show multiple liver cysts (**a–d**) and renal cysts (**d**) with wall calcification in some of them. Images (**a–d**) are nearly at the same levels of images Fig. 3.30a–d, respectively. Signs of infected cysts are not detectable

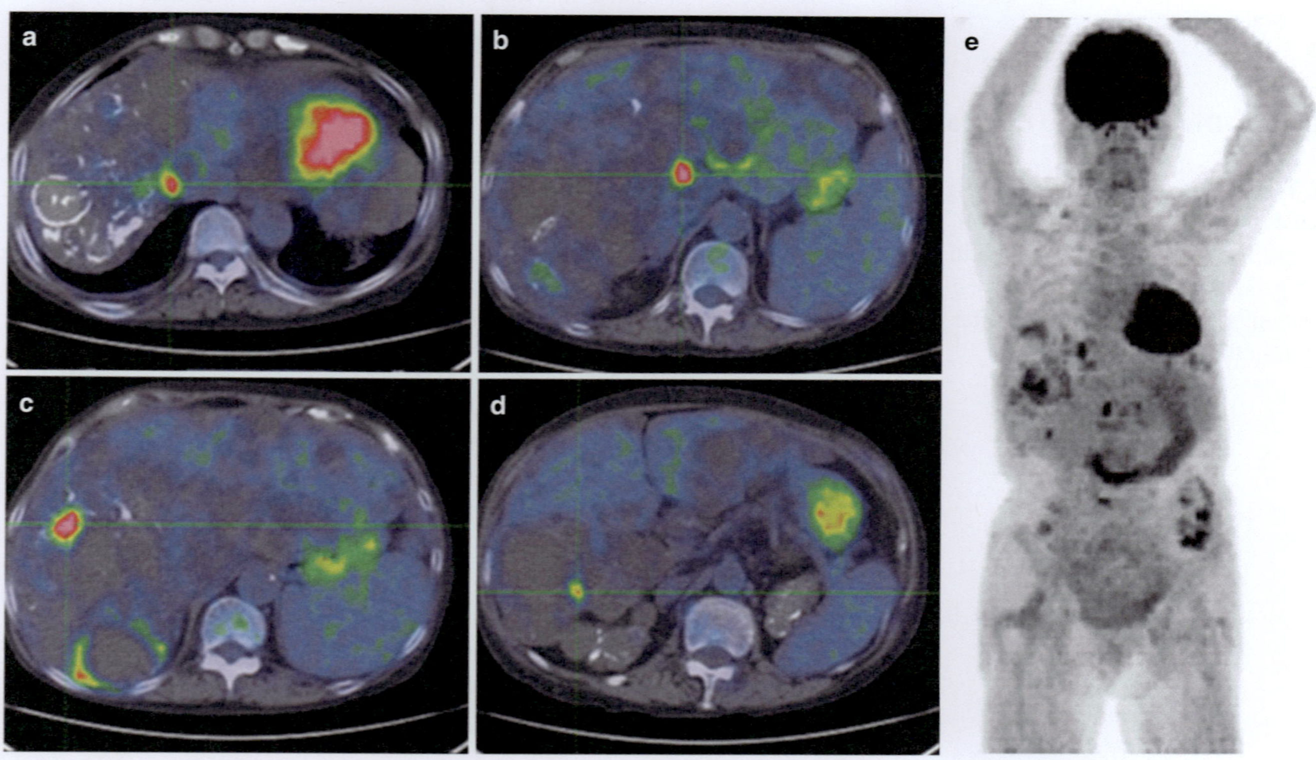

Fig. 3.30 Axial PET/CT images show multiple FDG-avid foci in the liver cysts (**a–d**). A maximum intensity projection image (**e**) shows no pathologic FDG uptakes except for those in the liver

3.12.3 Technique

- Patient preparation: the patient fasted for more than 6 h before FDG administration.
- 250 MBq of 18FDG administered intravenously.
- FDG PET/CT imaging performed at 90 min after FDG administration.
- Imaging device: whole-body PET/CT camera (Discovery STE (General Electrics)).
- Acquisition time: 3 min/1bed position.

3.12.4 Image Interpretation

Contrast-enhanced CT scans showed multiple liver cysts but otherwise unremarkable (Fig. 3.29). Axial fused FDG-PET/CT images (Fig. 3.30a–d) showed multiple pathologic FDG uptakes of the cyst wall in the liver, suggestive of hepatic cysts infection. No pathologic FDG-avid foci were detected elsewhere (Fig. 3.30e).

3.12.5 Differential Diagnosis

- Cyst infection
- Intracystic hemorrhage
- Malignancy

3.12.6 Diagnosis and Clinical Follow-Ups

CT-guided percutaneous drainage of possible infected cysts was performed based on the FDG-PET/CT findings. *Escherichia coli* was identified in cyst fluid from two (Fig. 3.30a, b) out of four drained cysts (Fig. 3.30a–d). The patient's condition improved after an appropriate change of antibiotic treatment.

3.12.7 Discussion

Cyst infection is a severe complication in patients with ADPKD. Identification of a renal or hepatic infected cyst is crucial to guide diagnostic and/or therapeutic percutaneous drainage [36, 37]. FDG-PET/CT is a powerful tool for diagnosing cyst infection compared to conventional imaging modalities [36–39], offering the ability to localize infected cysts.

3.13 Adrenal Histoplasmosis

Yuji Nakamoto

Abstract A 71-year-old woman complained of general malaise and body weight loss during her follow-up period for hypothyroidism. Abdominal ultrasound revealed bilateral adrenal masses. Subsequent enhanced CT showed heterogeneous masses in the bilateral adrenal glands. Thus, adrenal tumors, such as adrenal metastases or malignant lymphoma, were suspected. Although no tumor markers were elevated and the patient had no history of malignant disease, positron emission tomography (PET) with ^{18}F-fluorodeoxyglucose (FDG) was performed for whole-body screening. FDG-PET demonstrated a heterogeneous accumulation corresponding to the enlarged adrenal glands. An operation was performed and a final diagnosis of histoplasmosis was made.

Keywords: FDG, PET, Adrenal, Histoplasmosis

3.13.1 Clinical Presentation

A 71-year-old woman presented with general malaise and body weight loss during her follow-up period for hypothyroidism. Ultrasound and CT showed adrenal masses bilaterally. FDG-PET demonstrated heterogeneous accumulation corresponding to these masses.

3.13.2 Key Images

Fig. 3.31 Arterial phase (**a**) and equilibrium phase (**b**) of contrast-enhanced CT images, a maximum intensity projection image of FDG-PET (**c**), and a fused CT and PET image (**d**) are provided

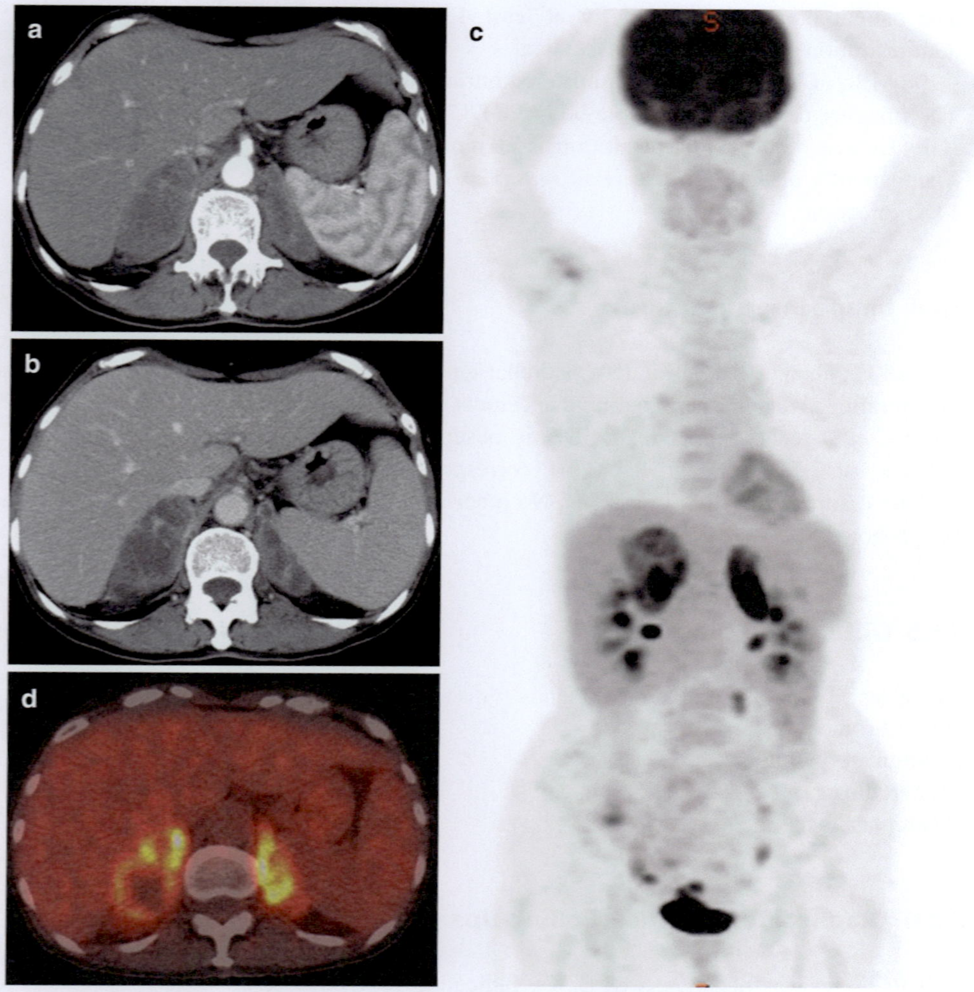

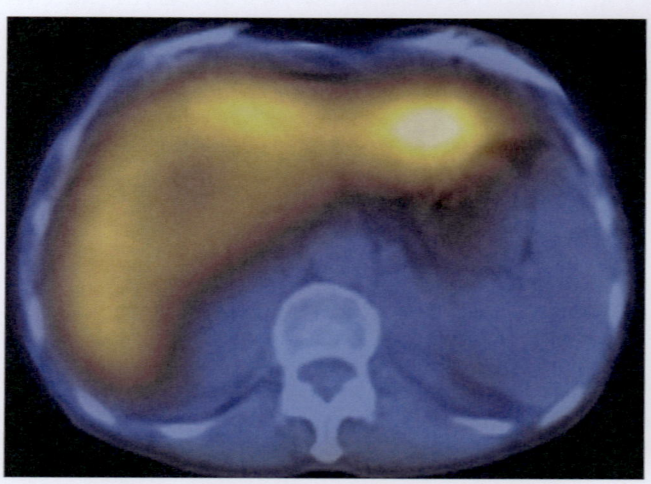

Fig. 3.32 A fused image between MIBG-SPECT and CT

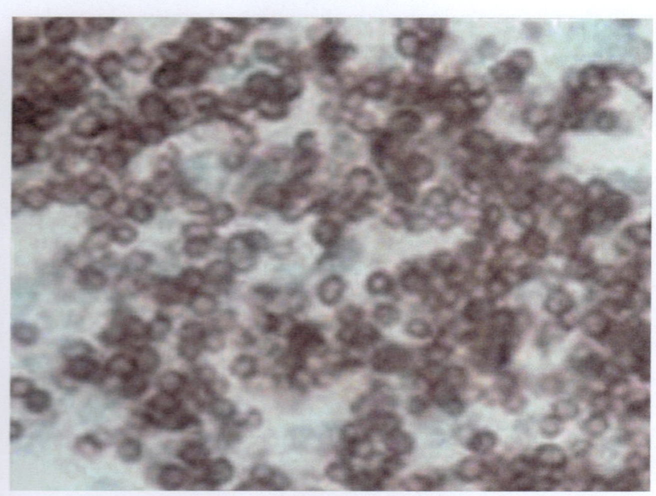

Fig. 3.33 Histopathology (Grocott staining) of resected specimen from the left adrenal gland is demonstrated

3.13.3 Technique

- The patient preparation fasted for at least 4 h before administration of the radiopharmaceutical.
- −208 MBq of 18F-FDG was administered intravenously.
- The imaging device was a whole-body PET/CT camera (GE Discovery STE) with a resolution of 5.0 mm FWHM.
- The patient's plasma glucose level was 120 mg/dL at FDG injection.

3.13.4 Image Interpretation

Enhanced CT images reveal bilateral- adrenal enlargement with central necrosis and peripheral enhancement. In FDG-PET/CT, heterogeneous uptake of FDG is observed with an SUV_{max} of 7.7 (right) and 8.4 (left), corresponding to the bilateral adrenal masses (Fig. 3.31). No other abnormal uptake is noted.

3.13.5 Differential Diagnosis

- Metastasis to the bilateral adrenal glands
- Pheochromocytoma
- Malignant lymphoma
- Tuberculosis
- Histoplasmosis

3.13.6 Diagnosis and Clinical Follow-Ups

^{123}I-MIBG scan was negative (Fig. 3.32), indicating pheochromocytoma less likely. Surgical resection was performed, with the histopathological confirmation of adrenal histoplasmosis (Fig. 3.33, Grocott staining). She was treated with antifungal drug, although her headache and general malaise persisted.

3.13.7 Discussion

Histoplasmosis is a systemic *fungal* infection caused by *Hisoplasma capsulatum*, mainly living in soil in North America (especially around the Ohio and Mississippi river valleys). Clinical manifestations are classified according to site (pulmonary or disseminated), duration (acute, subacute, or chronic), and pattern (primary or reactivation) of infection. FDG-PET is helpful for whole-body screening [40–44], but differentiation between a malignant tumor and active inflammation is difficult.

References

1. Assaf T, et al. Intraindividual comparison of preoperative 99mTc-MDP SPECT/CT and intraoperative and histopathological findings in patients with bisphosphonate- or denosumab-related osteonecrosis of the jaw. J Craniomaxillofac Surg. 2015;43(8):1461–9.
2. Fleisher KE, et al. Does fluorodeoxyglucose positron emission tomography with computed tomography facilitate treatment of medication-related osteonecrosis of the jaw? J Oral Maxillofac Surg. 2016;74(5):945–58.
3. Heye T, Stoijkovic M, Kauczor HU, Junghanss T, Hosch W. Extrapulmonary tuberculosis: radiological imaging of an almost forgotten transformation artist. Rofo. 2011;183(11):1019–29.
4. Ankrah AO, Glaudemans AWJM, et al. Tuberculosis. Seminars in nuclear medicine. Semin Nucl Med. 2018;48:108–30.
5. Martinez V, Castilla-Lievre MA, Guillet-Caruba C, et al. (18) F-FDG PET/CT in tuberculosis: an early non-invasive marker of therapeutic response. Int J Tuberc Lung Dis. 2012;16(9):1180–5.
6. Vorster M, Sathekge MM, Bomanji J. Advances in imaging of tuberculosis: the role of 18F-FDG PET and PET/CT. Curr Opin Pulm Med. 2014;20(3):287–93.
7. Ito K, et al. Imaging spectrum and pitfalls of ^{18}F-fluorodeoxyglucose positron emission tomography/computed tomography in patients with tuberculosis. Jpn J Radiol. 2013;31(8):511–20.
8. Testempassi E, et al. Constrictive tuberculous pericarditis diagnosed using 18F-fluorodeoxyglucose positron emission tomography: a report of two cases. Ann Nucl Med. 2010;24(5):421–5.
9. Global Tuberculosis Report World Health Organization, Geneva; 2018.
10. Zumla A, et al. Tuberculosis. N Engl J Med. 2013;368:745–55.
11. Douglas AP, Thursky KA, Worth LJ, Drummond E, Hogg A, Hicks RJ, Slavin MA. FDG PET/CT imaging in detecting and guiding management of invasive fungal infections: a retrospective comparison to conventional CT imaging. Eur J Nucl Med Mol Imaging. 2019;46(1):166–73.
12. Seban RD, Bonardel G, Guernou M, Lussato D, Queneau M. The use of FDG PET-CT imaging for the assessment of early antifungal treatment response in disseminated fusariosis. Clin Nucl Med. 2017;42(7):569–70.
13. Ankrah AO, Klein HC, Span LFR, de Vries EFJ, Dierckx RAJO, Sathekge MM, Glaudemans AWJM. The role of PET in monitoring therapy in fungal infections. Curr Pharm Des. 2018;24(7):795–805.
14. Leroy-Freschini B, Treglia G, Argemi X, Bund C, Kessler R, Herbrecht R, Imperiale A. 18F-FDG PET/CT for invasive fungal infection in immunocompromised patients. QJM. 2018;111(9):613–22.
15. Hohmann C, Michels G, Schmidt M, et al. Diagnostic challenges in infective endocarditis: is PET/CT the solution? Infection. 2019;47(4):579–87.
16. Chen W, Dilsizian V. FDG PET/CT for the diagnosis and management of infective endocarditis: expert consensus vs evidence-based practice. J Nucl Cardiol. 2019;26(1):313–5.
17. Mahmood M, Kendi AT, Ajmal S, et al. Meta-analysis of 18F-FDG PET/CT in the diagnosis of infective endocarditis. J Nucl Cardiol. 2019;26(3):922–35.
18. Pizzi MN, Roque A, Fernández-Hidalgo N, et al. Improving the diagnosis of infective endocarditis in prosthetic valves and intracardiac devices with 18F-fluordeoxyglucose positron emission tomography/computed tomography angiography. Circulation. 2015;132(12):1113–26.
19. Kouijzer IJE, Berrevoets MAH, Aarntzen EHJG, et al. 18F-fluorodeoxyglucose positron-emission tomography combined with computed tomography as a diagnostic tool in native valve endocarditis. Nucl Med Commun. 2018;39(8):747–52.

20. Smids C, Kouijzer IJ, Vos FJA, et al. Comparison of the diagnostic value of MRI and 18F-FDG-PET/CT in suspected spondylodiscitis. Infection. 2017;45(1):41–9.
21. Ioannou S, Chatziioannou S, Pneumaticos SG, Zormpala A, Sipsas NV. Fluorine-18 fluoro-2-deoxy-D-glucose positron emission tomography/computed tomography scan contributes to the diagnosis and management of brucellar spondylodiskitis. BMC Infect Dis. 2013;13:73.
22. Zhang T, Wang C, Niu R, Wang X. Pulmonary brucellosis on FDG PET/CT. Clin Nucl Med. 2014;39(2):222–3.
23. Alduraibi AK, Naddaf S, Alzayed MF. FDG PET/CT of spinal brucellosis. Clin Nucl Med. 2019;44(6):465–6.
24. Wang HH, Lin WR. Amebic liver abscess. N Engl J Med. 2018;379(23):2255.
25. Cavailloles FA, Mure A, Nasser H, et al. Multiple liver amoebic abscesses detected on FDG PET/CT. Clin Nucl Med. 2014;39:79–80.
26. Zhou W, Zhao J, Xing Y, et al. Diffuse hepatic amebiasis detected by FDG PET/CT. Clin Nucl Med. 2015;40:e167–70.
27. Yapar AF, Reyhan M, Canpolat ET. Interesting image. Ameboma mimicking lung cancer on FDG PET/CT. Clin Nucl Med. 2010;35:55–6.
28. Dong A, Wang Y, Zuo C, Zhu HFDGPET. CT findings in multiple splenic amebomas (amebic granulomas). Clin Nucl Med. 2016;41(5):379–81.
29. Scharko A, et al. Whole-body positron emission tomography in patients with HIV-1 infection. Lancet. 2003;20:959–61.
30. Sathekge M, et al. FDG-PET imaging in HIV infection and tuberculosis. Semin Nucl Med. 2013;43:349–66.
31. Scharko AM, et al. Whole-body positron emission tomography imaging of simian immunodeficiency virus-infected rhesus macaques. Proc Natl Acad Sci U S A. 1996;93(13):6425–30.
32. Lucignani G, et al. FDG-PET imaging in HIV-infected subjects: relation with therapy and immunovirological variables. Eur J Nucl Med Mol Imaging. 2009;36:640–7.
33. Lew DP, et al. Osteomyelitis. Lancet. 2004;364(9431):369–79.
34. van der Bruggen W, et al. PET and SPECT in osteromyelitis and prosthetic bone and joint infections: a systematic review. Semin Nucl Med. 2010;40(1):3–15.
35. Lemans JVC, et al. The diagnostic accuracy of 18F-FDG PET/CT in diagnosing fracture-related infections. Eur J Nucl Med Mol Imaging. 2018;46:999–1008. https://doi.org/10.1007/s00259-018-4218-6.
36. Sallée M, et al. Cyst infections in patients with autosomal dominant polycystic kidney disease. Clin J Am Soc Nephrol. 2009;4:1183–9.
37. Lantiga MA, et al. Diagnostic criteria in renal and hepatic cyst infection. Nephrol Dial Transplant. 2015;30:744–51.
38. Bleeker-Rovers CP, et al. Diagnosis of renal and hepatic cyst infections by 18-F-fluorodeoxyglucose positron emission tomography in autosomal dominant polycystic kidney disease. Am J Kidney Dis. 2003;41:E18–21.
39. Pijl JP, et al. FDG-PET/CT in autosomal dominant polycystic kidney disease patients with suspected cyst infection. J Nucl Med. 2018;59:1734–41.
40. Umeoka S, et al. High 18F-fluorodeoxyglocose uptake in adrenal histoplasmosis: a case report. Eur Radiol. 2005;15(12):2483–6.
41. Narang V, et al. Clinically inapparent bilateral adrenal masses due to histoplasmosis. Eur Urol. 2009;55(2):518–21.
42. Tsai YJ, et al. 18F-fluorodeoxyglucose positron emission tomography for the initial evaluation and monitoring of therapeutic response in bilateral adrenal histoplasmosis. Clin Imaging. 2013;37(4):791–3.
43. Shah SA, et al. [18F]Fluorodeoxyglucose-avid adrenal masses due to histoplasmosis. J Clin Oncol. 2009;27(5):827–8.
44. Kalathoorakath RR, et al. (18)F-FDG PET/CT imaging and PET-guided biopsy in evaluation and treatment decision in adrenal histoplasmosis. BJR Case Rep. 2016;2(3):20150451.

Suggested Readings

Igbinedion S, Mavuram MS, Boktor M, Bienvenu J. Pyogenic liver abscess caused by methicillin-susceptible Staphylococcus aureus in a 21-year-old male. Case Reports Hepatol. 2018; https://doi.org/10.1155/2018/9868701. E Collection 2018

Jolobe OMP. The special case of the left lobe amoebic liver abscess. QJM. 2019;112(1):67–8.

Hematological Diseases Mimic Inflammation

4

Hiroshi Toyama, Chao Cheng, Jun Zhou, Hongcheng Shi, Jingping Zhang, Xinzhong Hao, Zhifang Wu, and Sijin Li

4.1 Malignant Lymphoma

Chao Cheng

Abstract Lymphoma is a malignant tumor originated from the lymphatic hematopoietic system. It is mainly manifested as painless lymph node enlargement, hepatosplenomegaly, the involvement of all tissues and organs of the body, accompanied by fever, night sweat, weight loss, itching, and other systemic symptoms. The tumor cells are classified into non-Hodgkin's lymphoma (NHL) and Hodgkin's lymphoma (HL). The incidence of NHL is much higher than that of HL, which is the sum of a group of independent diseases with strong heterogeneity. Pathologically, it is mainly lymphocytes, tissue cells, or reticular cells with different degrees of differentiation. Depending on the origin of the lymphocytes, they can be classified as B-cell, T-cell, and NK-cell lymphomas.

Keywords: Lymphoma, FDG, PET/CT

4.1.1 Clinical Presentation

4.1.1.1 Case One

A 58-year-old woman known with Intermittent fever for more than 1 month without obvious incentives, with multiple lymph node enlargement for 1 month. Blood routine examination suggested decreased blood routine of the third line. Laboratory examination found: WBC, 4.97×10^9/L, RBC, 1.61×10^{12}/L, PLT, 37×10^9/L. The levels of tumor markers were normal.

4.1.1.2 Case Two

A 75-year-old woman known with recurrent fever with mild distension pain in the lower abdomen for 2 months. Laboratory examination found: WBC, 16.64×10^9/L; RBC, 2.97×10^{12}/L, CEA (−), CA199(−), CRP, 11.61 ng/mL.

H. Toyama (✉)
Department of Radiology, Fujita Health University, Toyoake, Aichi, Japan
e-mail: htoyama@fujita-hu.ac.jp

C. Cheng
Shanghai Changhai Hospital, Shanghai, China
e-mail: chao_cheng_1999@163.com

J. Zhou
Department of Nuclear Medicine, Xuhui District Central Hospital of Shanghai, Shanghai, China

Department of Nuclear Medicine, Zhongshan Hospital, Fudan University, Shanghai, China
e-mail: dr_zhoujun@163.com

H. Shi
Department of Nuclear Medicine, Zhongshan Hospital, Fudan University, Shanghai, China
e-mail: shi.hongcheng@zs-hospital.sh.cn

J. Zhang
The First Hospital of China Medical University, Shenyang, China
e-mail: zjp809302@163.com

X. Hao · Z. Wu · S. Li
The First Hospital of Shanxi Medical University, Shanxi, China
e-mail: history139@163.com; wuzhifang01@163.com; lisjnm123@163.com

H. Toyama et al. (eds.), *PET/CT for Inflammatory Diseases*, https://doi.org/10.1007/978-981-15-0810-3_4

4.1.2 Key Images

4.1.2.1 Case One

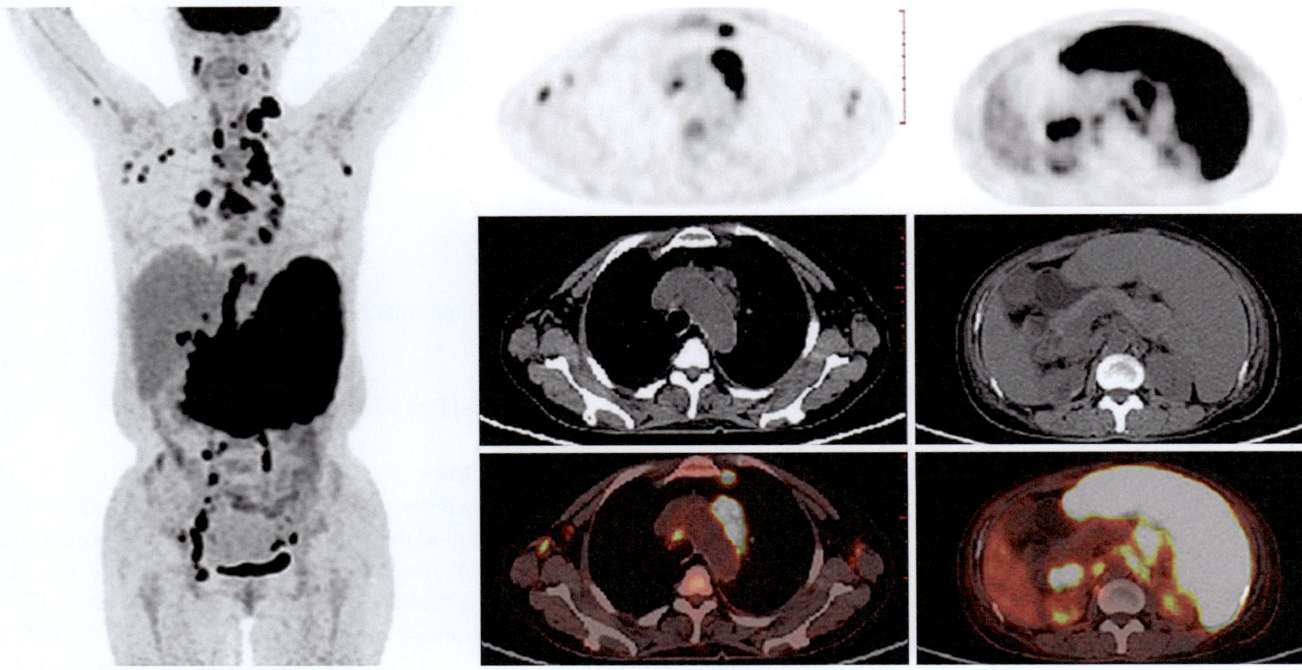

Fig. 4.1 Left parapharyngeal space, bilateral neck, and cervical root, mediastinum and bilateral hilum of the lung, bilateral pelvic wall and right inguinal multiple lymph node enlargements with FDG concentration, left cervical root lymph node (SUV_{max} = 20.6); Splenomegaly with diffuse FDG concentration (SUV_{max} = 20.3)

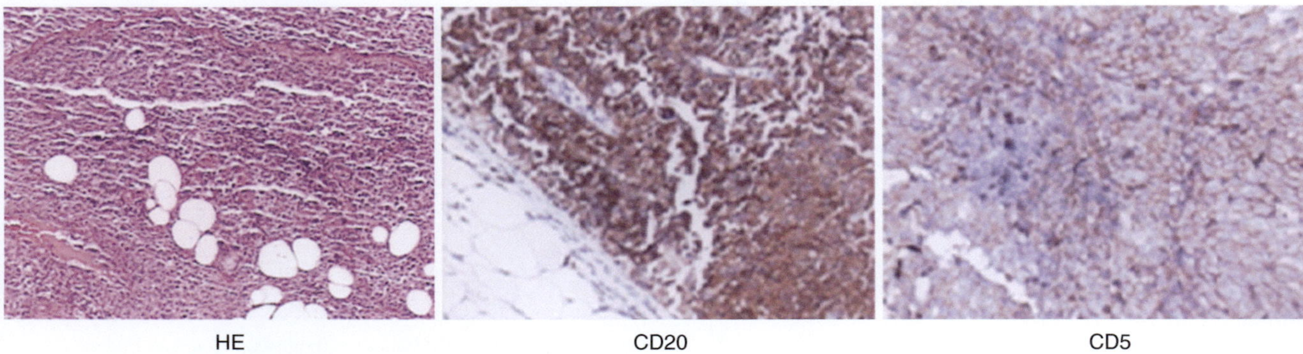

Fig. 4.2 The pathological results suggested that the nucleus is enlarged and deeply stained, and the abnormal morphology is obvious. Immunohistochemical results showed CD20 and CD5 positive

4.1.2.2 Case Two

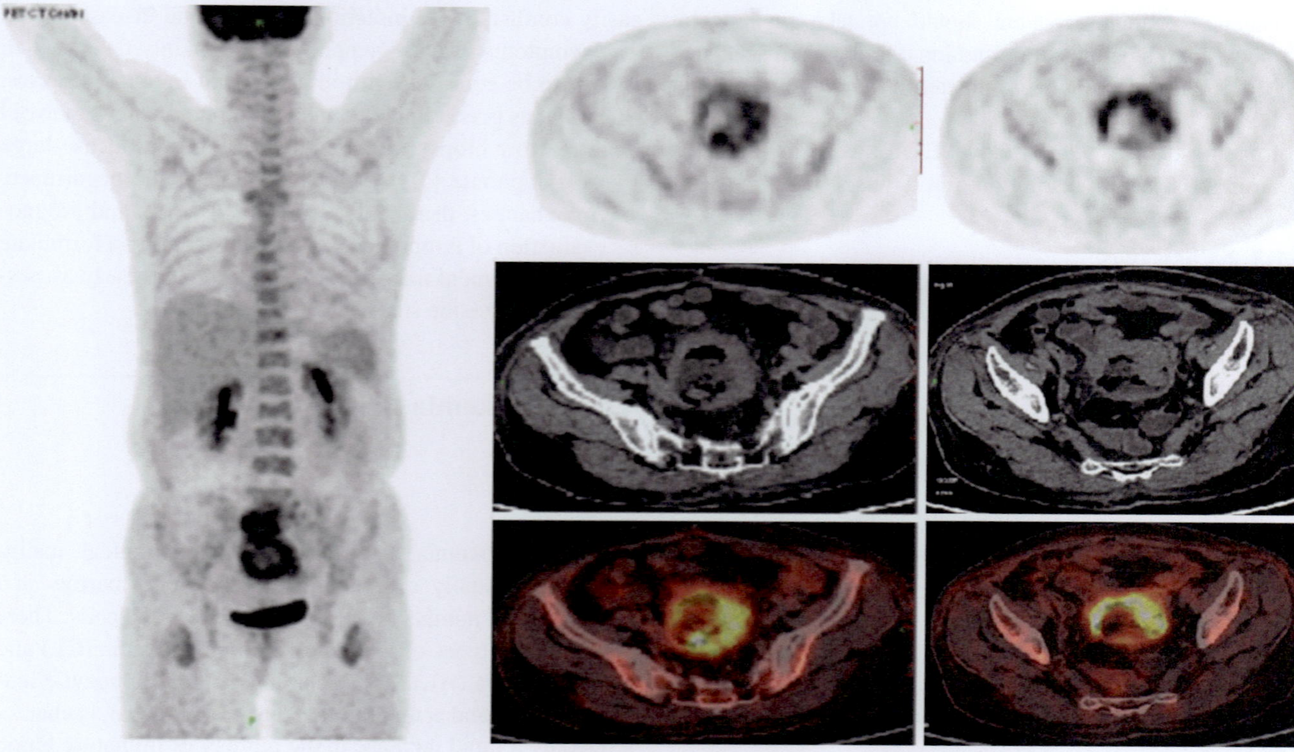

Fig. 4.3 In the pelvic cavity, thickening of the wall of the small intestine was observed, and lumen dilation was accompanied by increased FDG uptake (SUV_{max} = 7.7)

Fig. 4.4 Multiple lymph nodes were observed around the lesion intestine, with a mild increase of FDG metabolism. The immunohistochemical results showed LAT and TIA-1 positive

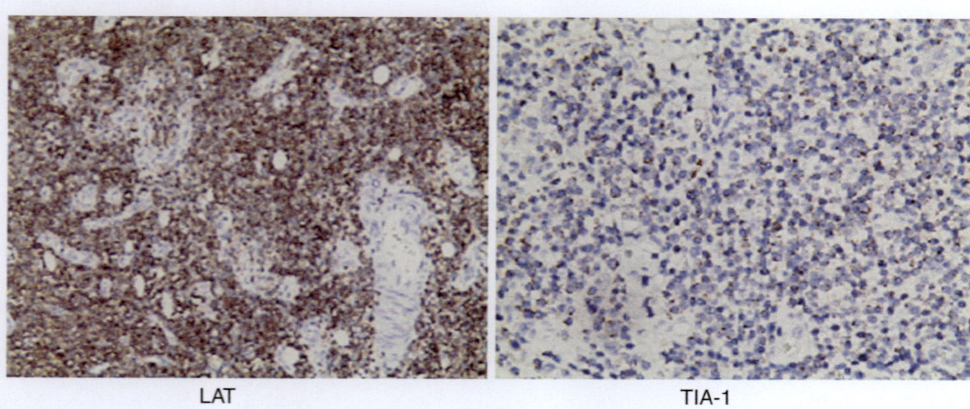

4.1.3 Technique

4.1.3.1 Case One

- Patient preparation: patient should not take anything by mouth for 6 h before administration of radiopharmaceutical.
- 314.5 MBq of 18FDG administered intravenously (body weight = 48 kg).
- Imaging device: whole-body PET/CT camera (Siemens biograph 64) with resolution of 4.0 mm FWHM.

4.1.3.2 Case Two

- Patient preparation: patient should not take anything by mouth for 6 h before administration of radiopharmaceutical.
- 248 MBq of 18FDG administered intravenously (body weight = 45 kg).
- Imaging device: whole-body PET/CT camera (Siemens biograph 64) with resolution of 4.0 mm FWHM.

4.1.4 Differential Diagnosis

4.1.4.1 Case One

- Tuberculous lymphadenitis
- Necrotizing lymphadenitis
- Sarcoidosis

4.1.4.2 Case Two

- Intestinal cancer
- Intestinal tuberculosis

4.1.5 Diagnosis and Clinical Follow-Ups

4.1.5.1 Case One

The middle-aged female presented with fever without obvious inducement, accompanied by painless progressive superficial lymphadenopathy. Biopsy report: (right cervical lymph node) peripheral B-cell lymphoma tends to be a diffuse large CD5-positive B-cell lymphoma (Fig. 4.2).

4.1.5.2 Case Two

The old-age female presented with fever without obvious inducement, accompanied by painless progressive superficial lymphadenopathy. Biopsy report: (ileal) peripheral T-cell lymphoma, which predisposes to enteropathic T-cell lymphoma (Fig. 4.4).

4.1.6 Discussion

Most lymphoma, led by fever in dispute, clinical symptoms, easily confused with infection, autoimmune disease [1, 2]. The symptoms of most lymphomas are mainly fever, which is easy to be confused with infection and immune diseases. PET/CT has good clinical value in lymphoma and can avoid bone marrow biopsy in patients with HL and diffuse large B-cell lymphoma [3, 4]. Early warning of the occurrence, staging changes, therapeutic effect, recurrence, and prognosis evaluation of lymphoma, so that physicians can formulate or adjust treatment measures for lymphoma as early as possible to improve the survival of patients [5].

4.2 Leukemia 1

Chao Cheng

Abstract Leukemia is a common hematological malignancy that usually originates from the bone marrow and results in high numbers of abnormal white blood cells. There are two main types of leukemia, chronic leukemia (CL) and acute leukemia (AL). AL, including acute lymphocytic leukemia (ALL) and acute myeloid leukemia (AML), is characterized by a rapid increase in the number of immature blood cells. Due to improvements in treatment, more AL patients now can have a longer life. As a result, it has been reported that the incidence of extramedullary relapse is increasing, especially in the patients that have received HSCT. F18-FDG PET/CT has become a very important tool in the diagnosis and staging of hematological malignancies, especially of aggressive lymphoma. Some articles, mainly case reports, have suggested that 18F FDG PET/CT is useful for detecting extramedullary AL and guiding biopsies.

Keywords: Leukemia, FDG, PET/CT

4.2.1 Clinical Presentation

A 31-year-old man known with high fever (T_{max} of 39 °C) and cold for 1 month. Chest X-ray film was diagnosed as pneumonia, CT scan prompted inflammation of the right lower lobe. Laboratory examination found: WBC, 33.33 × 10^9/L; RBC, 2.48 × 10^{12}/L; PLT, 129 × 10^9/L; HGB, 80.2 g/L; CRP, 9.82 mg/L. Physical examination revealed lymph node enlargement in the left neck.

4.2.2 Key Images

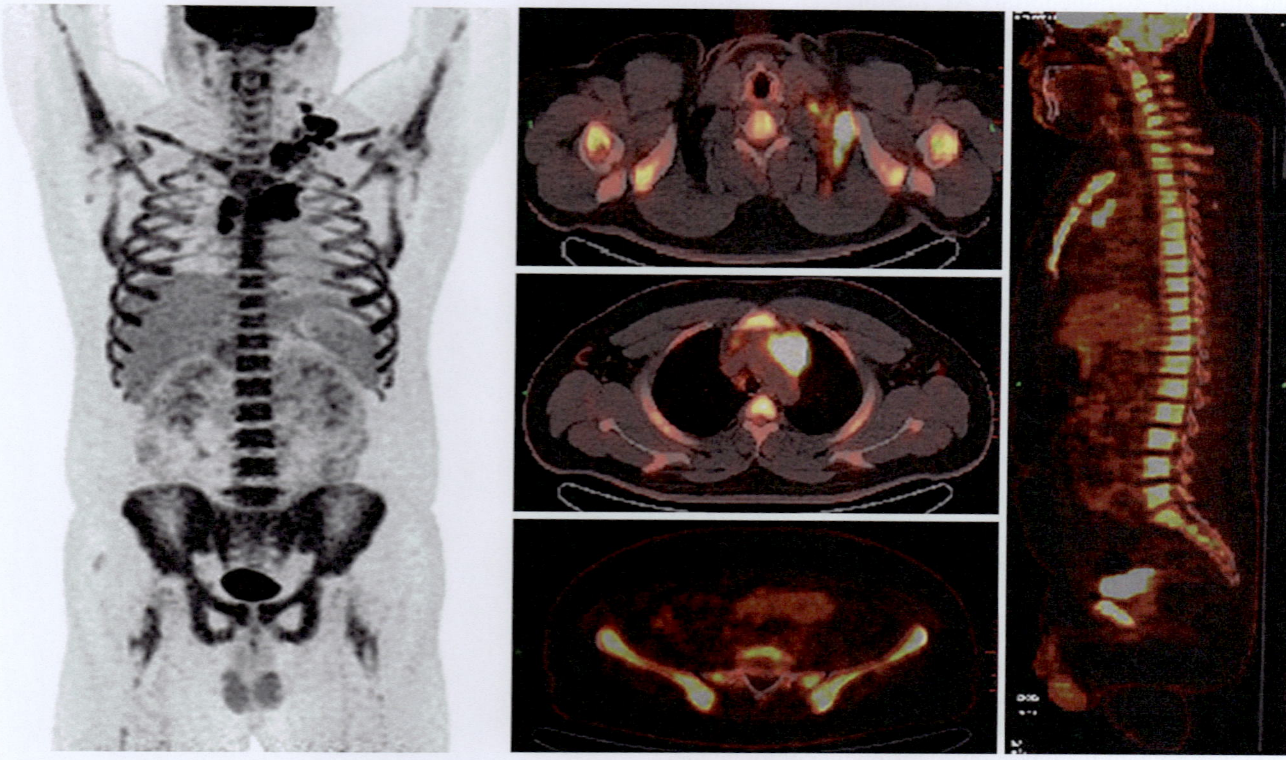

Fig. 4.5 Demonstrate multiple lymph node enlargement and abnormal increase of FDG uptake (SUV_{max} = 14.9). Systemic skull with high FDG metabolism (SUV_{max} = 9.5)

4.2.3 Technique

- Patient preparation: patient should not take anything by mouth for 6 h before administration of radiopharmaceutical.
- 518 MBq of 18FDG administered intravenously (body weight = 115 kg).
- Imaging device: whole-body PET/CT camera (Siemens biograph 64) with resolution of 4.0 mm FWHM.

4.2.4 Differential Diagnosis

- Lymphoma
- Infection
- Myelodysplastic syndrome
- Adult onset still's disease

4.2.5 Diagnosis and Clinical Follow-Ups

The result of this patient's bone marrow biopsy suggested acute leukemia. The patient received chemotherapy (dexamethasone) and transferred to other hospitals for further treatment.

4.2.6 Discussion

Extramedullary AL is when lesions occur at an anatomical site other than the bone marrow [6]. Identification of extramedullary involvement, especially recurrent extramedullary AL, has a major impact on treatment because some extramedullary lesions cannot be effectively treated by standard chemotherapy and require more intensive chemotherapy or allogeneic hematopoietic stem cell transplantation (HSCT). The data indicated that although extramedullary AL predominately involves certain sites such as the spleen, soft tissue, lymph nodes, and CNS, as reported in other studies, it can potentially occur at numerous sites in the body. With its ability to scan the whole body and high sensitivity, the present study demonstrated that 18F FDG PET/CT might be a useful imaging modality for patients with suspected extramedullary AL [7–9].

4.3 Leukemia 2

Jun Zhou and Hongcheng Shi

Abstract Acute myeloid leukemia (AML) with granulocytic maturation (M2) is one subtype of AML, which is a common life-threatening malignancy that originates from bone marrow. Here we presented a 69-year-old man diagnosed as AML-M2 with widespread chest and abdomen involvement (e.g., myeloid sarcoma of the duodenum) on the baseline PET/CT scan. After three cycles of chemotherapy, the patient's clinical manifestations disappeared, and the dominant lesions showed excellent complete metabolic response and good complete or partial morphologic remissions on the follow-up PET/CT scan.

Keywords: PET/CT, Acute myeloid leukemia, Myeloid sarcoma

4.3.1 Clinical Presentation

A 69-year-old man presenting with abdominal distension and discomfort, aggravation after each meal, and over 3 kg of weight loss around 1 month. As the disease progresses, the patient began to experience yellowed skin and sclera and could only eat liquid foods.

4.3.2 Key Images

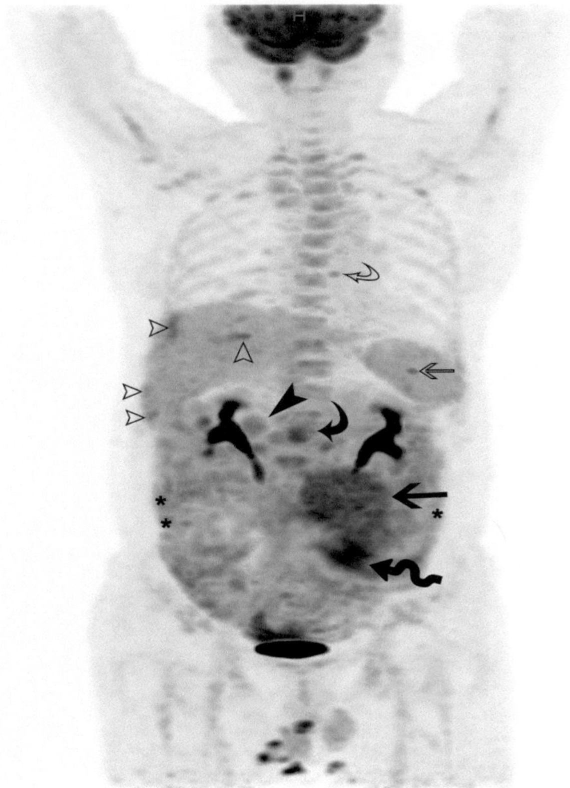

Fig. 4.6 Acute myeloid leukemia (AML) with granulocytic maturation (M2) with extramedullary presentations. The maximum intensity projection (MIP) image of the baseline PET scan demonstrates marked accumulation of 18FDG in the descending part of the duodenum (myeloid sarcoma; SUV_{max} 6.7; solid arrowhead), localized walls of the small intestine (the left middle abdomen: SUV_{max} 11.4; solid wave arrow), mesenteries (the left middle abdomen: SUV_{max} 9.1; solid arrow; the middle abdomen: solid curved arrow), greater omentum (asterisk), peritoneum (the perihepatic area: open arrowhead), rectovesical pouch, the left anterior intercostal region between the sixth and seventh ribs (open arrow), multiple lymphadenopathies in the retroperitoneal cavity, the right pleura, the area of the bilateral internal mammary arteries (the left side: open curved arrow), and the bilateral supraphrenic regions, and diffuse increased accumulation of 18FDG in the thoracic and lumbar vertebrae, the proximal ends of the bilateral humeri, multiple bilateral ribs and thoracic and lumbar vertebrae, and pelvis (AML). Note: urine contamination of 18FDG in the perineal region

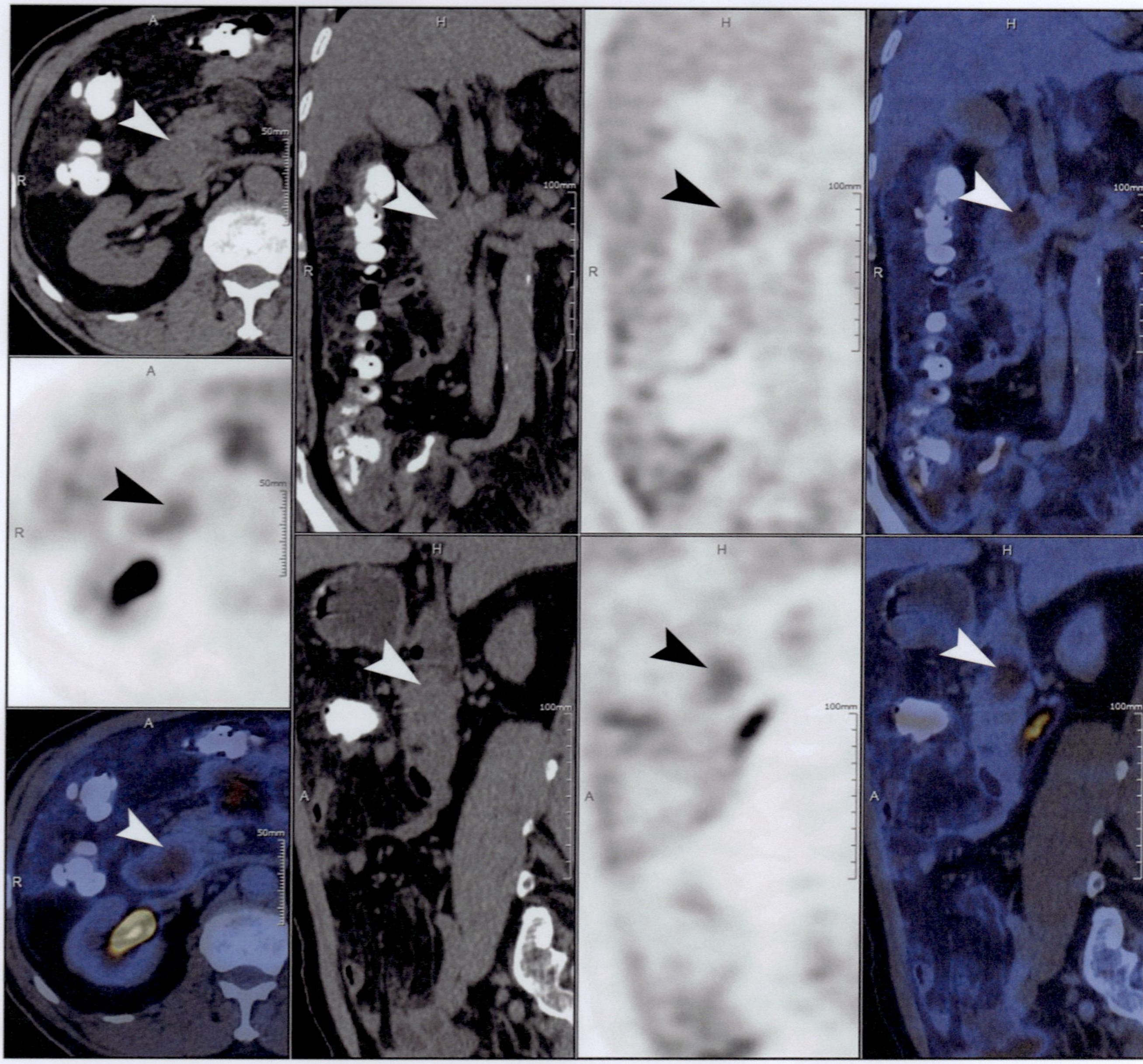

Fig. 4.7 Myeloid sarcoma of the descending part of the duodenum. The PET/CT images demonstrate a 34.4 × 26.4-mm soft-tissue mass with intense accumulation of 18FDG (myeloid sarcoma; SUV_{max} 6.7) within the lumen of the descending part of the duodenum (solid arrowhead)

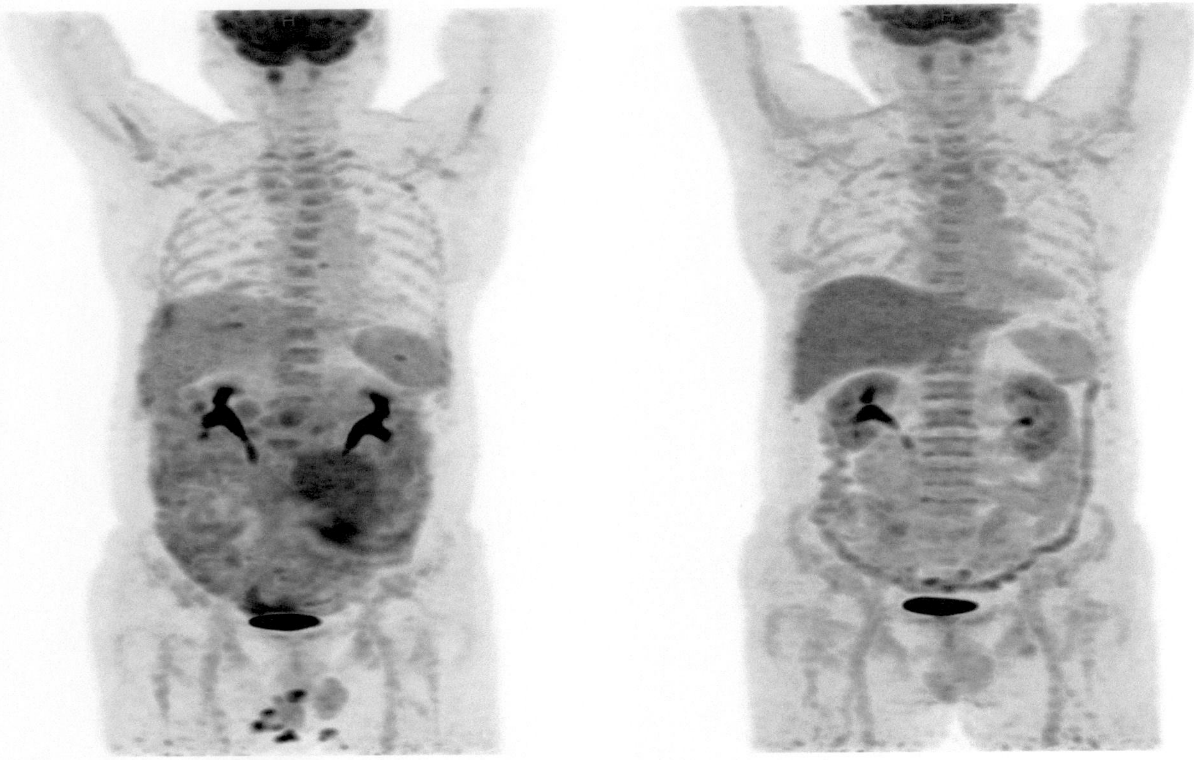

Fig. 4.8 Rapid response to three cycles of chemotherapy in the patient with AML-M2 and its extramedullary involvements. One and a half months after the third cycle of chemotherapy, the patient underwent a follow-up PET/CT scan. Compared with the baseline PET scan, the maximum intensity projection (MIP) image of the follow-up PET/CT scan shows complete metabolic response. The follow-up PET/CT scan also reveals disappearance of most of the lesions, and significant decrease in size and number of the rest lesions (not shown)

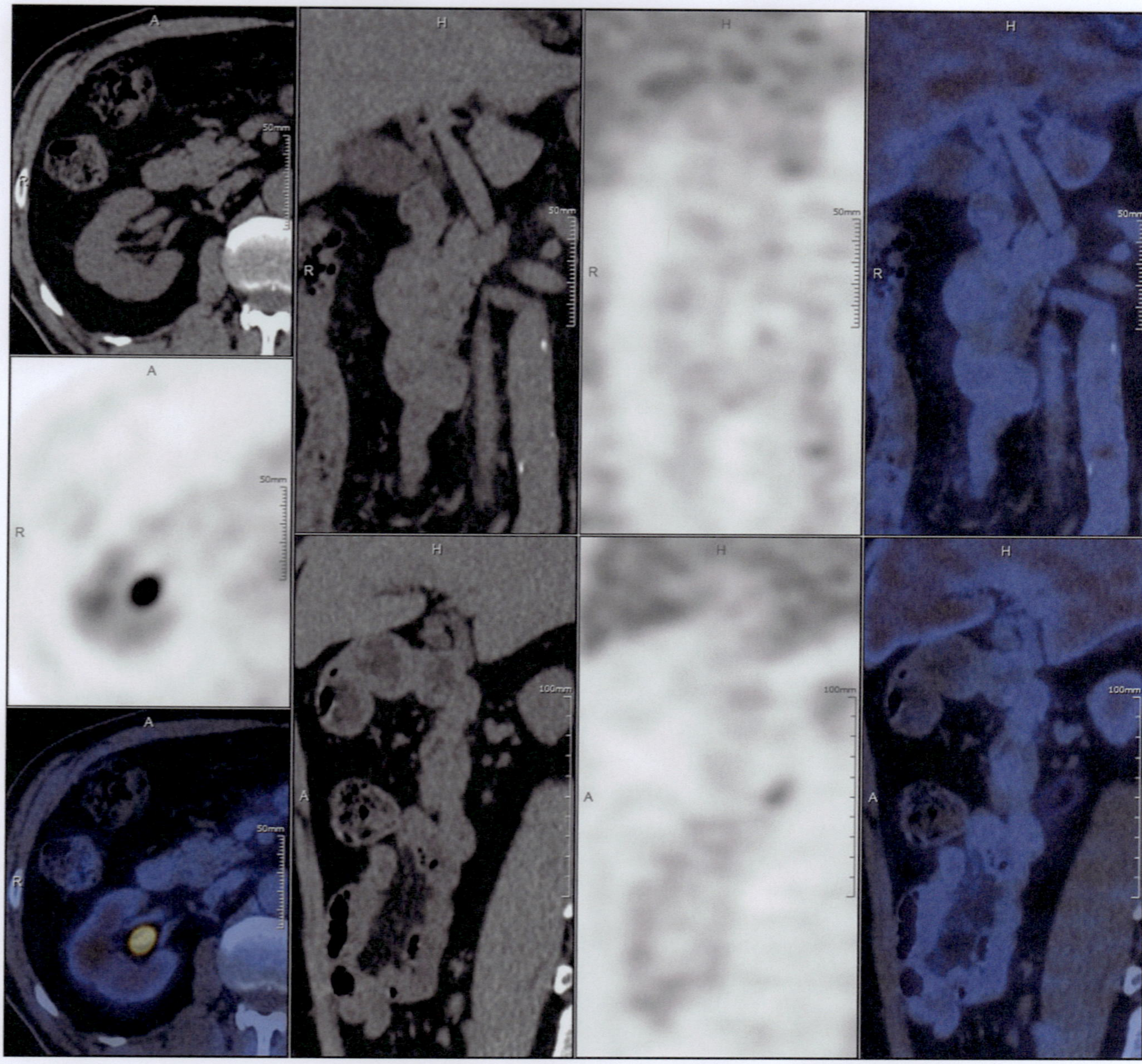

Fig. 4.9 Complete morphologic and metabolic responses of the myeloid sarcoma in the descending part of the duodenum. The follow-up PET/CT scan demonstrates disappearance of the mass in the descending part of the duodenum

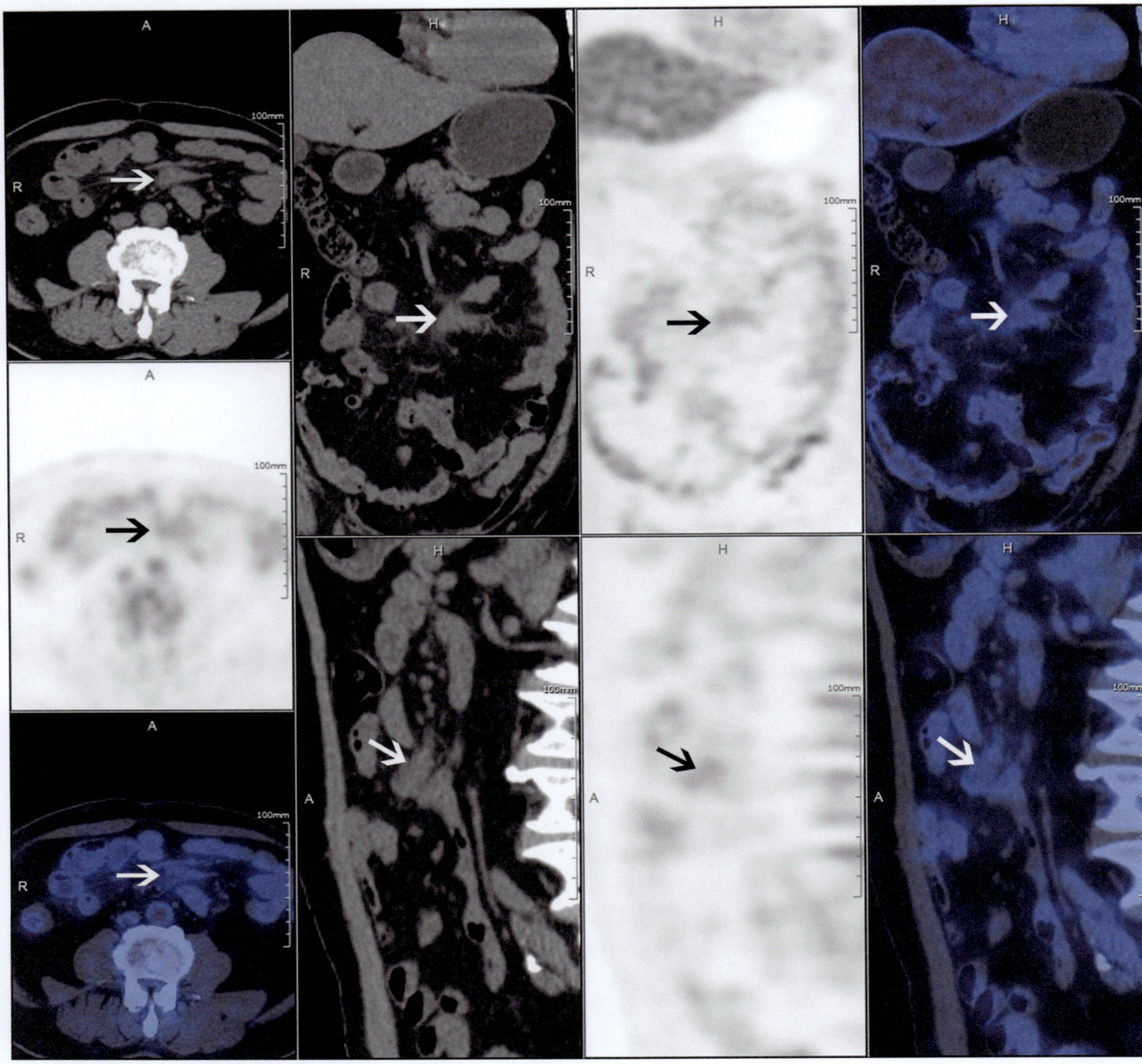

Fig. 4.10 Complete metabolic response and partial morphologic response of the acute myeloid leukemia with granulocytic maturation (AML-M2) with extramedullary involvement in the mesentery and the small intestine. The follow-up PET/CT scan reveals that the involved walls of the small intestine return to normal scale and the mass of the mesentery in the left middle abdomen have markedly shrunk (solid arrow)

4.3.3 Technique

- Patient preparation: patient fasted for more than 6 h prior to administration of radiopharmaceutical, and his serum blood glucose level was 5.5 mmol/L.
- Patient was administered intravenously with 306 MBq of 18FDG and rested quietly around 60 min.
- Imaging device: a whole-body high-resolution time-of-flight PET/CT scanner (Shanghai United Imaging Healthcare Co., Ltd., uMI510) with a PET scanner with lutetium-yttrium oxyorthosilicate (LYSO) crystal with size of 2.35 × 2.35 mm and FWHM of 3.0 and a 16-multi-detector row helical CT scanner with collimation of 1.2 mm.
- Scan parameters: a high-resolution time-of-flight body PET with ordered set expectation maximization (OSEM) iterative reconstruction algorithm (2 iterations, 24 subsets) and slice thickness of 2.44 mm, and a 16-multi-detector row helical CT scanner for body with tube voltage of 120 kV, tube current of 140 mAs, pitch of 0.9375, tube rotation speed of 0.6 s/r, and slice thickness of 1.5 mm.
- A whole-body PET/CT was acquired separately from the head to the inlet of thoracic cage (not shown) and from the base of skull to the mid-thigh.

4.3.4 Image Interpretation

The PET/CT images (Figs. 4.6 and 4.7) demonstrate intense accumulation of 18FDG in the descending part of the duodenum, localized walls of the small intestine, greater omentum, mesenteries, peritoneum, rectovesical pouch, multiple lymphadenopathies in the abdomen and the chest, and diffuse increased accumulation of 18FDG in the thoracolumbar vertebrae, pelvis, and multiple ribs.

4.3.5 Differential Diagnosis

- Acute myeloid leukemia with granulocytic maturation (AML-M2) with extramedullary involvements
- Lymphoma
- Duodenal carcinoma with widespread metastases
- IgG4-related disease

4.3.6 Diagnosis and Clinical Follow-Ups

Myeloid sarcoma of the duodenum and acute myeloid leukemia (AML) with granulocytic maturation (M2) were pathologically confirmed by endoscopic and bone biopsies, respectively. The surveillance PET/CT scan (Figs. 4.8, 4.9, and 4.10) showed AML-M2 and its extramedullary involvements had excellent complete metabolic response to chemotherapy with good complete or partial morphologic remissions.

4.3.7 Discussion

The advantage of 18FDG PET/CT of AML is to improve detection of bone marrow infiltration or monitoring subtle relapsed/refractory filtration [10, 11], and also to evaluate extramedullary presentations with more accurate in lesion detection and additional sites than CT and assess their morphologic and metabolic responses [12–16].

4.4 Myelodysplastic Syndromes

Chao Cheng

Abstract Myelodysplastic syndromes (MDS) comprise a heterogeneous group of clonal hematopoietic stem cell malignancies with significant morbidity and high mortality, which is typically diagnosed based on the presence of persistent cytopenia, dysplastic cells, and genetic markers. There is a relatively high rate of MDS patients in terms of acute myeloid leukemia (AML) evolution. Seventy-five percent of patients with MDS patients manifest as diffuse bone marrow hypermetabolism and enhanced spleen metabolism. It is difficult to differentiate the MDS from AML in PET/CT imaging. The heterogeneous nature of myelodysplastic syndromes (MDS) demands a complex and personalized variety of therapeutic approaches. Among them, allogeneic hematopoietic stem cell transplantation remains the only potentially curative option and is accessible to only a small number of fit patients.

Keywords: Myelodysplastic syndromes, FDG, PET/CT

4.4.1 Clinical Presentation

4.4.1.1 Case One

A 54-year-old man had a history of recurrent cough aggravated with chest tightness for more than 2 weeks. The temperature was as high as 38.8 °C. The CT scan of chest found the high-density shadow scattered in lungs. Laboratory examination found: WBC, 11.47 × 10^9/L; RBC, 1.80 × 10^{12} mg/L; BPC, 57 × 10^9/L; Hemoglobin, 56 g/L; ESR > 140 mm/H; CRP, 9.97 mg/L.

4.4.1.2 Case Two

A 61-year-old woman known with continued hyperpyrexia for 1 month. The temperature was as high as 40 °C. The antibiotic treatment did not work. Laboratory examination found panhematopenia: WBC, 2.55 × 10^9/L; RBC, 2.68 × 10^{12} mg/L; BPC, 41 × 10^9/L; Hemoglobin, 73 g/L. CRP, 175.0 mg/L; Plasma D-dimer, 2.58 μg/mL.

4.4.2 Key Images

4.4.2.1 Case One

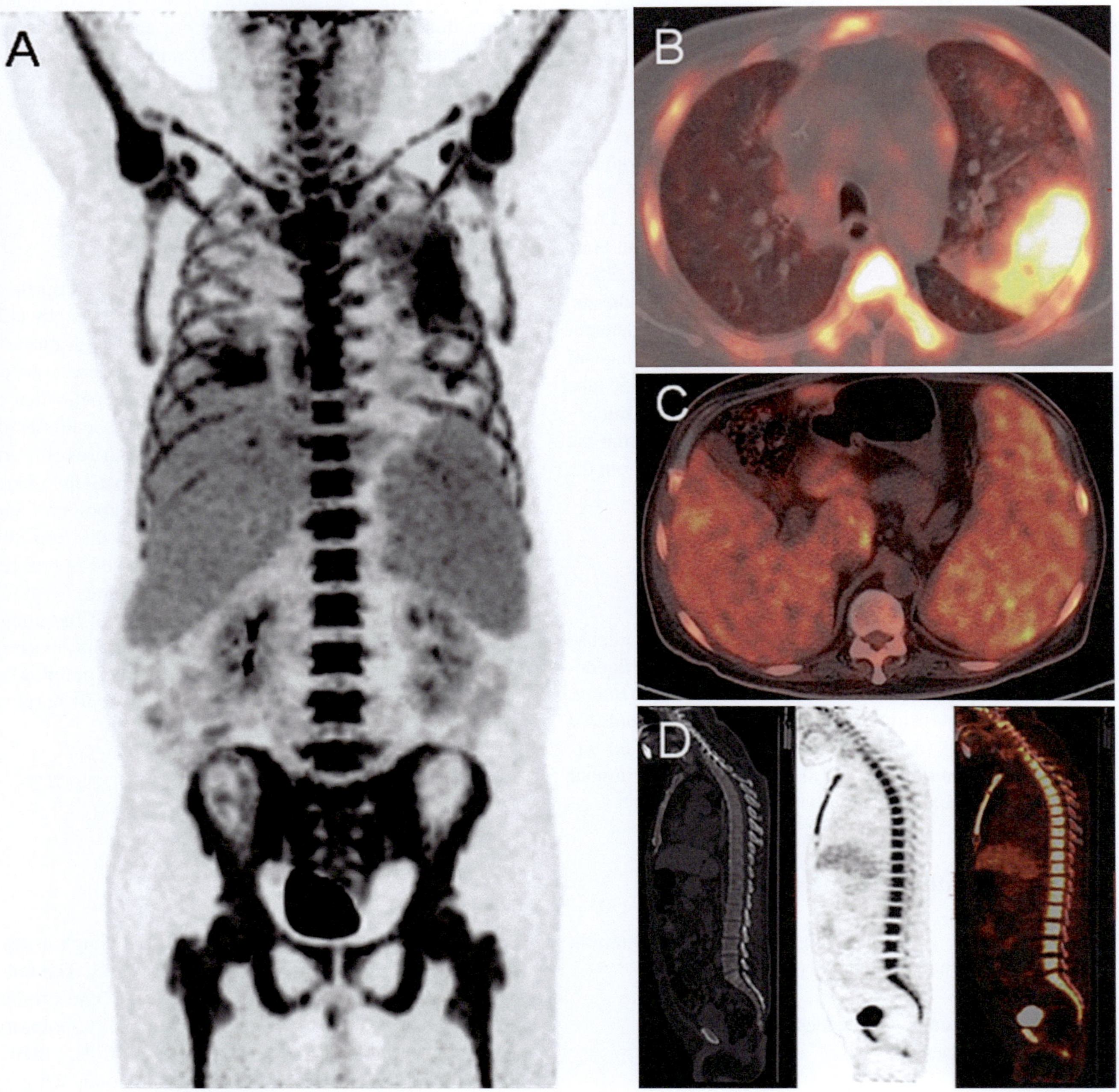

Fig. 4.11 Maximum intensity projection (MIP) PET image (**A**) and sagittal images (**D**) of patients with MDS showed diffuse bone marrow uptake in the central skeleton and proximal extremities (SUV_{max} = 11.4), (**C**) presented with mild spleen enlargement and moderate intake (SUV_{max} = 3.89), (**B**) the chest CT scan showed flaky high-density shadow in left upper lobe (SUV_{max} = 9.76)

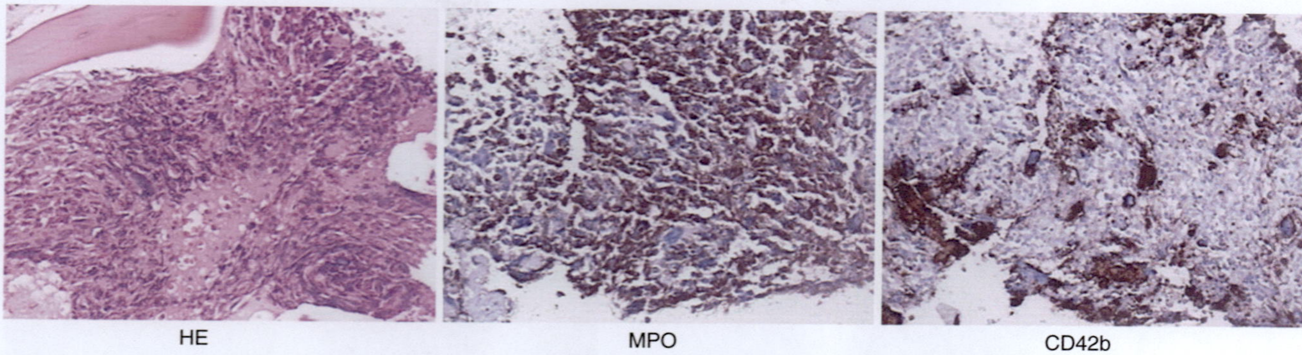

Fig. 4.12 Bone marrow biopsy immunohistochemical pathological results (Humerus). Myeloid hyperplasia is extremely active accompanied by abnormal megakaryocyte morphology, prone to myelodysplastic syndrome/myeloproliferative disease

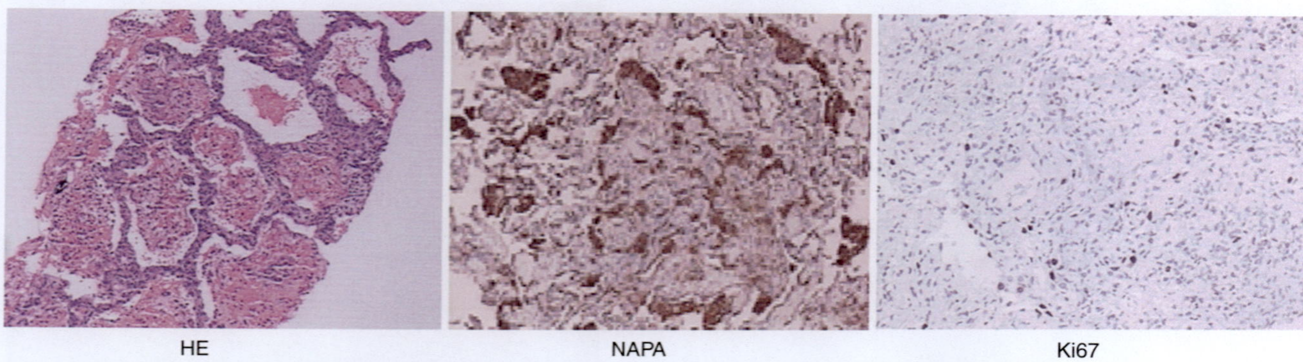

Fig. 4.13 This figure shows puncture tissue of left lung immunohistochemical pathological results: organizing pneumonia, chronic inflammation along with acute cellulitis

4.4.2.2 Case Two

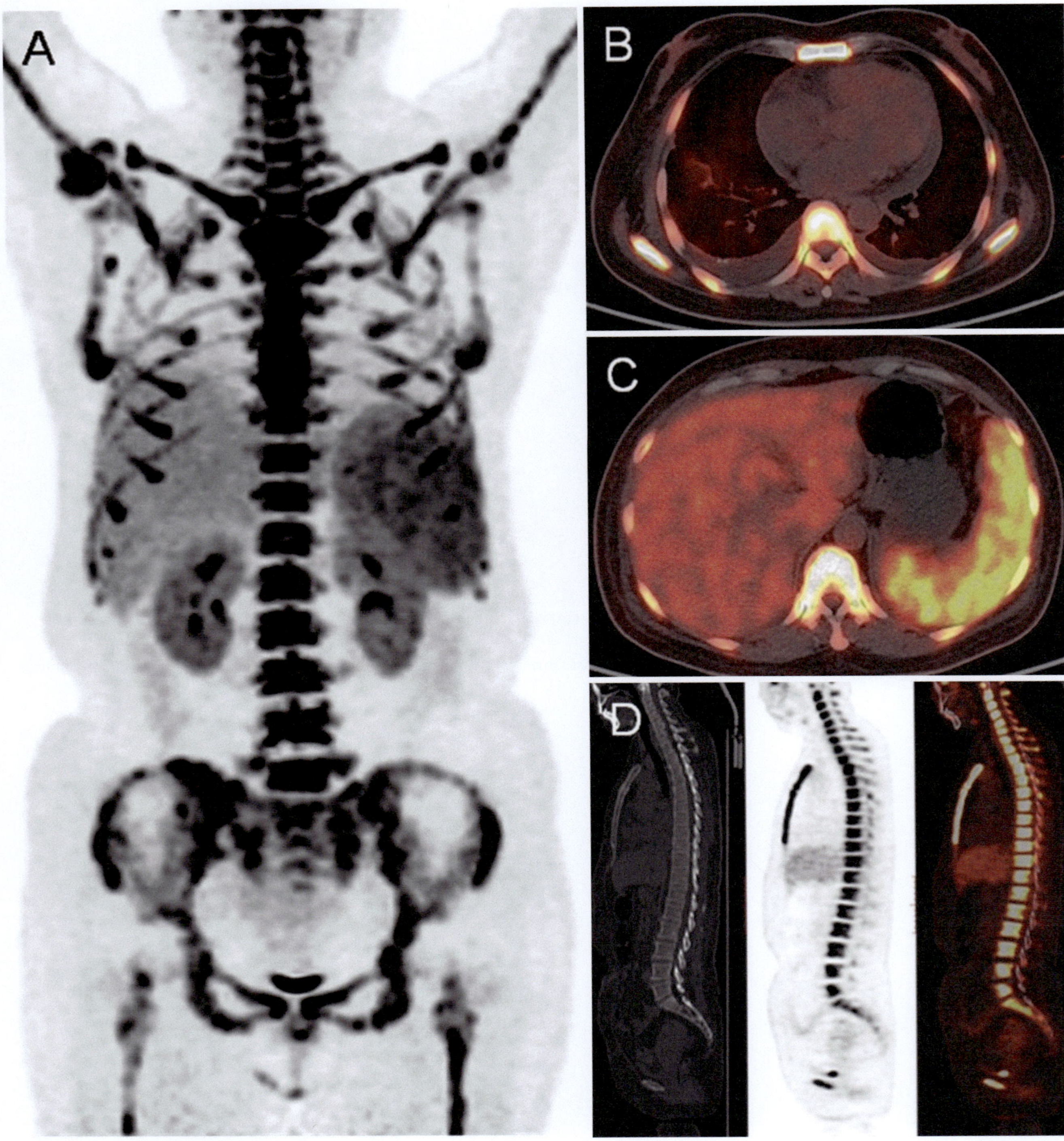

Fig. 4.14 Maximum intensity projection (MIP) PET image (**A**) and sagittal images (**D**) of patients with MDS showed diffuse bone marrow uptake in the central skeleton and proximal extremities ($SUV_{max} = 11.9$), (**C**) splenomegaly with mild accumulation ($SUV_{max} = 5.7$), (**B**) the chest CT scan showed pericardial and bilateral pleural effusion

4.4.3 Technique

4.4.3.1 Case One
- Patient preparation: patient should fast 6 h before administration of radiopharmaceutical.
- 390 MBq of 18FDG administered intravenously (body weight = 85 kg).
- Imaging device: whole-body PET/CT camera (Siemens biograph 64) with resolution of 4.0 mm FWHM.

4.4.3.2 Case Two
- Patient preparation: patient should fast 6 h before administration of radiopharmaceutical.
- 330 MBq of 18FDG administered intravenously (body weight = 55 kg).
- Imaging device: whole-body PET/CT camera (Siemens biograph 64) with resolution of 4.0 mm FWHM.

4.4.4 Differential Diagnosis

4.4.4.1 Case One
- Lung cancer
- Lymphoma
- Leukemia

4.4.4.2 Case Two
- Lymphoma
- Leukemia
- Aplastic anemia (AA)

4.4.5 Diagnosis and Clinical Follow-Ups

4.4.5.1 Case One
Sweet syndrome associated with MDS, severe anemia. During hospitalization, the patient received anti-infection and transfusion treatment, got better in the short term. But, he suffered the gastrointestinal bleeding and rescued invalid death in 2 months.

4.4.5.2 Case Two
Myelodysplastic syndrome (MDS). Bone marrow biopsy pathological results: myelodysplastic syndrome, noting the hemophilic cells, tend to define MDS and secondary haemophilus syndrome. During hospitalization, the patient suffered the sudden precordial pain and rescued invalid death. The possible cause of death was acute myocardial infarction, pulmonary embolism cannot be excluded (Plasma D-dimer, 12.03 μg/mL; IcTnI, 0.050 μg/L).

4.4.6 Discussion

There has been no systematic article to describe the utility of PET/CT in the diagnosis of MDS. MDS needs to be differentiated from acute myelocytic leukemia (AML). MEILAN CHEN's study revealed that the AML has a higher SUV value of bone marrow. MDS also needs to be differentiated from aplastic anemia (AA). The metabolism of MDS bone marrow is significantly increased and the spleen is mildly hypermetabolism while AA presents with the hypometabolism in bone marrow and spleen. It is occasionally difficult to differentiate AA with atypical manifestations from MDS [17, 18]. As reported in the literature, MDS induced the various types of infections sometimes, such as Sweet Syndrome and Behcet's disease, which should be noted in the diagnosis [19, 20]. It is meaningful of FDG PET/CT in describing the lesions of the whole body, choosing the biopsy site, predicting prognosis, and evaluating the therapy.

4.5 Hodgkin Lymphoma

Jingping Zhang

Abstract A 48-year-old woman was found lymph nodes enlarged for 7 months and diagnosed lymphoma for 8 days. Pathologic findings: classic Hodgkin's lymphoma. PET showed multiple FDG uptake increased shadows in bilateral parotid gland area, bilateral neck, submaxilla, and supraclavicular lymph node. Increasing FDG uptake in bilateral diaphragmatic feet, retroperitoneum, intraperitoneal and bilateral groin.

Keywords: ^{18}F-FDG PET/CT, Hodgkin lymphoma, fever

4.5.1 Clinical Presentation

A 48-year-old woman was found cervical lymph node enlargement 7 months ago, accompanied by low fever. After anti-inflammatory treatment, the body temperature returned to normal, and there was no other discomfort. One month ago, there was lymph node enlargement in the left neck, significant weight loss, and chest distress and shortness of breath. Pathologic findings: classic Hodgkin's lymphoma (Figs. 4.15 and 4.16).

4.5.2 Key Images

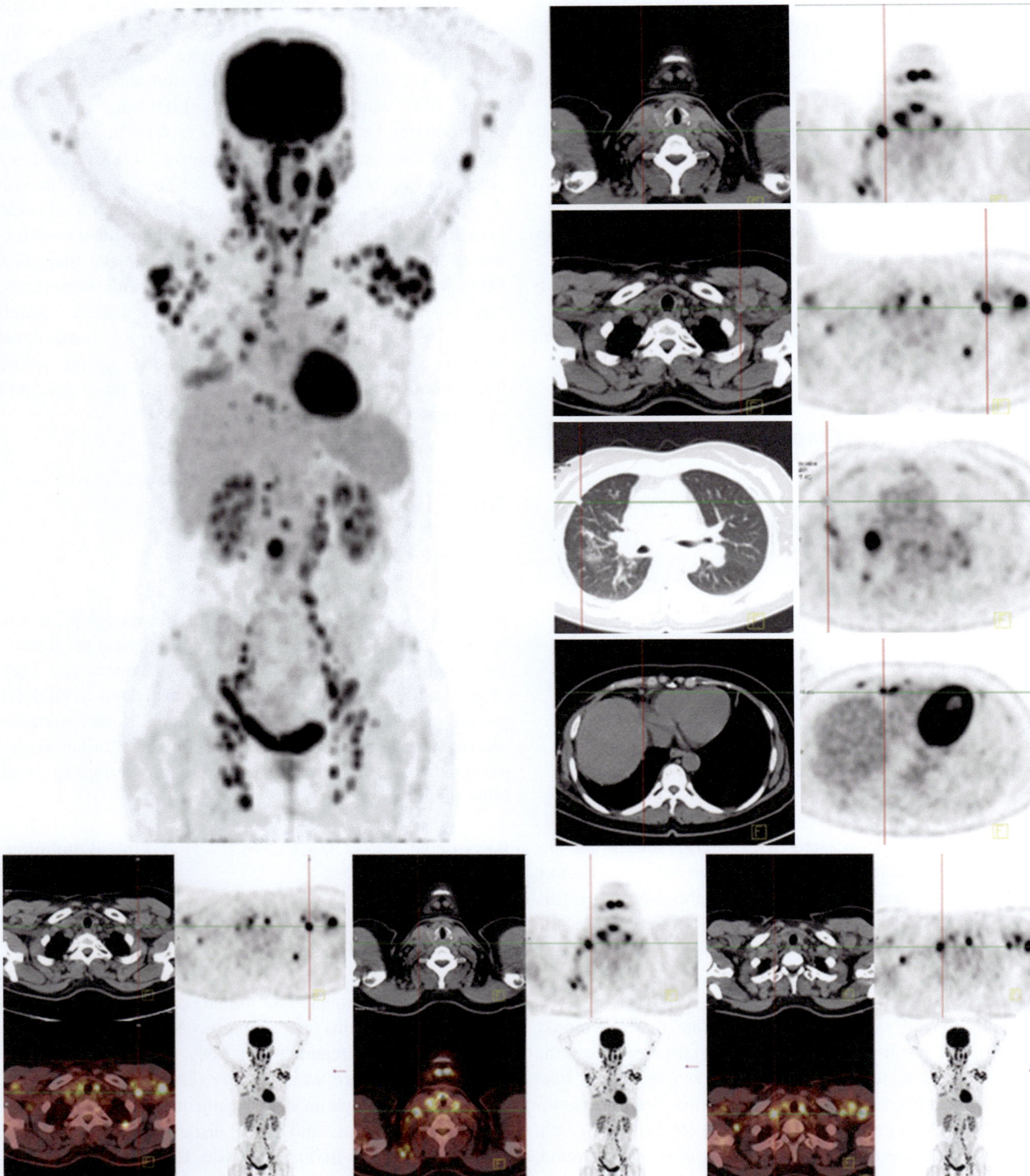

Fig. 4.15 PET/CT—multiple lymph node shadows, partial enlargement, increased metabolism

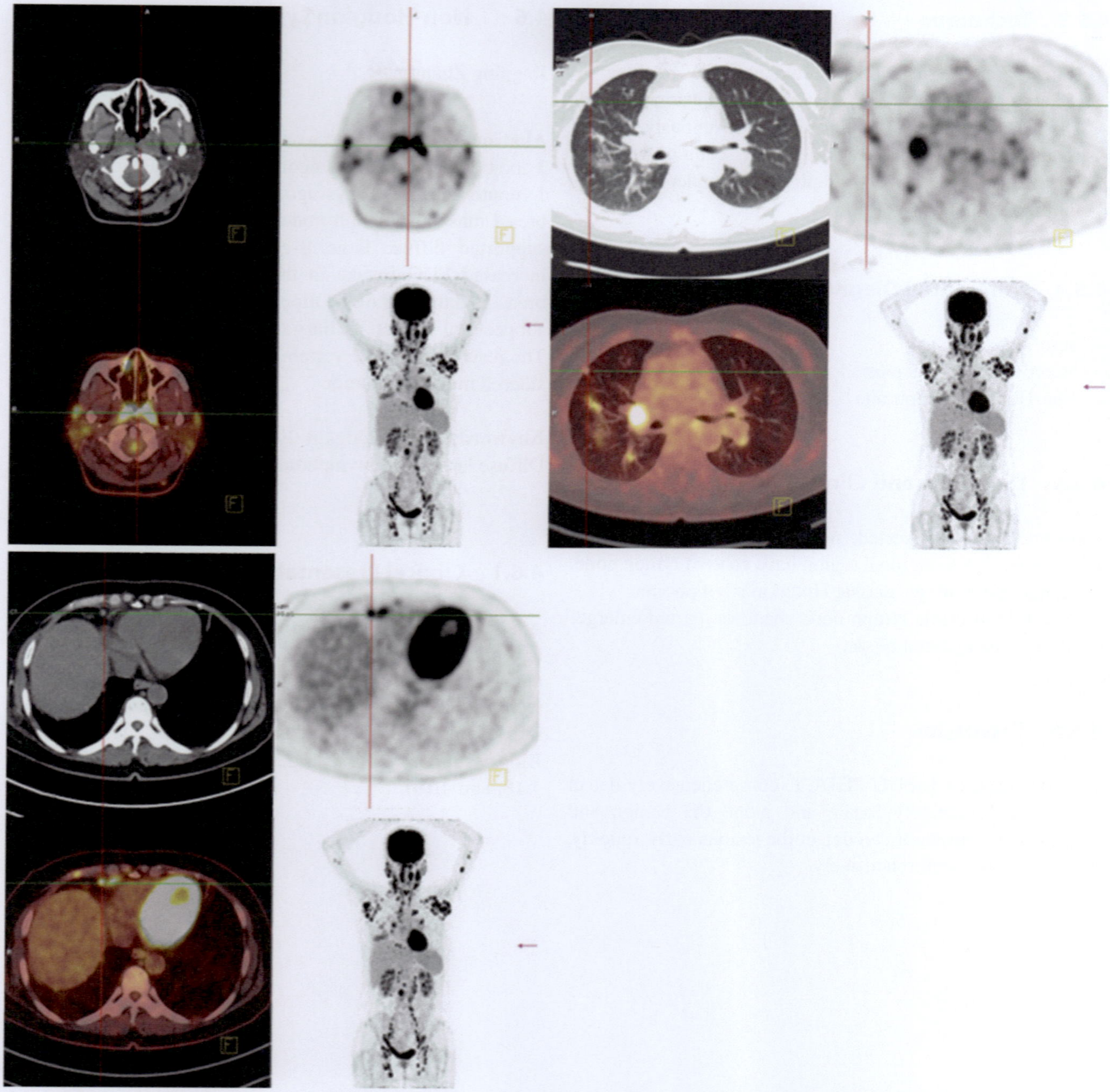

Fig. 4.16 PET/CT—density increased in right orbit and right nasal cavity with increased metabolism. Left-side ilium has nodule shadow, metabolism increased. Right-side pleura and right-side abdominal wall have nodule shadow, metabolism increased

4.5.3 Technique

- Patient preparation: patient should not take anything by mouth for 6 h before administration of radiopharmaceutical.
- 185 MBq of ^{18}F-FDG administered intravenously.
- Imaging device: Whole-body PET/CT scanning was performed using Siemens biograph mCT scanner with resolution of 5.0 mm FWHM.

4.5.4 Differential Diagnosis

- Scrofula
- Infectious mononucleosis
- Non-Hodgkin lymphoma

4.5.5 Diagnosis and Clinical Follow-Ups

Ultrasonography suggested: neck, clavicular fossa, axilla, suprasternal fossa, inguinal region have echo of lymph node.

Pathologic findings: classic Hodgkin's lymphoma.

PET/CT: Multiple lymph node shadows, partial enlargement, increasing metabolism.

4.5.6 Discussion

The advantage of 18FDG PET/CT: comprehensively detect the lesions, accurately locate and judge the benign and malignant lesions, so it can detect the lesions early, quickly, accurately, and comprehensively.

4.6 Non-Hodgkin Lymphoma

Jingping Zhang

Abstract A 52-year-old woman was found left breast mass 3 months ago and felt uncomfortable in her left shoulder 1 month ago. Two days ago, ultrasound-guided biopsy of breast mass and lymph nodes was performed: The results supported diffuse large B-cell lymphoma. PET showed increased FDG uptake in the upper quadrant of the left breast and the rear of the nipple. Multiple nodular in the left subpectoral and left axillary regions increased FDG uptake. The result of thoracic vertebral enhancement MR was considered metastatic tumor.

Keywords: Non-Hodgkin lymphoma, ^{18}F-FDG PET/CT, Diffuse large B-cell lymphoma

4.6.1 Clinical Presentation

A 52-year-old women was found left breast mass 3 months ago and felt uncomfortable in her left shoulder 1 month ago. No fever, normal weight, no diarrhea, and constipation were found. Ultrasound showed two parenchymal occupying lesions in the left breast are possible. The result of Biopsy supports diffuse large B-cell lymphoma (Figs. 4.17, 4.18, and 4.19).

4.6.2 Key Images

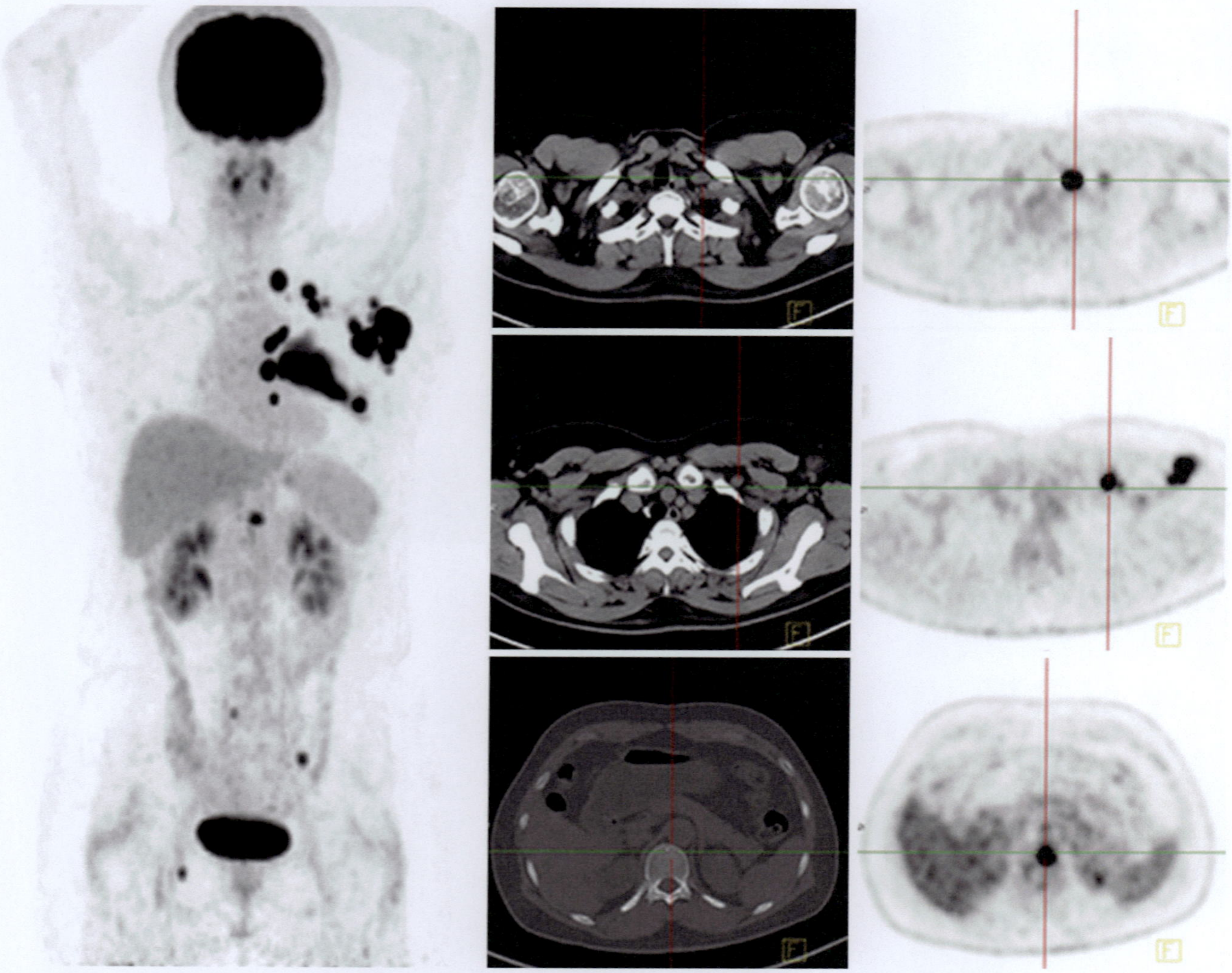

Fig. 4.17 PET/CT—soft-tissue density nodule shadow and mass shadow in the upper quadrant of the left breast and the rear of the nipple, metabolism increased, and malignant lesions were more considered

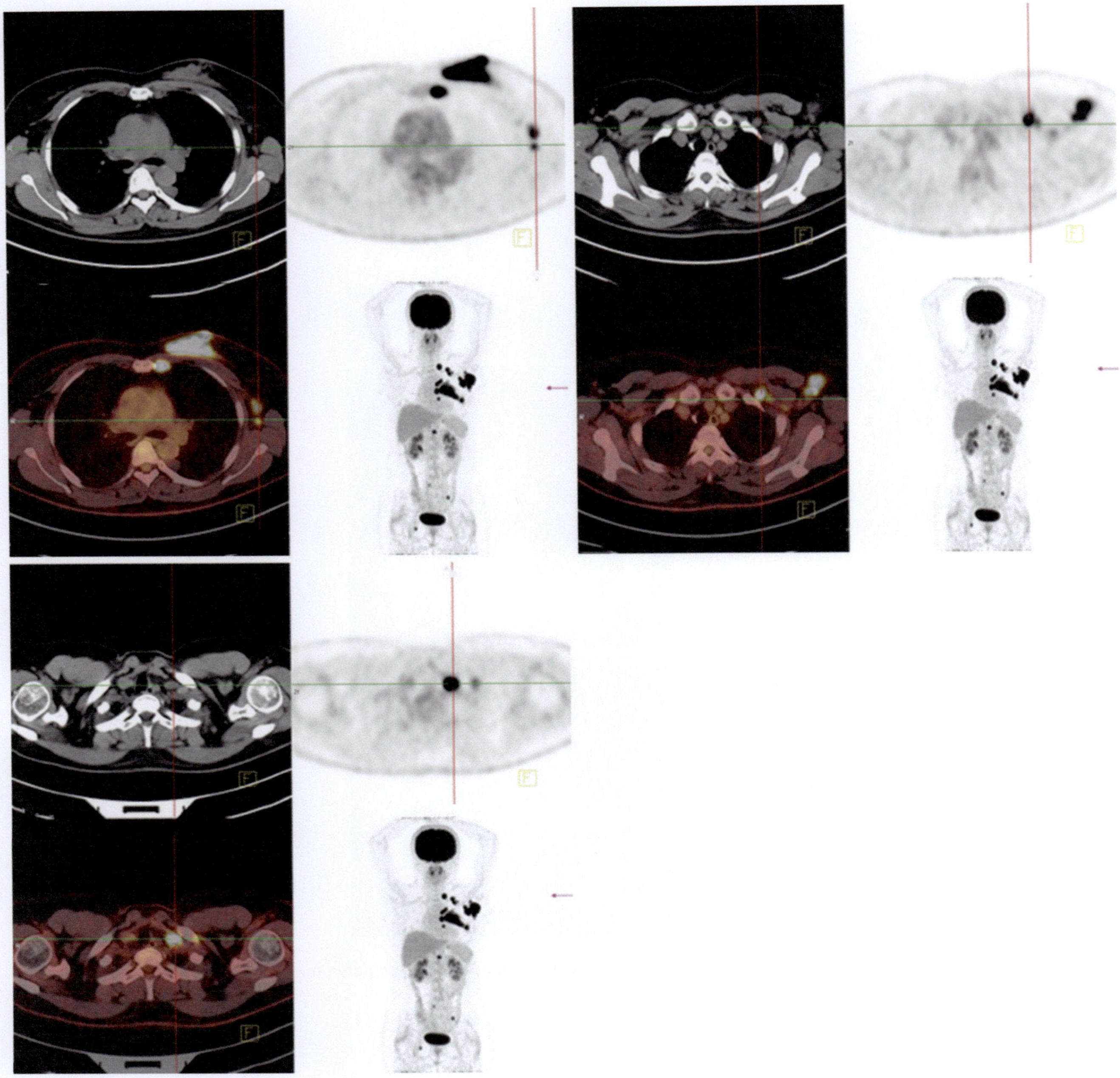

Fig. 4.18 PET/CT—multiple lymph node shadows were found in the left side of the sternum, the left side of the chest muscle and the left axilla, and the metabolism increased, malignant metastasis were more considered

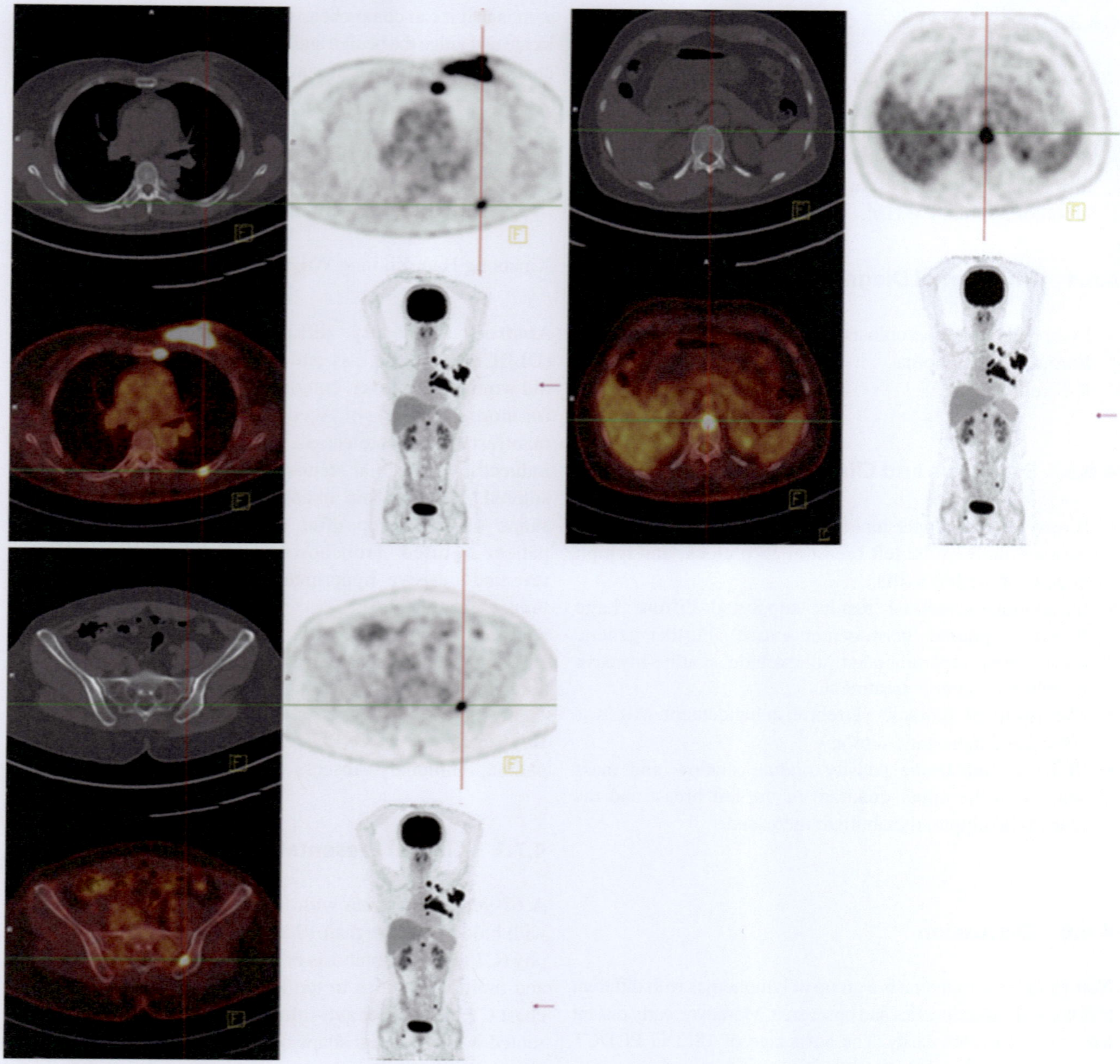

Fig. 4.19 PET/CT—multiple increasing metabolism of bone

4.6.3 Technique

- Patient preparation: patient should not take anything by mouth for 6 h before administration of radiopharmaceutical.
- 185 MBq of ^{18}F-FDG administered intravenously.
- Imaging device: Whole-body PET/CT scanning was performed using Siemens biograph mCT scanner with resolution of 5.0 mm FWHM.

4.6.4 Differential Diagnosis

- Lymphadenitis tuberculosis
- Extranidal lymphoma
- R-S cell

4.6.5 Diagnosis and Clinical Follow-Ups

- Biopsy shows: Upper inner quadrant A of the left breast, para-areola B of the left breast at 12 o'clock, and lymph node C of the left axilla.
- Immunohistochemical results supported diffuse large B-cell lymphoma (germ-center source). Further genetic testing was recommended to exclude double-invasive lymphoma to guide treatment.
- The result of thoracic vertebral enhancement MR was considered metastatic tumor.
- PET/CT: Soft-tissue density nodule shadow and mass shadow in the upper quadrant of the left breast and the rear of the nipple, metabolism increased.

4.6.6 Discussion

Non-Hodgkin lymphoma is a group of lymphomas with different histological characteristics and onset area. Moreover, early distant transmission occurs easily. The advantage of 18FDG PET/CT scan is that it can comprehensively detect the lesions, accurately locate and judge the benign and malignant lesions, so it can detect the lesions early, quickly, accurately, and comprehensively.

4.7 Pulmonary Diffuse Large B-Cell Lymphoma Mimicking Lung Abscess Induced by Bronchial Stenosis

Xinzhong Hao, Zhifang Wu, and Sijin Li

Abstract Pulmonary diffuse large B-cell lymphoma (DLBCL) with necrosis and atelectasis is rare. A 67-year-old woman with fever, cough up yellow phlegm with blood for more than 10 days. According to chest CT and clinical manifestations, atelectasis with pulmonary abscess induced by bronchial stenosis in left lower lobe was considered. However, no change presented in the size and shape of the lesion after anti-infective treatment. The patient refused bronchoscopy. Subsequently, PET/CT revealed massive hypermetabolic foci in the left lower lung with atelectasis. Two months later, the patient was admitted again with similar symptoms, the second PET/CT suggested disease progression. Then, DLBCL was confirmed by biopsy.

Keywords: ^{18}F-FDG PET/CT, Diffuse large B-cell lymphoma, Pulmonary, Abscess

4.7.1 Clinical Presentation

A 67-year-old woman with fever, cough up yellow phlegm with blood for more than 10 days. Chest computed tomography (CT) revealed stenosis of the basal bronchus, atelectasis, and multiple cavities in the left lower lung. On the second chest CT image after anti-infective treatment, no change presented in the size and shape of the lesion.

4.7.2 Key Images

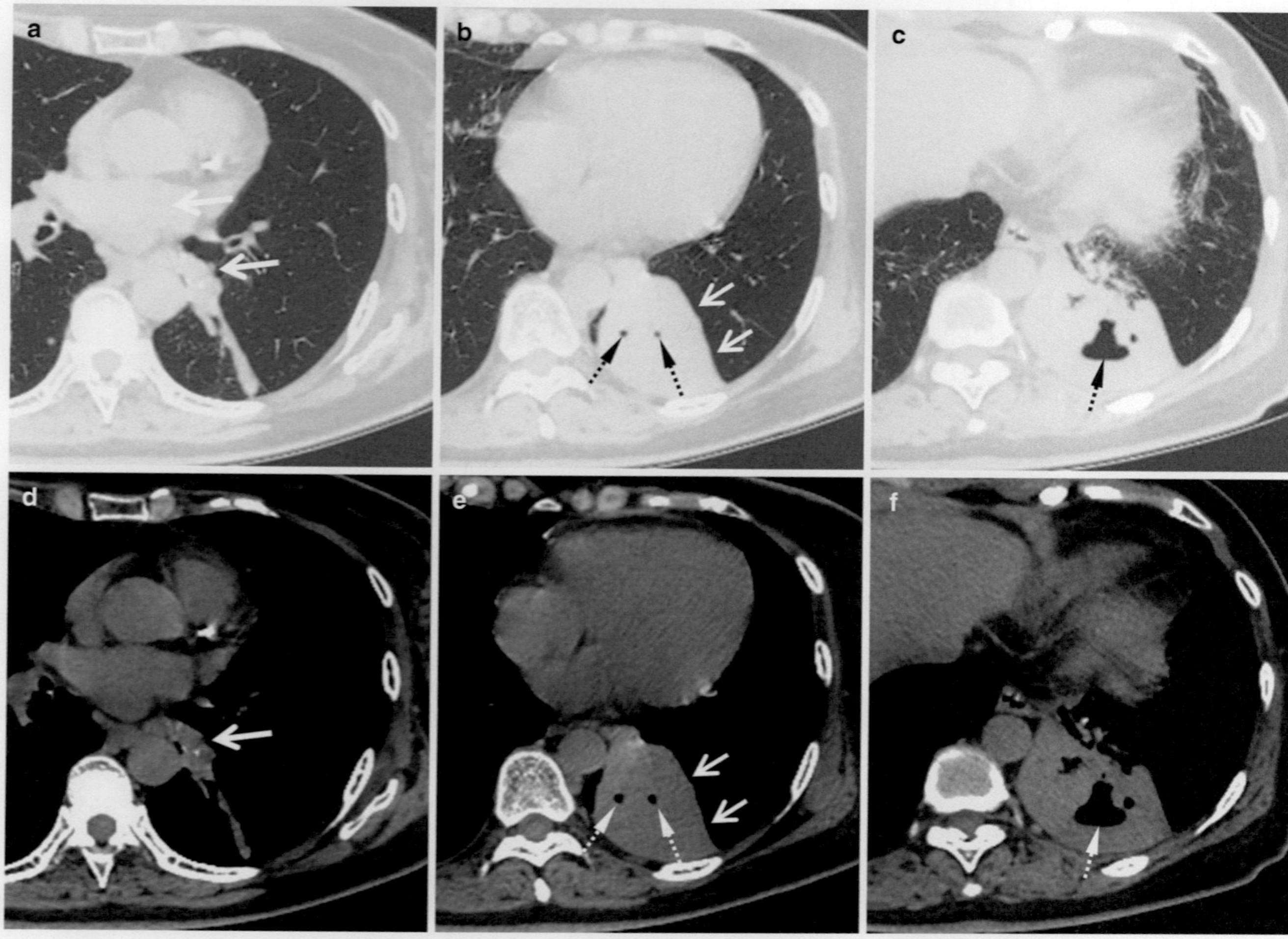

Fig. 4.20 The chest CT image after anti-infective therapy. (**a–c**) are axial CT images with lung window at different level in the left lower lung, (**d–f**) are the corresponding CT images with mediastinal window

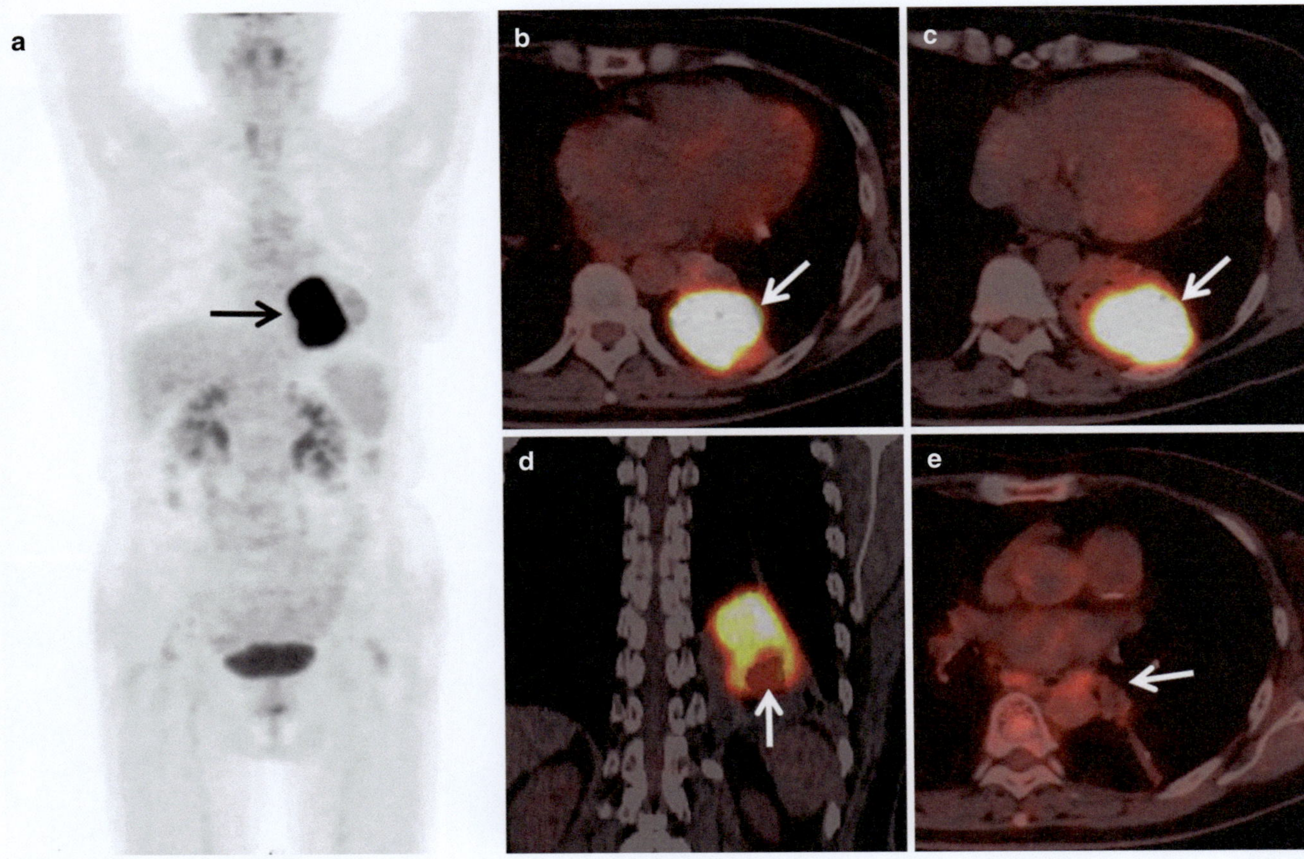

Fig. 4.21 The first PET/CT image after anti-infective therapy. (**a**) is the maximum intensity projection (MIP) image for positron emission tomography (PET), (**b**, **c**) are the axial fused PET/CT images at the level of active lesion, (**d**) is the coronal fused PET/CT image, (**e**) is the axial fused PET/CT image at the level of basal bronchus in the left lower lung

4.7.3 Technique

- Patient preparation: patient was asked to fast for more than 6 h before the PET/CT examination.
- 223 MBq of 18F-FDG administered intravenously and rested for 50 min.
- Imaging device: GE Discovery VCT64 PET/CT Scanner.
- Image acquisition: Data acquisition began with CT at 120 kVp, 60 mA, 1.98 cm pitch, and 0.8 s tube rotation; this was followed by PET with resolution of 6.0 mm FWHM and 3D acquisition mode.
- PET image reconstruction: The images were reconstructed by means of the standardized ordered-subset expectation maximization (OSEM) technique using 20 subsets and 2 iterations with a 128 × 128 matrix.

4.7.4 Image Interpretation

Chest CT (Fig. 4.20) revealed basal trunk bronchial stenosis (a and d, arrow), atelectasis (b and e, solid arrow) and multiple cavities (b–c and e–f, dotted arrow) in the left lower lung.

PET/CT (Fig. 4.21) demonstrates apparent and increased FDG uptake with a lump-like profile in collapsed left lower lung (a–c, arrow), SUV_{max} = 35.1, no increased FDG uptake in necrotic area (d, arrow) and stenosed basal trunk bronchus (e, arrow).

4.7.5 Differential Diagnosis

- Bronchial stenosis-induced obstructive pulmonary abscess
- Lung cancer
- Tuberculosis

4.7.6 Diagnosis and Clinical Follow-Ups

No treatment was performed after the first PET/CT examination. Two months later, the patient was hospitalized for recurrent cough and hemoptysis.

The second PET/CT (Fig. 4.22) was performed, suggested hypermetabolic mass in left lower lung enlarged (a, b, and e, thick solid arrow), and new lesions appeared in the left lung (a, c, and f, thin solid arrow), the right lobe of thyroid (a, d, and g, dashed arrow), and bilateral neck lymph nodes (a, dotted arrows). In addition, increased diffuse FDG uptake was seen in spleen, the effusion appeared in the left pleural cavity. Compared with the first PET/CT, it showed disease progression.

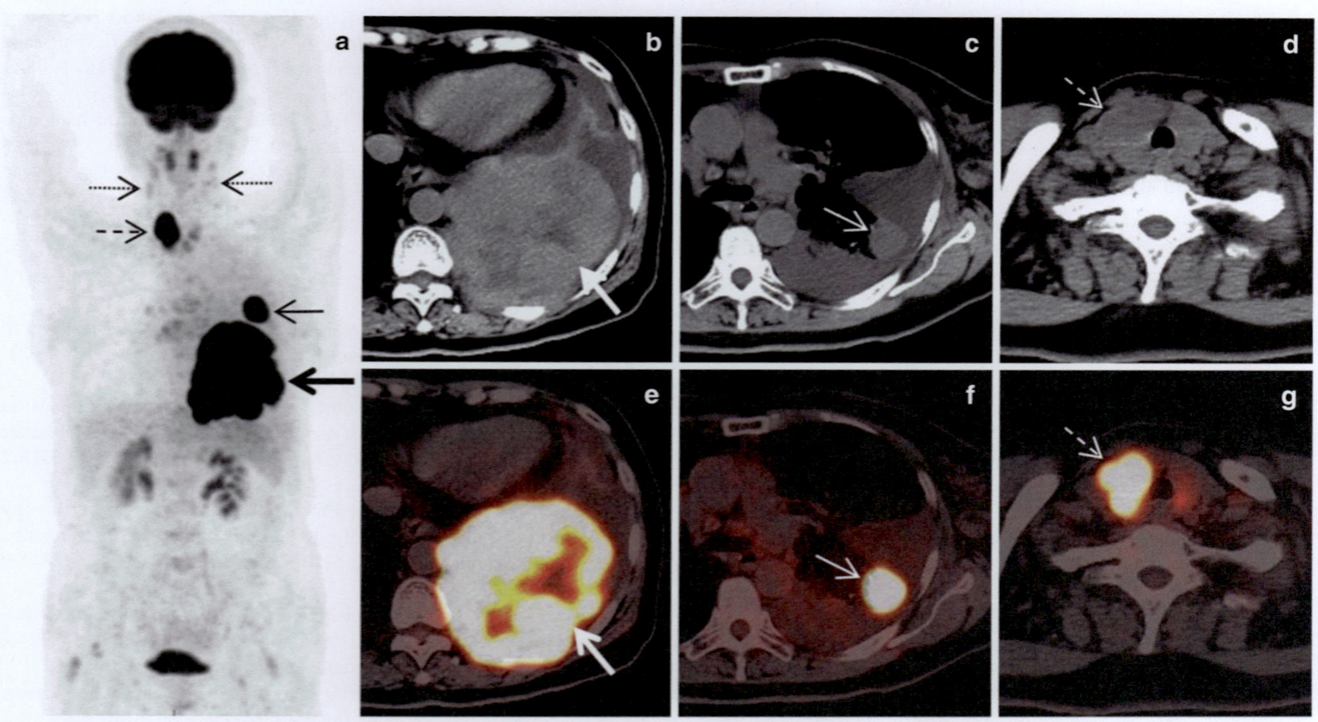

Fig. 4.22 The second PET/CT image. (**a**) is the MIP PET image, (**b–d**) are the axial CT images, (**e, f**) are the corresponding fused PET/CT images

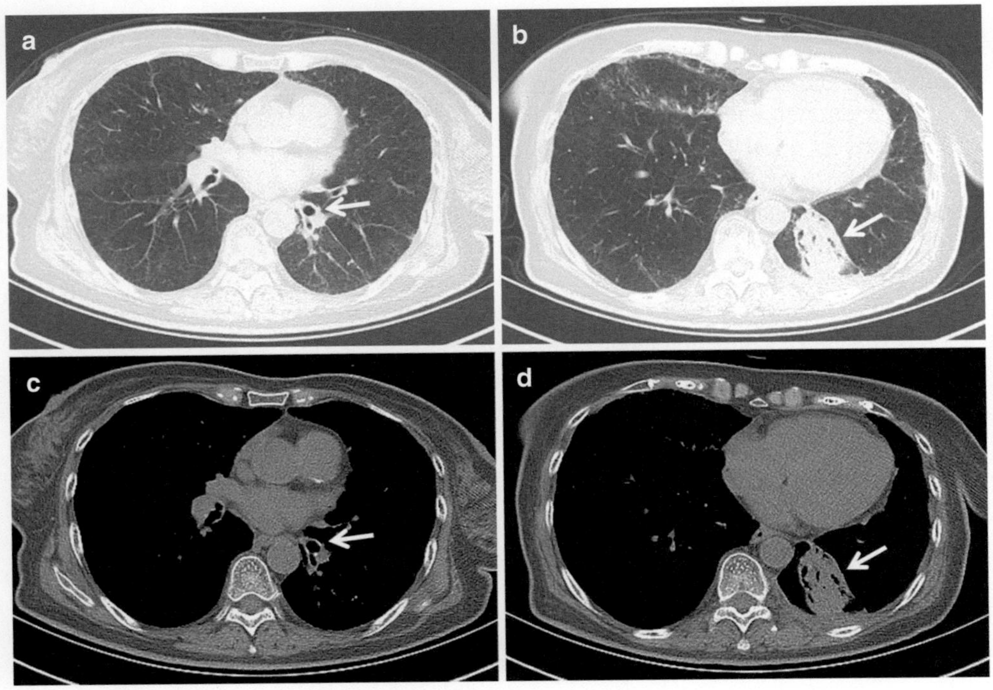

Fig. 4.23 The chest CT image after chemotherapy. (**a**, **b**) are axial CT images at the level of basal bronchus, (**b–d**) are axial CT images at the level of active lesion in the left lower lung

Subsequently, DLBCL was confirmed by core needle biopsy of the left lower lung lesion.

After four cycles of chemotherapy, chest CT (Fig. 4.23) showed that the left lower lung basal bronchus reopened (a and c, arrow), and the left lower lung lesion shrined (b and d, arrow).

4.7.7 Discussion

Pulmonary diffuse large B-cell lymphoma (DLBCL) is rare [21]. Internal necrosis in lymphoma is also uncommon [22], when it coexists with bronchial obstruction and atelectasis, it is more likely to be misdiagnosed as abscess, tuberculosis, or lung cancer. A significant, high FDG uptake may be the primary feature for DLBCL [23, 24], which contributes to distinguish DLBCL from other disease.

References

1. Jiang M, Bennani NN, Feldman AL. Lymphoma classification update: T-cell lymphomas, Hodgkin lymphomas, and histiocytic/dendritic cell neoplasms. Expert Rev Hematol. 2017;10(3):239–49. https://doi.org/10.1080/17474086.2017.1281122.
2. Yudistiro R, Arisaka Y, Tokue A, Nakajima T. Differentiation of sarcoidosis-lymphoma syndrome lesions: a case report on the use of two different positron emission tomography tracers. BMC Med Imaging. 2016;16:1. https://doi.org/10.1186/s12880-015-0104-x.
3. Valls L, Badve C, Avril S, et al. FDG-PET imaging in hematological malignancies. Blood Rev. 2016;30(4):317–31. https://doi.org/10.1016/j.blre.2016.02.003.
4. Teagle AR, Barton H, Charles-Edwards E, Dizdarevic S, Chevassut T. Acta Radiol. 2017;58(12):1476–84. https://doi.org/10.1177/0284185117701305. Epub 2017 Apr 6
5. Chin V, Fulham M, Hertzberg M, Jackson M, Lindeman R, Brighton T, Kidson-Gerber G, Wegner EA, Cheung C, MacCallum S, Williams J, Thompson SR. J Med Imaging Radiat Oncol. 2018;62(3):432–9. https://doi.org/10.1111/1754-9485.12719.
6. Cribe AS, Steenhof M, Marcher CW, et al. Extramedullary disease in patients with acute myeloid leukemia assessed by (18) F-FDG PET. Eur J Haematol. 2013;90:273–8.
7. Hutchings M, Specht L. PET/CT in the management of haematological malignancies. Eur J Haematol. 2008;80:369–80.
8. Cribe AS, Steenhof M, Marcher CW, et al. Extramedullary disease in patients with acute myeloid leukemia assessed by (18) F-FDG PET. Eur J Haematol. 2013;90:273–8.
9. Zhou W-l, Wu H-b, Wang L-j, et al. Usefulness and pitfalls of F-18-FDG PET/CT for diagnosing extramedullary acute leukemia. Eur J Radiol. 2016;85:205–10.
10. Arimoto MK, et al. Increased bone marrow uptake of 18F-FDG in leukemia patients: preliminary findings. Springerplus. 2015;4:521. https://doi.org/10.1186/s40064-015-1339-2.
11. Kaya Z, et al. Utility of 18-fluorodeoxyglucose positron emission tomography in children with relapsed/refractory leukemia. Pediatr Hematol Oncol. 2019;35:1–14. https://doi.org/10.1080/08880018.2018.1557306.
12. Aschoff P, et al. Integrated FDG-PET/CT for detection, therapy monitoring and follow-up of granulocytic sarcoma. Initial results. Nuklearmedizin. 2009;48(5):185–91. https://doi.org/10.3413/nukmed-0236.
13. Stolzel F, et al. (1)(8)F-FDG-PET/CT for detection of extramedullary acute myeloid leukemia. Haematologica. 2011;96(10):1552–6. https://doi.org/10.3324/haematol.2011.045047.
14. Schliemann C, et al. Targeting interleukin-2 to the bone marrow stroma for therapy of acute myeloid leukemia relapsing after allogeneic hematopoietic stem cell transplantation. Cancer Immunol Res. 2015;3(5):547–56. https://doi.org/10.1158/2326-6066.CIR-14-0179.

15. Zhou WL, et al. Usefulness and pitfalls of F-18-FDG PET/CT for diagnosing extramedullary acute leukemia. Eur J Radiol. 2016;85(1):205–10. https://doi.org/10.1016/j.ejrad.2015.11.019.
16. O'Donnell MR, et al. Acute myeloid leukemia, Version 3.2017, NCCN Clinical Practice Guidelines in Oncology. J Natl Compr Cancer Netw. 2017;15(7):926–57. https://doi.org/10.6004/jnccn.2017.0116.
17. Chen M, Lu L, Li J, et al. Value of systemic PET/CT in the diagnosis and differential diagnosis of aplastic anemia. Oncol Lett. 2018;16(3):3215–22.
18. van der Bruggen W, Glaudemans AWJM, Vellenga E, Slart RHJA. PET in benign bone marrow disorders. Semin Nucl Med. 2017;47(4):397–407.
19. Dong A, Wang Y, Gao L, Zuo C. 18F-FDG PET/CT findings in a patient with Sweet syndrome associated with myelodysplastic syndrome. Clin Nucl Med. 2013;38(12):e454–7.
20. Ito K, Kubota K. 18F-FDG PET/CT findings in two cases with myelodysplastic syndrome accompanied by Behçet's disease. Clin Nucl Med. 2016;41(8):e392–3.
21. Neri N, Jesus Nambo M, Aviles A. Diffuse large B-cell lymphoma primary of lung. Hematology. 2011;16:110–2.
22. Baratto L, Davidzon GA, Moghbel M, et al. Comparison between different PET and CT-based imaging interpretation criteria at interim imaging in patients with diffuse large B-cell lymphoma. Clin Nucl Med. 2018;43:1–8.
23. Bai Y, Liang W. CT and PET/CT findings of primary pulmonary diffuse large B-cell lymphoma: one case report and literature review. Medicine (Baltimore). 2017;96:e8876.
24. Foderaro AE, Reagan JL. Hodgkin lymphoma mimicking lung abscess. Blood. 2016;128:3011.

Further Readings

Bailly C, Carlier T, Touzeau C, Arlicot N, Kraeber-Bodere F, Le Gouill S, Bodet-Milin C. Interest of FDG-PET in the management of mantle cell lymphoma. Front Med (Lausanne). 2019;6:70. https://doi.org/10.3389/fmed.2019.00070. ECollection 2019

Daruwalla ZJ, Razak AR, Duke D, Grogan L. Acute upper arm ischemia: a rare presentation of non-Hodgkin's lymphoma. Ir J Med Sci. 2010;179(4):589–92. https://doi.org/10.1007/s11845-008-0206-3. Epub 2008 Aug 12

Hua FC, Liu YC, Zhao J, et al. The value of ^{18}F-FDG PET/CT or PET/CT imaging in fever of unknown origin for screening lymphoma. Chin J Nucl Med. 2004;24(1):11–3.

Reske SN. PET and restaging of malignant lymphoma including residual masses and relapse. Eur J Nucl Med Mol Imaging. 2003;30(1):S89–96.

FDG-PET/CT for Large-Vessel Vasculitis

5

Junichi Tsuchiya, Ukihide Tateishi, Hajime Yoshifuji, Hideo Onizawa, Yukio Sato, Masatoshi Itoh, Takeshi Sasaki, Tadashi Watabe, Tetsuya Higuchi, Shinro Matsuo, Chao Cheng, Zhang Jingping, Jun Hashimoto, Yuri Yamada, Toshiki Kazama, Takakiyo Nomura, Yutaka Imai, Xuena Li, and Kazuo Kubota

5.1 Role of FDG PET/CT in Diagnosis of Inflammation of Vessels

Junichi Tsuchiya and Ukihide Tateishi

Abstract Patients with large-vessel vasculitis (LVV) may present with nonspecific clinical symptoms and increased inflammatory markers, including C-reactive protein and erythrocyte sedimentation rate. Due to these nonspecific characteristics, routine diagnostic tests may be inconclusive for such patients. FDG-PET/CT is a functional imaging modality that can be a useful tool for diagnosis in inflammatory diseases, as well as in oncology assessments. Functional FDG-PET, when combined with anatomical CT, may be of synergistic value for optimal diagnosis, monitoring of disease activity, and evaluation of damage progression in LVV. Diagnostic delay in patients with LVV may cause severe aortic complications, thereby leading to surgery or angioplasty for occlusive lesions. Thus, early diagnosis and detection of relapse are imperative in clinical practice with respect to LVV. 18F-FDG-PET/CT is a promising modality for use in the assessment of patients with LVV.

Keywords: FDG, PET, Takayasu arteritis, Giant-cell arteritis

5.1.1 Introduction

Vasculitis is a heterogeneous group of disorders, characterized by inflammation and fibrinoid necrosis of blood vessel walls. Patients with large-vessel vasculitis (LVV) show nonspecific or multifocal constitutional symptoms including

J. Tsuchiya · U. Tateishi (✉)
Department of Diagnostic Imaging and Nuclear Medicine, Tokyo Medical and Dental University, Tokyo, Japan
e-mail: tcymrad@tmd.ac.jp; ttisdrnm@tmd.ac.jp

H. Yoshifuji · H. Onizawa
Department of Rheumatology and Clinical Immunology, Graduate School of Medicine, Kyoto University, Kyoto, Japan
e-mail: yossii@kuhp.kyoto-u.ac.jp; honizawa@kuhp.kyoto-u.ac.jp

Y. Sato · M. Itoh
Sendai Medical Imaging Clinic, Sendai, Miyagi, Japan
e-mail: yukiosato@mrj.biglobe.ne.jp; itomsts@gmail.com

T. Sasaki
Department of Rheumatology, Tohoku Medical and Pharmaceutical University Wakabayashi Hospital, Sendai, Miyagi, Japan

T. Watabe
Osaka University Graduate School of Medicine, Osaka, Japan
e-mail: watabe@tracer.med.osaka-u.ac.jp

T. Higuchi
Department of Diagnostic Radiology and Nuclear Medicine, Gunma University Graduate School of Medicine, Maebashi, Gunma, Japan
e-mail: tetsuyah92md@gmail.com

S. Matsuo
Department of Nuclear Medicine, Kanazawa University, Kanazawa, Japan
e-mail: smatsuo@med.kanazawa-u.ac.jp

C. Cheng
Shanghai Changhai Hospital, Shanghai, China
e-mail: 13501925757@163.com

Z. Jingping
The First Hospital of China Medical University, Shenyang, China
e-mail: zjp809302@163.com

J. Hashimoto · Y. Yamada · T. Kazama · T. Nomura · Y. Imai
Tokai University School of Medicine, Hiratsuka-shi, Kanagawa, Japan
e-mail: junhashi@tokai-u.jp; yy805443@tsc.u-tokai.ac.jp; kazamat@fg7.so-net.ne.jp; yh_4amm1208@yahoo.co.jp; imaiy@is.icc.u-tokai.ac.jp

X. Li
Department of Nuclear Medicine, The First Hospital of China Medical University, Shenyang, Liaoning Province, China
e-mail: lixuenacmunm@163.com

K. Kubota
Department of Radiology, Southern TOHOKU General Hospital, Koriyama, Fukushima, Japan
e-mail: kkubota@cpost.plala.or.jp

H. Toyama et al. (eds.), *PET/CT for Inflammatory Diseases*, https://doi.org/10.1007/978-981-15-0810-3_5

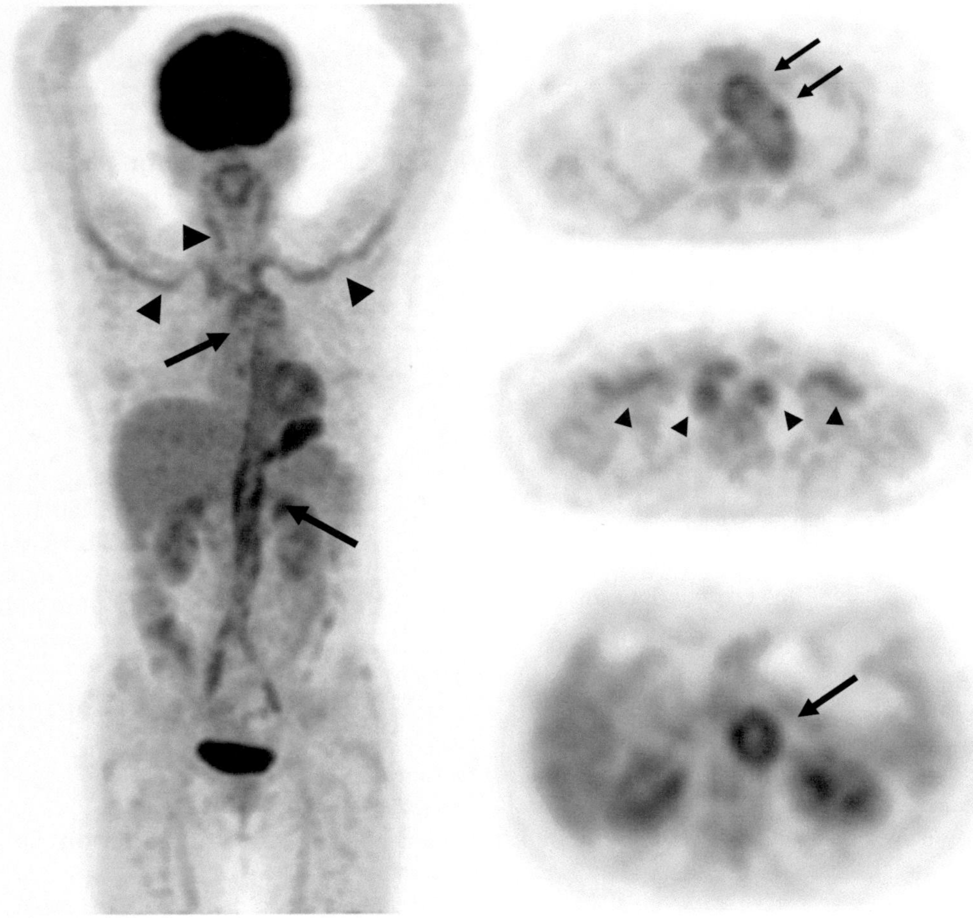

Fig. 5.1 Anterior MIP images of FDG-PET in a patient with Takayasu arteritis show F-18 uptake in the region of the ascending aorta, aortic arch, and abdominal aorta (arrows), as well as the right carotid artery and the right and left subclavian arteries (arrowheads). Axial PET images show FDG uptake in the walls of the thoracic and abdominal aorta (arrows) and its branches (arrowheads)

fatigue, malaise, weight loss, anorexia, fever, night sweats, and changes in inflammatory indices (e.g., C-reactive protein (CRP) levels and erythrocyte sedimentation rate (ESR)) [1]. This nonspecificity may lead to an extensive diagnostic workup and delay in diagnosis. LVV predominantly affects the large arteries and main branches; this disease includes two major variants, Takayasu arteritis (TA) and giant-cell arteritis (GCA). Although TA and GCA are different diseases with different ages of onset, these two diseases share inflammatory pathways, in which T lymphocytes and monocytes/macrophages play a main role. Due to histopathological similarity, arterial lesions in GCA and TA are challenging to distinguish. GCA is characterized by arterial injuries with female predominance, which affect the media with lymphocyte-monocyte transmural infiltration [2]. The incidence rate of GCA is estimated at 15–25 per 100,000 persons over 50 years of age, and the mean age of onset is 76 years [3]. Approximately 40% of patients with GCA have polymyalgia rheumatica (PMR) [4, 5]. TA is a rare granulomatous pan-arteritis, which also exhibits female predominance [6]. The incidence of TA has been estimated as 2 per one million persons, and the mean age of onset is 35 years. The disease occurs worldwide, but is most prevalent in Asia. TA can cause late complications including stenoses, occlusions, and aneurysms in the vessel; consequently, TA can be life-threating, leading to high mortality rates as high as 35% at 5 years after diagnosis [7].

Routine diagnostic procedures, including CT, MRI, and angiography, may yield inconclusive results for patients with LVV. FDG-PET imaging can detect increased metabolism and functional changes before morphological transformations become apparent. Thus, FDG-PET/CT is a useful tool in both inflammatory diseases and oncology. FDG-PET/CT can detect the onset of inflammation in the arterial wall by visualizing enhanced glycolytic activity of inflammatory cells [8] (Fig. 5.1). FDG-PET may be valuable for optimal diagnosis, monitoring of disease activity, and evaluation of damage progression in LVV [9]. Although there have been no guidelines on FDG-PET in LVV, a joint procedural recommendation regarding FDG-PET/CT imaging in LVV and PMR was made by several European and American associations and groups [10].

5.1.2 FDG-PET Protocol in LVV

The impact of high glucose level on FDG uptake in inflammatory lesions is not fully understood. One study

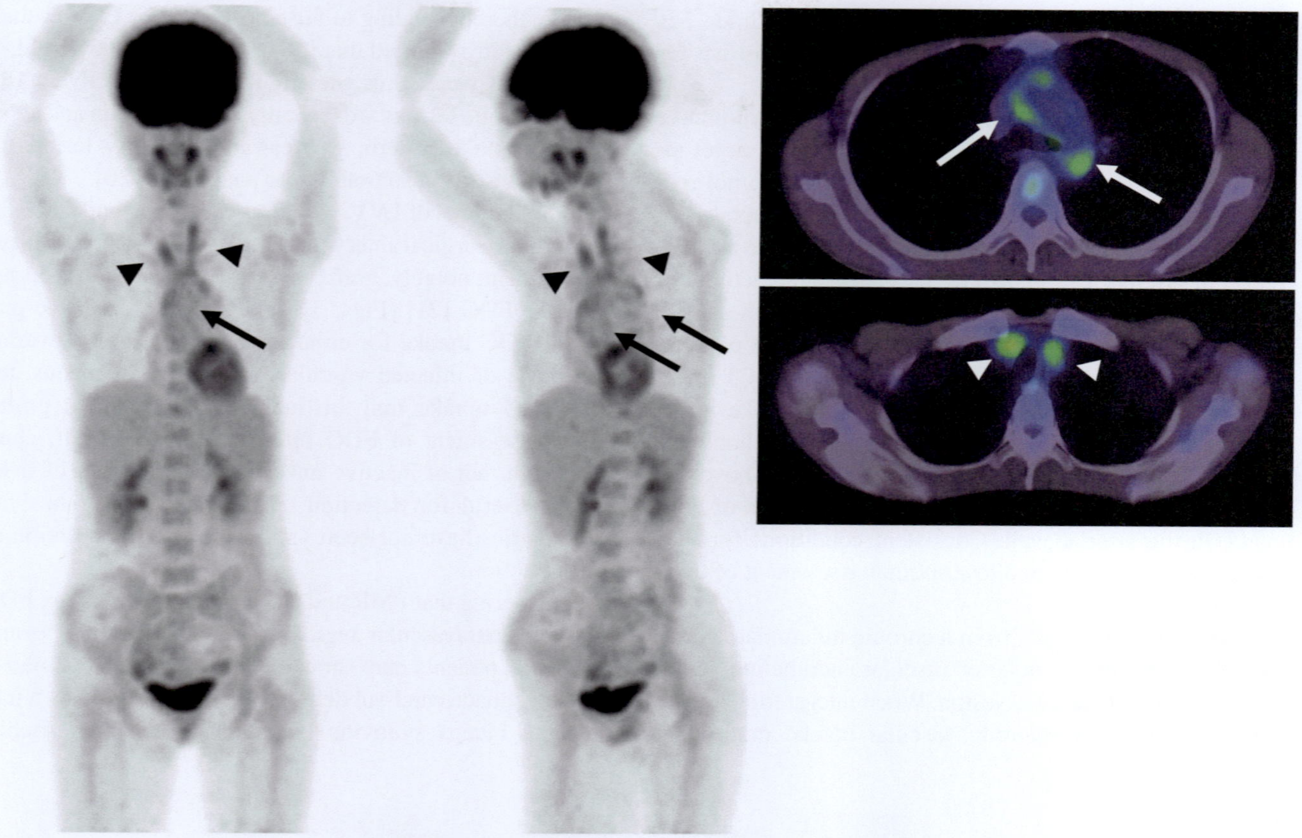

Fig. 5.2 Anterior MIP images of FDG-PET in a patient with Takayasu arteritis show F-18 uptake in the region of the ascending aorta and aortic arch (arrows), as well as the right and left carotid arteries (arrowheads). Axial fused F-18 PET/CT images show uptake in the aortic arch (arrows) and right and left carotid arteries (arrowheads)

reported that fasting glucose levels had a negative correlation with FDG uptake in the arterial walls, as well as positive correlation with blood pool activity [11]. To suppress mediastinal blood pool activity, which is an obstacle for the assessment of FDG uptake in the vessel walls, glucose levels below 7 mmol/L (126 mg/dL) are recommended [10].

Glucocorticoid (GC) is a mainstay of treatment for LVV: GC may decrease FDG uptake in the vessels, and thus FDG-PET should be taken within 3 days of the initiation of GC therapy. Moreover, GC can increase FDG uptake in the liver, leading to possible underscoring of FDG uptake after extended administration of GC [12]. Performing FDG-PET as early as possible and before the start of GC therapy is recommended if the clinical situation permits without critical symptoms [10].

Delayed acquisition at 2.5–3 h after FDG injection reportedly renders a detailed image of arterial wall uptake due to decreased blood pool activity [11, 13]. However, the evidence is insufficient to confirm that this is an appropriate time interval for LVV; currently, an uptake interval of at least 60 min is recommended [10].

Resolution of the PET scanner limits the detection of an inflammatory process in the vascular system to that within larger arteries. For high-resolution image reconstruction, the time-of-flight (TOF) reconstruction method is recommended. TOF imaging can depict vessels differently, relative to that in non-TOF imaging (Fig. 5.2). Thus, TOF settings should be carefully considered when interpreting PET images for LVV. PET scanners with semiconductor detectors, which have been shown to render high-resolution images, are expected to enable improved detection of arterial lesions.

5.1.3 Interpretation of FDG-PET in LVV

FDG-PET assessment of vascular disease can be challenging because FDG accumulates in the blood pool. For the interpretation of FDG-PET in patients with LVV, many criteria have been proposed for visual analysis and semiquantitative analysis. Among these methods, studies currently support the use of a visual grading scale (vascular to liver uptake), which is structured as follows: 0 = no uptake (≤ mediastinum); 1 = low-grade uptake (< liver); 2 = intermediate-grade uptake (= liver), 3 = high-grade uptake (> liver). Grade 2 is possibly indicative, and grade 3 is considered positive for active LVV [14, 15].

Several methods have been proposed for semiquantitative analysis, including basic SUV parameters and target-to-background ratio (TBR). Simple SUV metrics are not recommended because of the overlap between FDG uptakes of intact and inflammatory arterial walls [16, 17]. The normalization of arterial wall uptake to the background activity of the venous blood pool yields a good reference for assessment of vascular inflammation [12]. For the evaluation of treatment response, it is vital to compare baseline PET/CT imaging and posttreatment imaging. Slight FDG uptake in the region where a lesion was identified initially should be regarded as residual inflammation. As described above, the resolution of PET imaging can affect the depiction of FDG uptake in the arterial wall. Consistent conditions for PET imaging are preferable to allow optimal assessment of treatment response.

Atherosclerosis results from a chronic inflammatory process within the intimal layer of vascular endothelium and is the most common vascular lesion. When interpreting arterial FDG uptakes, atherosclerotic vascular uptake may be an obstacle, thereby leading to false positivity for LVV evaluation. One study reported that 9% of all plaques showed FDG uptake and were thus determined to be active [18]. Atherosclerotic lesions are typically skipped lesion and show a patchy uptake pattern, whereas inflammatory lesions of LVV demonstrate a smooth linear pattern [19, 20].

Complications of LVV, including aneurysm and stenosis, may require surgical intervention. Graft stenting is a possible treatment; notably, grafts themselves have been reported to uptake FDG [21] (Figs. 5.3 and 5.4). Although the patterns of FDG uptake for uninfected vascular grafts overlap with those of infected vascular grafts, heterogeneous and focal FDG uptake may be indicative of infected grafts. Visual assessment of FDG uptake within the graft, compared with that of inactive muscle and fat, or that of liver, may be useful for detection of infected grafts. Thus far, SUV metrics have not been validated for differentiation of graft infection.

Considering that PMR and GCA frequently overlap, FDG uptake in extravascular regions should be carefully examined. PMR patients may show FDG uptake in glenohumeral synovia, subacromial-subdeltoid bursa, supraspinatus tendinitis and biceps synovitis (shoulder), trochanteric/ischial

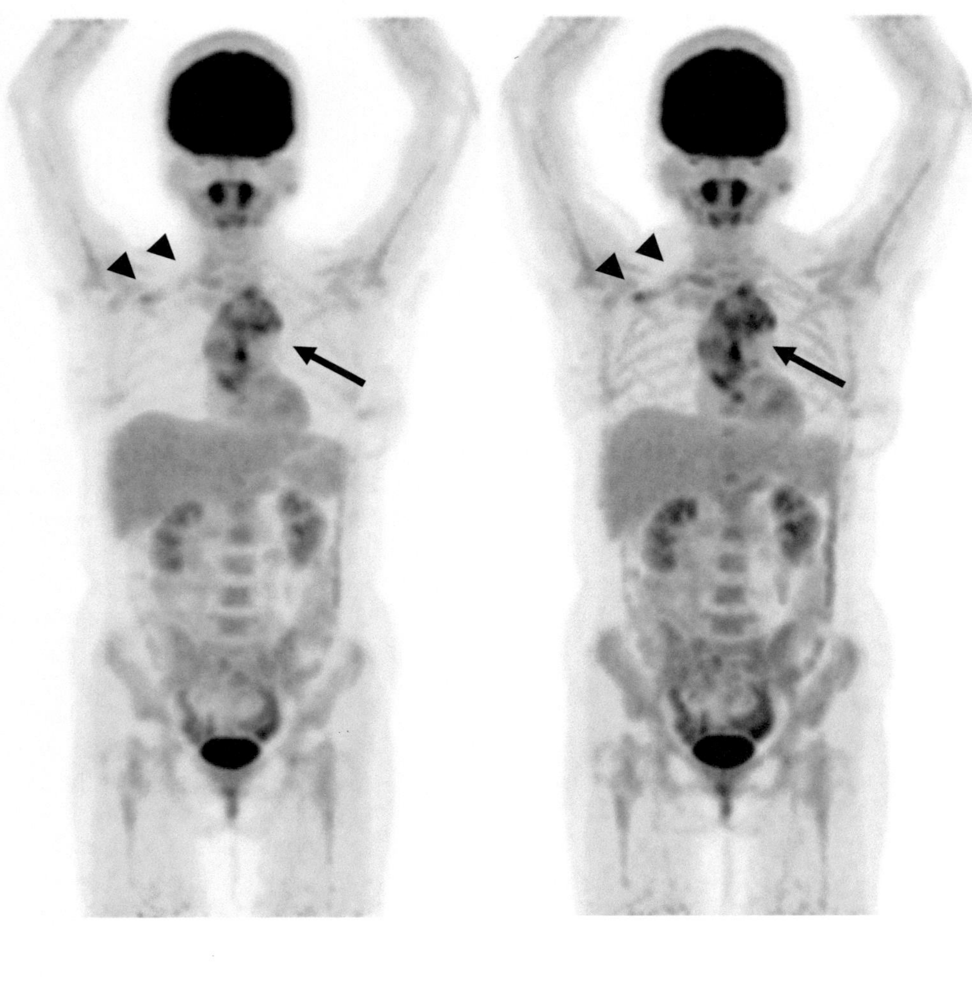

Fig. 5.3 Anterior MIP images of FDG-PET in a patient with Takayasu arteritis show F-18 uptake in the region of the ascending aorta, aortic arch, and right subclavian artery. The time-of-flight image (right) depicts FDG uptake more clearly than the image without time-of-flight (left)

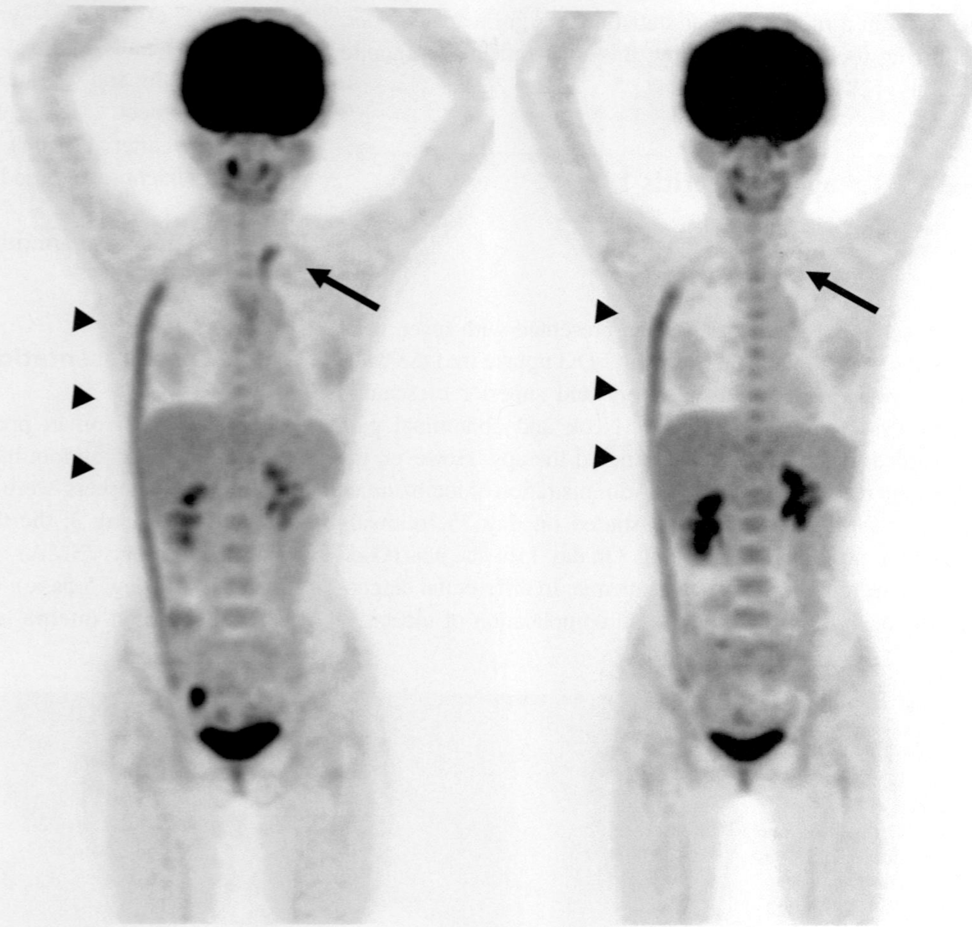

Fig. 5.4 Anterior MIP images of FDG-PET in a patient with Takayasu arteritis show F-18 uptake in the region of the left subclavian artery with active inflammation (left). After glucocorticoid therapy, this uptake disappeared (right). Note the uptake in the right subclavian to iliac artery graft, which does not change with treatment

bursa, hip synovia, interspinous regions of the cervical and lumbar vertebrae, or the synovial tissue of the knees [22, 23]. One study of 130 GCA patients reported that extravascular uptake was observed in 32, including 15 with coexisting vascular uptakes. Among 20 patients in that study, extravascular uptake was indicative of cancer in 5 (lung, colon, prostate, mandible, and uterus), subacromial bursitis in 8, colic polyps in 3, mediastinal lymphadenopathy in 2, uterus leiomyoma in 1, and benign nodule in the thyroid gland in 1 [24]. Among TA patients who underwent FDG-PET in our institution, extravascular uptake was detected in vertebra and thyroid glands (data not shown). Further studies are needed to verify the clinical significance of this uptake.

A previous meta-analysis of GCA patients evaluated by FDG-PET showed pooled sensitivity and specificity of 80% and 89%, respectively [25]. FDG-PET demonstrated pooled sensitivity of 87% and specificity of 73% for the assessment of disease activity in patients with TA [15]. However, there are several challenges related to the precise evaluation of the diagnostic accuracy of FDG-PET for the diagnosis of LVV. FDG-PET is affected by the delay of imaging after the initiation of GC therapy. Some patients cannot undergo diagnostic tests other than FDG-PET; this situation has thus far resulted in a lack of a gold standard. However, FDG-PET imaging is of considerable diagnostic value for LVV, based on the available data.

5.1.4 Treatment Response Assessment with FDG-PET for LVV

FDG-PET is considered to be useful for monitoring the treatment response because it can detect metabolic changes indicative of active or inactive disease before morphological changes become apparent on CT or MRI scans. The optimal interval of FDG-PET in PMR after treatment with GC remains unknown. A prior study found that the FDG-PET/CT score, based on the semiquantitative approach described by Meller et al. [26] (score < 3), remained positive for vasculitis after 3 days of GC treatment; however, it became negative after 10 days [27]. It is unclear whether GCA disease activity can be monitored by FDG-PET in patients receiving tumor necrosis factor α (TNF-α)-blocking agents for TA or interleukin-6 receptor blockade (tocilizumab) for GCA. In a study of the use of FDG-PET for the assessment of tocilizumab in patients with PMR, FDG uptake was shown to decrease in a moderate, but statistically significant manner, following tocilizumab therapy; this may reflect therapeutic response [28].

5.2 Takayasu Arteritis 1

Hajime Yoshifuji and Hideo Onizawa

Abstract An 18-year-old woman presented with fever, neck pain, and abdominal pain, showing FDG uptake into the walls of her right internal carotid artery and superior mesenteric artery (SMA) in FDG-PET/CT. Neck and abdominal pain responded to the initial glucocorticoid therapy. However, the neck pain reemerged on day 67. Administration of tocilizumab, an interleukin-6 inhibitor, was started on day 75 following which the neck pain disappeared. On day 116, she was hospitalized due to bloody stools and anemia. In differential diagnosis, the occlusion of the SMA and complication of ulcerative colitis were excluded by enhanced CT and colonoscopy, respectively. Finally, she was diagnosed as having a nonspecific enteropathy and was successfully treated with conservative management. Here, we discuss the characteristic distribution of arterial lesions, the efficacy of biologics, and the differential diagnosis of bloody stool in Takayasu arteritis.

Keywords: Takayasu arteritis, Mesenteric artery, CT, FDG, FDG-PET/CT

5.2.1 Case Presentation

An 18-year-old woman presented with fever, right neck pain, and lower abdominal pain to a medical center. Inflammatory markers were elevated: ESR 57 mm/h, CRP 4.4 mg/dL. On day 3, the thickened walls of her superior mesenteric artery (SMA) were highlighted as seen on enhanced CT (Fig. 5.5a–c). On day 5, FDG uptake into the walls of her right internal carotid artery (ICA) and SMA

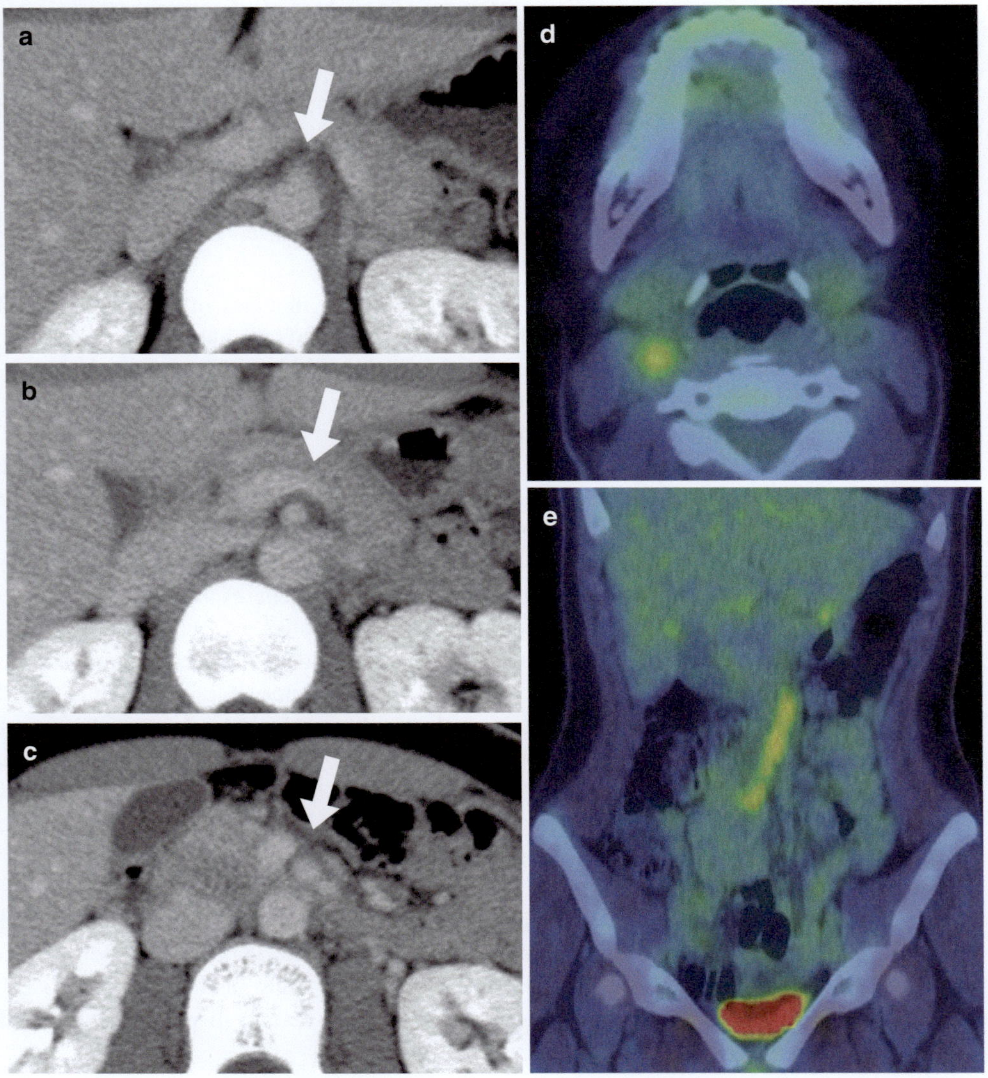

Fig. 5.5 (**a–c**) Horizontal sections of the superior mesenteric artery in the late phase of enhanced CT on day 3. (**d** and **e**) Horizontal section of the lower jaw (**d**) and coronal sections of the abdomen (**e**) in FDG-PET/CT on day 5

was detected using FDG-PET/CT (Fig. 5.5d, e). She was diagnosed with Takayasu arteritis, and 30 mg/day of oral prednisolone (PSL) was started on day 7 (Fig. 5.6). The neck and abdominal pain subsided on day 10. Inflammatory markers were reduced: ESR 17 mm/h, CRP 0.1 mg/dL. Low-dose aspirin and vonoprazan were initiated for prophylaxis of arterial occlusion and gastric mucosal injury, respectively. She was referred to our hospital on day 25, and the tapering of PSL was started.

She had fever on day 48, when the dose of PSL was 18 mg/day. The inflammatory markers were elevated again: ESR 32 mm/h, CRP 1.2 mg/dL. She was suspected of having an upper respiratory tract infection, and oral cephem (cefcapene) was administered from day 53 to 58. However, she felt intense neck pain on day 67. The series of symptoms were reconsidered as a relapse of Takayasu arteritis, and biweekly administration of tocilizumab (TCZ), an interleukin-6 inhibitor, was started subcutaneously on day 75. The neck pain disappeared promptly following the treatment, accompanied by a reduction of inflammatory markers.

On day 111, she felt faintness, and on day 116, she was hospitalized due to right abdominal pain and bloody stools. Progressing anemia without elevated inflammatory markers was noted: HGB 7.8 mg/dL, ESR 12 mm/h, CRP 0.1 mg/dL. Although vasculitic occlusion of the SMA was suspected, her SMA was patent in the early phase of enhanced CT (Fig. 5.7a–c). The thickened walls of the SMA were improved, compared to day 3. In colonoscopy, a punched-out ulcer and several small ulcers were detected in the terminal ileum (Fig. 5.7d, e) without any further findings in the whole colon. Cytomegaloviral (CMV) antigenemia and CMV-DNA in the mucosal samples were negative. Finally, she was diagnosed as having a nonspecific enteropathy. Tocilizumab, low-dose aspirin, and vonoprazan were discontinued. The bloody stools subsided only by conservative management without the use of antibiotics or antivirals. Iron supplements were started, and she was discharged from the hospital on day 129.

After the discontinuation of TCZ, glucocorticoid monotherapy was continued for the treatment of vasculitis. The tapering of PSL was resumed with careful observation for signs of relapse. On day 215, the terminal ileal ulcers were in a healing stage as detected on a follow-up colonoscopy. No further recurrences of vasculitis were observed until the last visit on day 340 (PSL 9 mg/day).

5.2.2 Discussion

Takayasu arteritis often occurs in young women. In histopathology, media of the aorta and large arteries are eroded by granulomatous inflammation [29], and the destruction of media causes remodeling of the arteries, namely dilation and stenosis, leading to outcomes such as aortic aneurysms, aortic regurgitation, myocardial infarction, cerebral infarction, and visual disturbance.

Fever and neck pain, which appeared first in the present case, are common symptoms during the onset of Takayasu arteritis [30]. Since a biopsy is difficult to perform in Takayasu arteritis, imaging is pivotal for the diagnosis of Takayasu arteritis. Especially, enhanced CT and ultrasound are used for screening, while FDG-PET/CT has shown high sensitivity and specificity [31]. In the present study, enhanced CT contributed to an early diagnosis, while FDG-PET/CT contributed to a definitive diagnosis of vasculitis.

Since vasculitic findings in ICA and SMA were detected by imaging in the present case, a differential diagnosis would

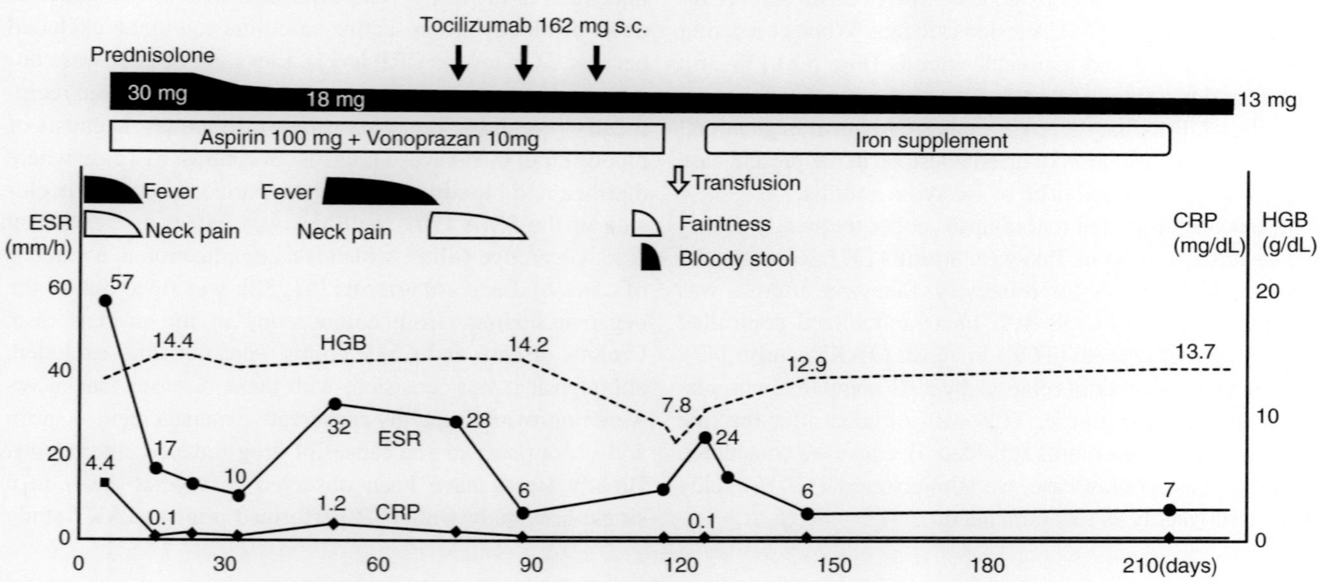

Fig. 5.6 The clinical course. Scale for erythrocyte sedimentation rate (ESR) is indicated on the left vertical axis. Scales for hemoglobin (HGB) and C-reactive protein (CRP) are indicated on the right vertical axis

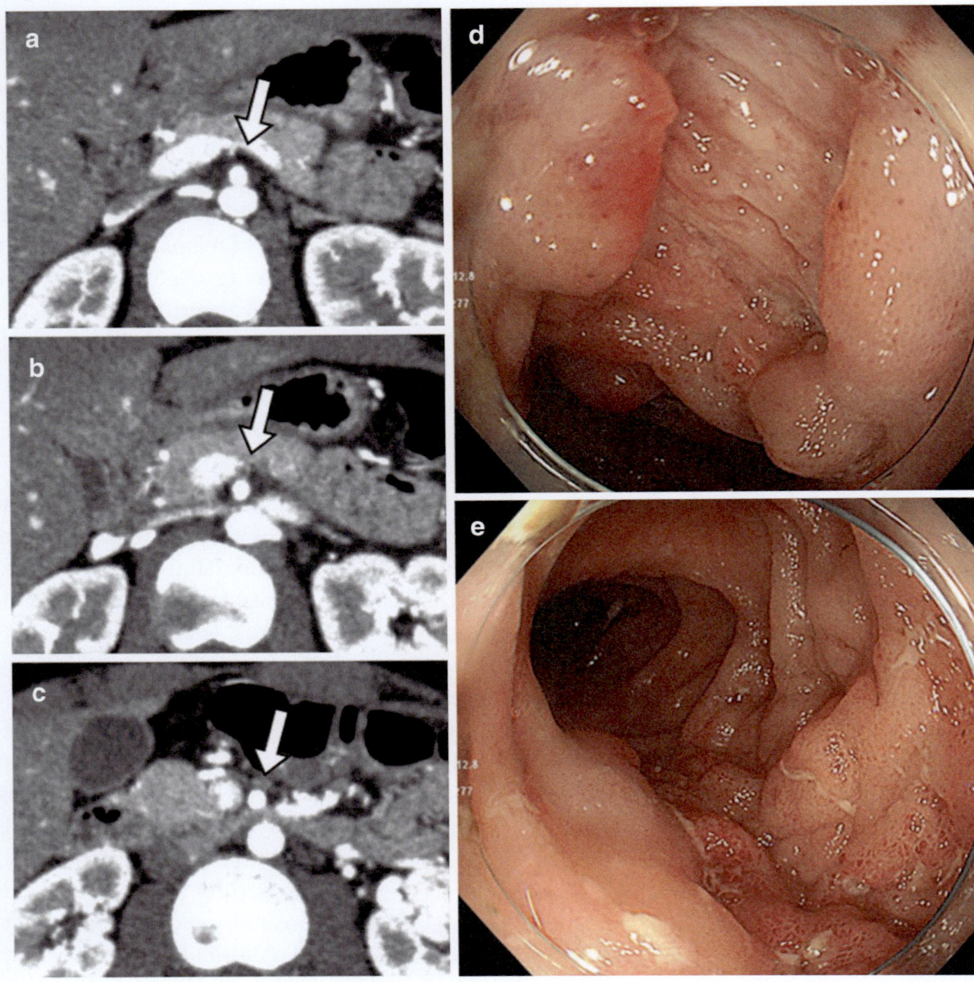

Fig. 5.7 (**a–c**) Horizontal sections of the superior mesenteric artery in the early phase of enhanced CT on day 116. (**d–e**) A punched-out ulcer (**d**) and multiple small ulcers (**e**) in terminal ileum on day 117

have been polyarteritis nodosa, Takayasu arteritis, and giant-cell arteritis. In polyarteritis nodosa, SMA branch lesions are frequent [32], although ICA lesions are rare. When comparing Takayasu arteritis and giant-cell arteritis (Fig. 5.8) [33–36], carotid and mesenteric artery lesions are frequent in Takayasu arteritis, while axillary artery lesions are frequent in giant-cell arteritis. The distribution of arterial lesions in the present case is considered a characteristic of Takayasu arteritis.

It has been reported that relapses occur frequently during the treatment course of Takayasu arteritis [37]. Recently, the efficacy of biologics for refractory Takayasu arteritis was reported (Table 5.1) [38–49]. In a randomized controlled trial using tocilizumab (TCZ) in Japan (TAKT study) [47], TCZ reduced the risk of relapses by 59% compared with placebo. In the present case, TCZ was initiated after the first relapse, and the symptoms subsided. Because we considered the relapse as a minor case, we administered TCZ biweekly instead of weekly as recommended.

In the present case, bloody stools appeared after three injections of biweekly TCZ. Although CRP was negative at onset of bloody stools, active vasculitis cannot be excluded because TCZ lowers CRP levels. Elevation of ESR was considered due to anemia, because ESR and HGB moved reciprocally (Fig. 5.6). Table 5.2 shows differential diagnosis of bloody stool in Takayasu arteritis. In contrast to a case where diarrhea and bloody stools were reported due to the occlusion of the SMA [50], the SMA was patent in the present case. Ulcerative colitis, which is a complication in about 6% of cases of Takayasu arteritis [51, 52], was ruled out by the negative findings from colonoscopy in the present case. Crohn's disease and CMV colitis were not fully excluded, although it is not consistent with these diseases that ulcers were improved simply by conservative management. Aspirin and vonoprazan can be causes of drug-induced enteropathy. Bloody stools have been observed in several cases in a single-arm study with TCZ performed prior to TAKT study

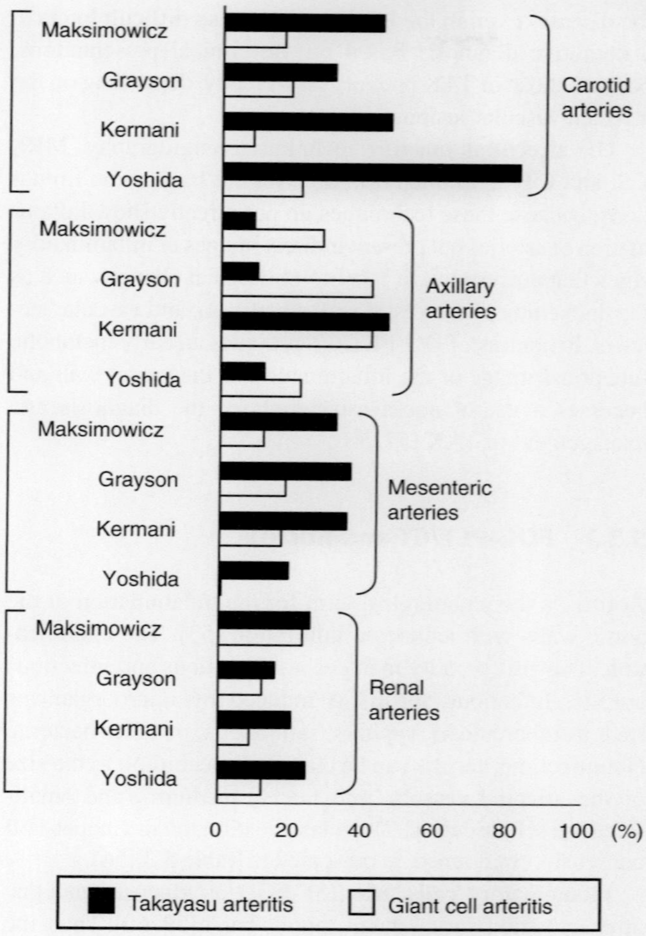

Fig. 5.8 Frequencies of various arterial lesions in the comparison between Takayasu arteritis and giant arteritis. Created from four reports [33–36]

(unpublished), so that the history of periodic melena is listed in the exclusion criteria of TAKT study [47] (Supplementary Materials). The mechanism of bleeding induced by TCZ is unclear, although it may be caused by an infection due to the immunosuppressive effects of TCZ.

In the present case, we have considered the tumor necrosis factor (TNF) inhibitors as possible next candidates of treatment after TCZ because TNF inhibitors have been reported to be effective for refractory Takayasu arteritis (Table 5.1) and are also effective for inflammatory bowel diseases. However, we have not used them since no relapses have occurred.

In conclusion, enhanced CT and FDG-PET/CT are useful in the diagnosis of Takayasu arteritis. Lesions in carotid and mesenteric arteries are characteristics of Takayasu arteritis. The efficacy of biologics for refractory Takayasu arteritis has been shown. Bloody stool in Takayasu arteritis should be carefully examined as it can be caused by various mechanisms.

Table 5.2 Differential diagnosis of bloody stool in Takayasu arteritis

Differential diagnosis	Causes	Backgrounds
Ischemic enteropathy	SMA, IMA stenosis	Vasculitic lesions of Takayasu arteritis
Inflammatory bowel diseases	Autoimmunity	Comorbidities of Takayasu arteritis
Infectious enteropathy	Virus, bacteria	Compromised state due to treatments or ischemia
Drug-associated enteropathy	NSAIDs, antibiotics, tocilizumab(?)	Medications
Nonspecific enteropathy	Unknown	Association with Takayasu arteritis is uncertain

IMA inferior mesenteric artery, *NSAID* nonsteroidal anti-inflammatory drug, *SMA* superior mesenteric artery

Table 5.1 Efficacy of biologics in Takayasu arteritis

Biologics	Design	Case no.	Outcomes	Author, year
IFX, ETN	Retrospective	15	Remission induction: 93%, remission maintenance: 67%	Hoffman, 2004
IFX, ETN	Retrospective	25	Remission induction: 88%, remission maintenance: 60%	Molloy, 2008
IFX, ETN, ADA	Retrospective	20	Remission induction: 90%, remission maintenance: 50%	Schmidt, 2012
IFX	Retrospective	5	Reduction of inflammatory markers, reduction of GC dose	Comarmond, 2012
IFX	Retrospective	11	Remission maintenance: 87%	Mekinian, 2012
IFX, ETN	Retrospective	32	Higher event-free survival rate compared with DMARDs group	Gudbrandsson, 2017
CZP	Retrospective	10	Reduction of activity score, reduction of GC/MTX dose	Novikov, 2018
TCZ	Single arm	4	Regression of inflamed arteries, reduction of GC dose	Nakaoka, 2013
TCZ	Retrospective	46	Higher event-free survival rate compared with DMARDs group	Mekinian, 2018
TCZ	Randomized controlled	36	Higher relapse-free survival rate compared with placebo group	Nakaoka, 2018
UST	Single arm	3	Alleviation of symptoms, reduction of inflammatory markers	Terao, 2016
ABT	Randomized controlled	34	No difference in relapse-free survival compared with placebo group	Langford, 2017

Created from 12 reports [38–49]

ABT abatacept, *ADA* adalimumab, *CZP* certolizumab pegol, *DMARD* disease-modifying antirheumatic drug, *ETN* etanercept, *GC* glucocorticoid, *IFX* infliximab, *MTX* methotrexate, *TCZ* tocilizumab, *UST* ustekinumab

5.3 Takayasu Arteritis 2

Yukio Sato, Masatoshi Itoh, and Takeshi Sasaki

Abstract Takayasu arteritis (TAK) is an intractable disease with an unidentifiable cause involving inflammation of the aorta and its major branches and, without an appropriate treatment, leads to fatal occlusive or aneurysmal degeneration of the arteries. However, the signs/symptoms of TAK patients vary greatly, depending on the vascular involvements, and markers of inflammation such as serum C-reactive protein (CRP) and erythrocyte sedimentation rate (ESR) are not specific for TAK. These conditions make definitive diagnosis difficult and delayed. Recently, FDG-PET/CT is playing an increasing role as a noninvasive tool for the diagnosis and management of TAK by providing an early metabolic functional image of the inflammation of the vessel wall that precedes morphological changes such as an aortic wall thickening or edema on MRI or CT.

Keywords: Positron emission tomography, Vasculitis, Takayasu arteritis, Giant-cell arteritis, Ulcerative colitis

5.3.1 Introduction

Takayasu arteritis (TAK), known also as pulseless disease, is a chronic progressive vasculitis of unknown etiology, predominantly affecting the aorta, its primary branches, the coronary arteries, and pulmonary arteries. TAK affects 2–3 patients per million per year in worldwide population, with predilection to young Asian female aged 15–20 years. In Japan, this disease is five to ten times more frequent among females than males [30, 53].

The early stage of TAK is manifested by nonspecific systemic symptoms/signs, such as fever, malaise, night sweats, weakness and pain, and increased levels of C-reactive protein (CRP) or erythrocyte sedimentation rate (ESR) [54]. In this stage, granulomas and infiltration of mononuclear cells occur in the adventitia and media. In the late stage of the disease, known as occlusive or pulseless phase, the prolonged inflammation of the aorta and its major branches causes progressive fibrosis of the arterial wall, leading to occlusive degeneration of the affected arteries [55, 56]. Less frequently, the inflammatory destruction of the media of vessel walls leads to aneurysmal dilatation of artery. These complications cause ischemic organ damages such as ischemic heart disease and/or aortic aneurysm and increase mortality. To prevent these complications, an early diagnosis and appropriate treatments of TAK are necessary. However, the diagnosis of aortitis remains a challenge because of its nonspecific symptoms and laboratory data in the early stage of the disease. Even in the late stage, it is also difficult to make a definitive diagnosis based on the clinical presentations, because those of TAK patients vary greatly, depending on the affected vascular lesions.

The structural imaging techniques (angiography, MRI, US, and CT) help diagnosis of TAK but have some limitations, because these techniques do not directly show inflammation of arteries but present indirect images of inflammatory signs that correspond to late morphological changes such as the thickening of the vessel wall, aneurysm, and vascular stenosis. In contrast, FDG-PET/CT provides an early metabolic functional image of the inflammation of the vessel wall and becomes a useful noninvasive tool for the diagnosis and management of TAK [57, 58].

5.3.2 FDG-PET/CT and Aortitis

Aortitis is the pathological term for the inflammation of the aortic walls with leukocyte infiltration [53]. The classification of aortitis broadly includes noninfectious and infectious aortitis. Infectious aortitis is induced by microorganisms such as tuberculosis, syphilis, salmonella, or other bacteria. Noninfectious aortitis can be classified, according to the size of the affected vessels, into large-, medium-, and small-sized-vessel vasculitis. This classification, as in Chapel-Hill consensus conference, is presented in Table 5.3 [56].

Inflammatory cells take 18F-FGD as glucose analogue after activation during the metabolic burst [59, 60]. Thus, the accumulation of 18F-FDG in activated inflammatory cells enables the imaging of inflammation. Hence, FDG-PET/CT can detect early inflammation of arteries that precedes morphological changes such as an aortic wall thickening or edema on MRI or CT. However, most PET/CT studies have focused on the visualized inflammation of the aorta and the larger arteries but not on the medium- and small-sized vasculitides due to the disadvantage of limited spatial resolution. TAK and giant-cell arteritis are the most common causes of

Table 5.3 Names for vasculitides adopted by the 2012 International Chapel Hill Consensus Conference on the Nomenclature of Vasculitides [56].

Large-vessel vasculitis (LVV)
Takayasu arteritis (TAK)
Giant-cell arteritis (GCA)
Medium-vessel vasculitis (MVV)
Polyarteritis nodosa (PAN)
Kawasaki disease (KD)
Small-vessel vasculitis (SVV)
Antineutrophil cytoplasmic antibody (ANCA)-associated vasculitis (AAV)
Microscopic polyangiitis (MPA)
Granulomatosis with polyangiitis (Wegener's) (GPA)
Eosinophilic granulomatosis with polyangiitis (Churg-Strauss) (EGPA)

large-vessel vasculitis and have been thoroughly studied using FDG-PET/CT.

In contrast to large-vessel vasculitis, vasculitis of medium and small vessels has been less thoroughly studied due to limited spatial resolution. However, there are sporadic reports on the use of FDG PET in a variety of vasculitides of small- and medium-size vessels such as polyarteritis nodosa [61], Wegener's granulomatosis [62], Churg-Strauss syndrome [63], or relapsing polychondritis [64]. PET technique has not been established as a reliable tool for the assessment of the medium and small-sized-vessel vasculitis. In summary, FDG-PET/CT is useful in noninfectious aortitis involving especially large vessels such as TAK (Fig. 5.9). It aids in diagnosis, differential diagnosis, the exclusion of other inflammatory diseases, and the identification of affected arteries.

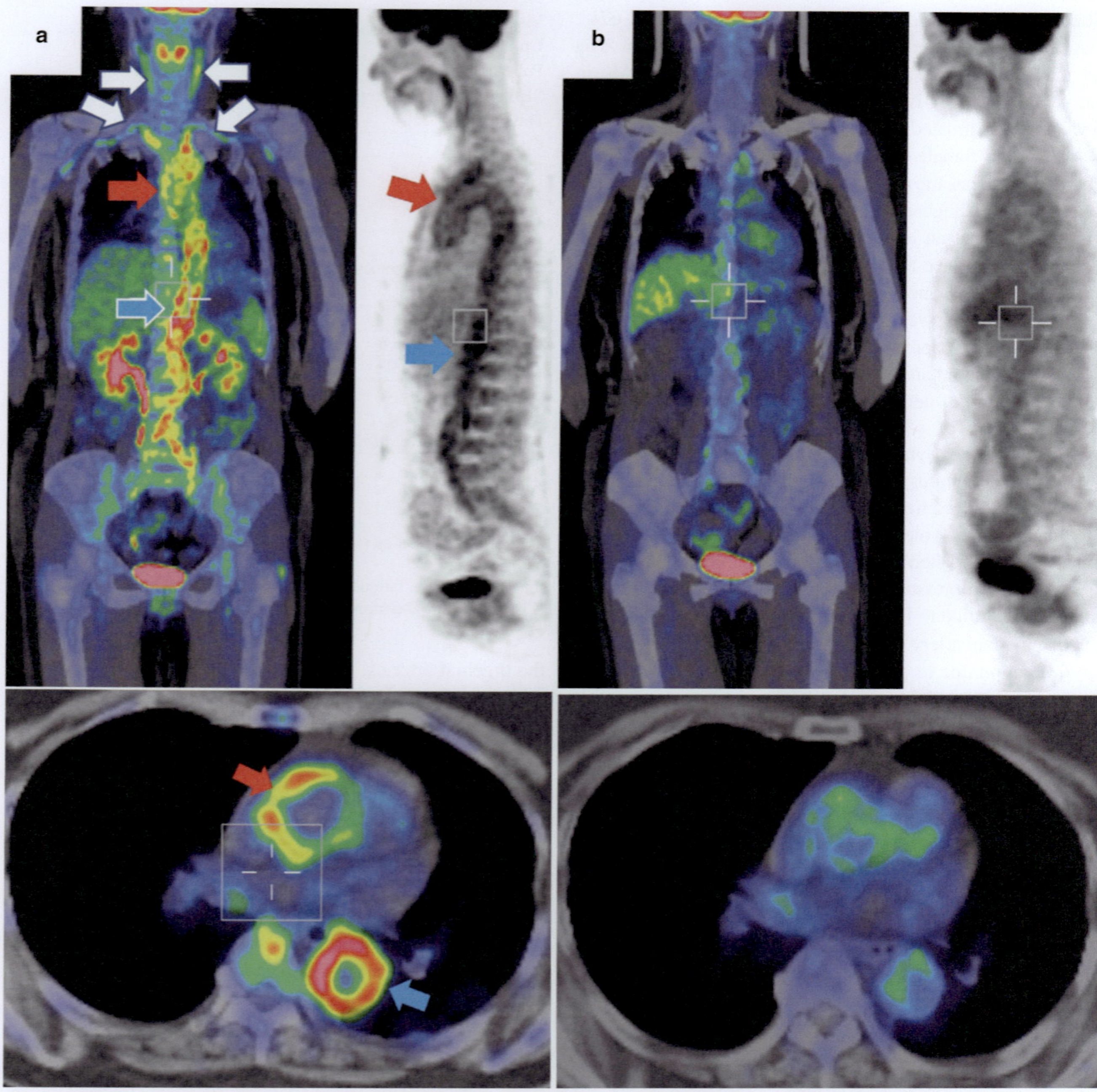

Fig. 5.9 Takayasu arteritis in a 62-year-old female patient. (**a**) FDG-PET/CT (coronal and axial slices) and PET (sagittal slice) images before treatment. High accumulation of FDG in the subclavian and carotid arteries (white arrows on coronal view) and the ascending (red arrows on coronal, sagittal and axial views) and descending aorta (blue arrows on sagittal and axial views). (**b**). FDG-PET/CT examination 4 months after treatment. Normalization of vascular metabolism is seen in the affected arteries and aorta

5.3.3 Takayasu Arteritis

TAK is a chronic progressive vasculitis of unknown etiology, predominantly affecting the aorta and its primary branches in women aged from 20 to 40 years. The age at onset of ≤40 years was an obligatory criterion in the first clinical diagnostic criteria suggested by Ishikawa [65]. The early onset is still a criterion used favorably for TAK diagnosis, the mandatory criterion of age was removed, because patients with elderly onset have recently been reported [30, 66, 67].

As for the global epidemiology, TAK is prevalent in Asia and the Middle East. The estimated incidence of TAK in Europe and the USA is 0.4–2.6 per million people, while the prevalence is estimated to be over 0.003% in Asian countries [68]. Although female patients tend to be predominant in all geographical areas, the percentage of female patients is highest in Japan. The pathogenesis of this disease remains elusive, but it is assumed that an autoimmunity targets the arterial wall, leading to progressive wall fibrosis, which ultimately results in luminal stenosis or aneurysmal formation since good clinical responses were observed in most patients treated with corticosteroids, immunosuppressive drugs, and biological agents.

The initial signs and symptoms of TAK include fever of unknown origin, neck pain, and generalized malaise (Table 5.4), all of which are nonspecific for TAK [30]. Subsequently, signs/symptoms due to vascular lesions develop, but the clinical features of TAK patients may differ, depending on the involved arteries. For example, stenotic lesions may often cause signs/symptoms of cerebral ischemia and visual impairment due to stenosis of branches of the aortic arch; difference in blood pressure between the right and left arms and lack of a pulse due to ischemia in the upper limbs; hypertension due to renal artery stenosis and aortic coarctation; pulmonary infarction due to pulmonary artery stenosis; and angina due to coronary ostial stenosis. Dilatated lesions may often cause aortic aneurysms/dissection and heart failure due to aortic insufficiency secondary to aortic annular dilatation. These nonspecific and various signs/symptoms make the definitive diagnosis of TAK difficult. If the diagnosis of TAK is delayed, as frequently occurs, vascular inflammation can progress, leading to stenosis, aneurysms, and end-organ ischemia. In a recent report, the median age at death of patients with TAK was 38 (25–47) years, especially due to vascular mesenteric ischemia and aortic aneurysm rupture [69]. Hence, early inflammation control and vascular injury relief are the crucial goals of TAK management.

Table 5.4 Details of chief complaints at onset of Takayasu aortitis in Japan (*n* = 1372) [30]

Head and neck, *n* (%)	365 (22.6)
Dizziness/vertigo	129 (9.4)
Headache	113 (8.2)
Syncope	36 (2.6)
Masseter claudication	5 (0.4)
Neck pain	133 (9.7)
Eyes, *n* (%)	45 (3.3)
Sight loss	2 (0.1)
Visual disorder	37 (2.7)
Upper limbs, *n* (%)	238 (17.3)
Pulselessness	67 (4.9)
SBP difference (≥10 mm Hg)	53 (3.9)
Fatigue	63 (4.6)
Coldness	23 (1.7)
Numbness	49 (3.6)
Heart, *n* (%)	153 (11.1)
Breathlessness	61 (4.4)
Palpitation	29 (2.1)
Feeling of chest tightness	21 (1.5)
Lung, *n* (%)	92 (6.7)
Hemosputum	11 (0.8)
Sensation of dyspnea	61 (4.4)
Hypertension, *n* (%)	54 (4.0)
Lower limbs,[a] *n* (%)	49 (3.6)
Body pain,[b] *n* (%)	218 (15.9)
Systemic manifestation, *n* (%)	562 (41.0)
Fever	476 (34.7)
Malaise	166 (12.1)
Fatigue	23 (1.7)

Data are expressed as *n* (% of 1372 patients). SBP indicates systolic blood pressure

[a]Leg claudication, fatigue, coldness, numbness, or pain

[b]Chest, back, or abdominal pain

5.3.4 FDG-PET/CT for Takayasu Arteritis

FDG-PET/CT is not a component of the criteria of American College of Rheumatology that included: (1) age at disease onset ≤40 years; (2) limb claudication; (3) pulse deficits over the brachial arteries; (4) blood pressure asymmetry between arms; (5) bruits over the subclavian arteries or aorta; and (6) angiographic abnormalities [70]. However, FDG-PET/CT may play a role in diagnosis, differential diagnosis, the exclusion of other causes of arteritis, and the identification of affected arteries (Fig. 5.9a).

Although MRI and CT help diagnosis by showing the early morphological changes such as the thickening of the vessel wall, FDG-PET/CT is more useful in the early diagnosis than these imaging techniques since FDG-PET/CT can detect metabolic changes that precede anatomical changes.

FDG-PET/CT allows differentiation between active and inactive TAK and is useful in the evaluation of disease activity. Usually, disease activity of TAK is assessed using conventional inflammatory markers such as a high ESR and CRP which reflect systemic inflammation. However, these markers are nonspecific for TAK, and immunomodulatory agents such as biologic agents can modify these parameters. In contrast, the accumulation of FDG that reflects the inflammation is specific for TAK activity. An example of active phase of TAK before treatment and 4 months after glucocorticoid treatment with some normalization of wall vessel activity is shown in Fig. 5.9. In the active phase of TA high uptake of 18F-FDG in PET/CT study is observed, whereas in inactive disease this uptake is decreased.

Estimation of the biodistribution of FDG is based on visual assessment or/and semiquantitative analysis, for example, by evaluating the maximum standardized uptake value (SUV_{max}). Tezuka et al. proposed the cutoff values of $SUV_{max} \geq 2.1$, CRP > 0.2 mg/dL, and ESR ≥ 19 mm/h for active stage TAK [71]. FDG-FDG-PET/CT was shown to be high sensitivity for detecting active diseases during immunosuppression [72]. It was also reported that FDG-PET/CT could identify the distribution of inflammation in some TAK patients with inactive stage according to the NIH criteria [73, 74]. Taken together, FDG-PET/CT may be useful in guiding therapy and in assessing the response to immunosuppressive therapy.

TAK is often associated with ulcerative colitis, which is an inflammatory bowel disease [75]. This complication affects the treatment and prognosis of patients with TAK since anticoagulants used for stenosis of arteries may promote the bleeding from the inflamed colonic mucosa. Since FDG-PET/CT facilitates the detection of remote sites of inflammation, FDG-PET/CT can also be useful in the diagnosis of ulcerative colitis by visualizing the affected colon. Hence FDG-PET/CT is recommended for the diagnosis of TAK and detection of its complications. In summary, FDG PET/CT is useful in early diagnosis of TAK. Moreover, it is helpful for evaluating disease extent and activity, detecting the remote inflammatory lesions, monitoring the response to therapy, and evaluating therapeutic effectiveness.

5.4 Takayasu Arteritis 3

Tadashi Watabe

Abstract A 59-year-old female patient with Takayasu arteritis showed increased uptakes in the left common carotid, bilateral subclavian, and right brachiocephalic arteries on FDG-PET; in contrast, no significant uptake was observed in the thoracic or abdominal aorta. Contrast-enhanced CT revealed aortic dissection in the abdominal aorta. According to a previous study, high uptakes are usually observed in the thoracic or abdominal aorta in Takayasu arteritis. However, involvement of the carotid, left subclavian, and mesenteric arteries is a typical finding of Takayasu arteritis.

Keywords: Takayasu arteritis, Aortic dissection, Fever of unknown origin

5.4.1 Clinical Presentation

A 59-year-old woman presented with fever of unknown origin and an elevated white blood cell level count. The patient showed no response to antibiotic treatment. Upper gastrointestinal endoscopy revealed a duodenal ulcer with bleeding.

5.4.2 Key Images

5.4.3 Technique

- Patient preparation: the patient was instructed to fast for 4 h before administration of radiopharmaceutical.
- Approximately 227 MBq of ^{18}F-FDG was administered intravenously.
- Imaging device: Whole body PET/CT camera (GE Discovery710) with resolution of 4.9 mm FWHM.
- Image reconstruction: 3D OSEM(Vue Point FX), TOF(+), PSF(+), Iteration: 8, Subset: 3, Gaussian Filter: 4 mm, FOV: 700 mm, matrix: 192∗192.

5.4.4 Image Interpretation

Increased uptake was observed in the right bilateral subclavian and right brachiocephalic arteries (Fig. 5.10) and in the left common carotid artery (Fig. 5.11, right). No significant uptake was observed in the thoracic or abdominal aorta. Uptakes in the abdominal area were considered to be on account of inflammatory lesions, as there was no tumor evident in the previous contrast enhanced CT.

5.4.5 Differential Diagnosis

- Arteriosclerosis
- Vascular Behcet's disease
- Syphilitic mediasmiths
- Giant-cell arteritis

5.4.6 Diagnosis and Clinical Follow-ups

This patient showed negative results of tests for antinuclear antibody and infectious diseases, and was diagnosed as having Takayasu arteritis (type V), as there was an aortic dissection in the abdominal aorta. The patient was treated with steroids and antihypertensive drugs.

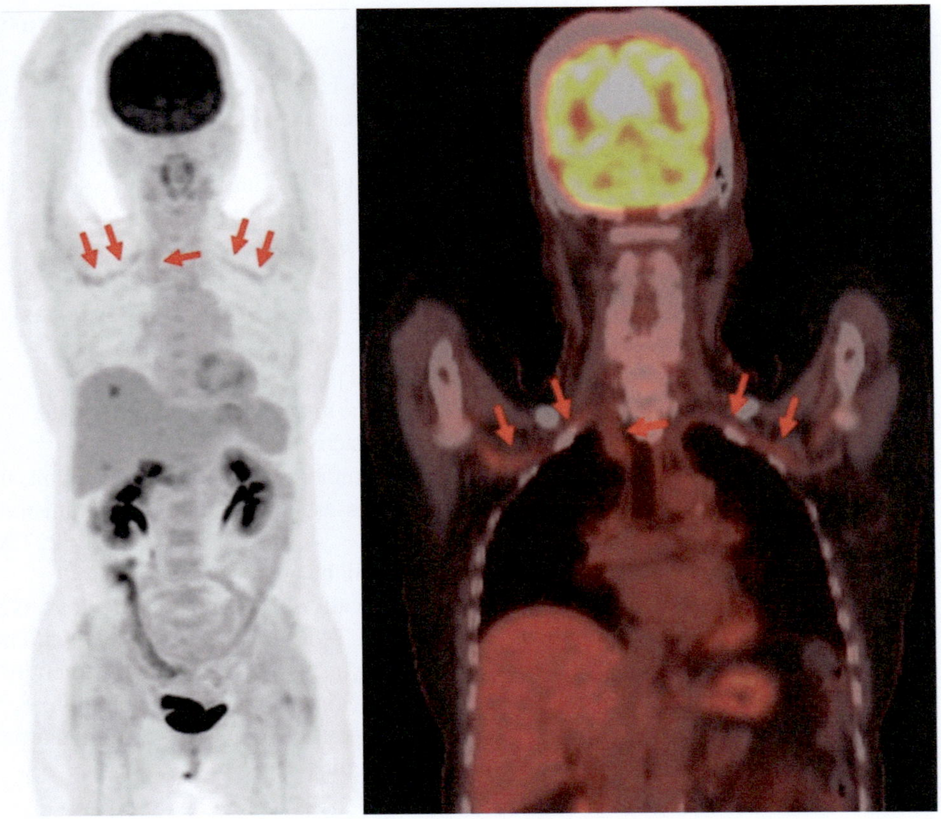

Fig. 5.10 Maximum-intensity projection image of FDG-PET (left) and coronal fused PET/CT image (right) showing increased uptake in the arteries

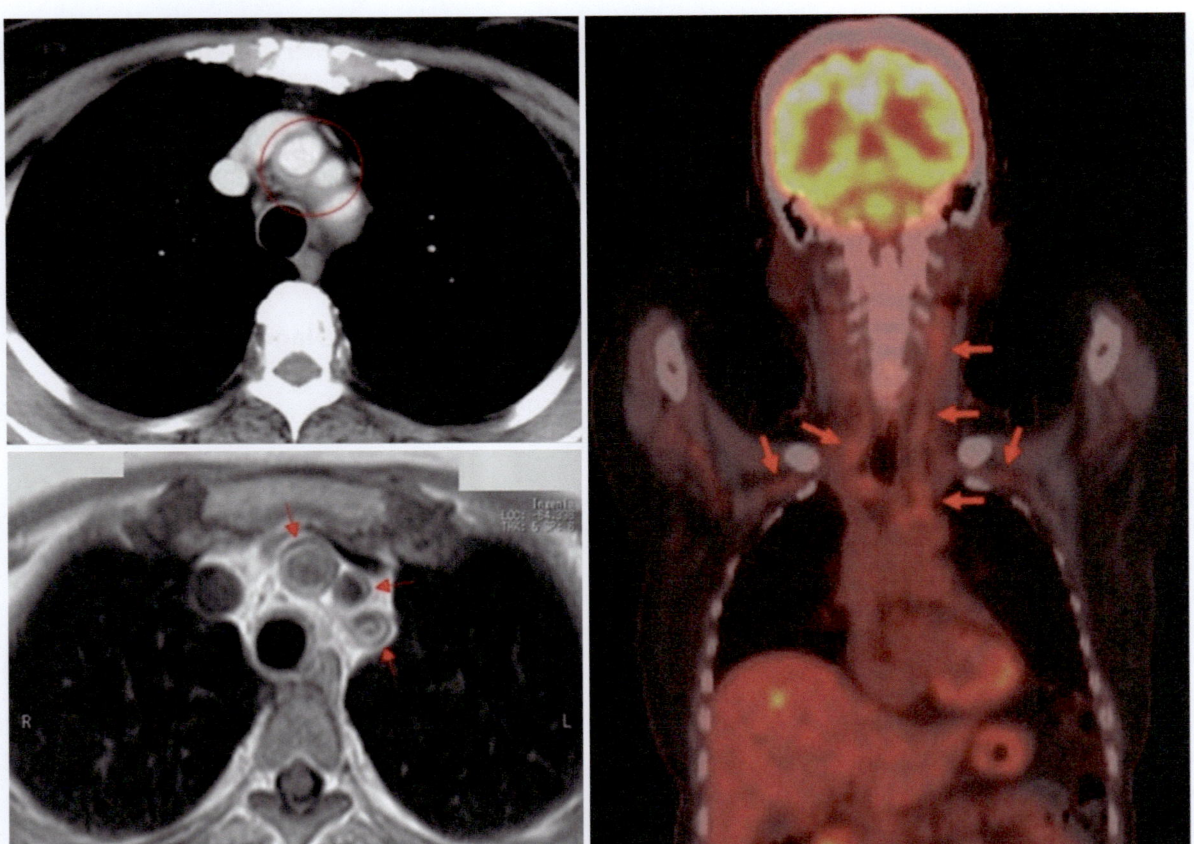

Fig. 5.11 Contrast-enhanced CT and MRI (left) images showing wall thickening and mild enhancement in the right brachiocephalic artery and left common carotid artery. Fused FDG-PET/CT images revealed mildly increased uptake in the arteries

5.4.7 Discussion

In this patient, no significant uptake was observed in the thoracic or abdominal aorta, while mildly increased uptakes were observed in the left common carotid, bilateral subclavian, and right brachiocephalic arteries. According to previous reports, high uptakes are usually observed in the aorta in Takayasu arteritis [76]. However, involvement of the subclavian artery and carotid artery is a typical finding [77].

5.5 Takayasu Arteritis 4

Tetsuya Higuchi

Abstract Takayasu disease is an idiopathic systemic granulomatous disease of large- and medium-sized vessels that may lead to vascular lesions such as segmental stenosis, occlusion, dilatation, and aneurysm formation in the aorta and its main branches [78]. It is well known that about 70% of the patients with Takayasu disease undergo recurrence of active aortitis after treatment with steroids; therefore, aggressive surveillance is important. The use of FDG-PET/CT in the patient with suspected large-vessel aortitis including Takayasu disease has recently been included in Japanese medical insurance coverage and the localization of active arteritis has become easier [79].

Keywords: Takayasu disease, FDG, Inflammatory activity

5.5.1 Clinical Presentation

Male aged 50s, developed left common iliac artery (CIA) stenosis and treated with endovascular treatment. Follow-up CT and first FDG-PET/CT indicated the clinical diagnosis of Takayasu aortitis, and oral prednisolone of 20 mg dose was started and tapered to 2.5 mg after 5 months. Fever up and back pain was noted.

5.5.2 Key Images

Figures 5.12–5.14.

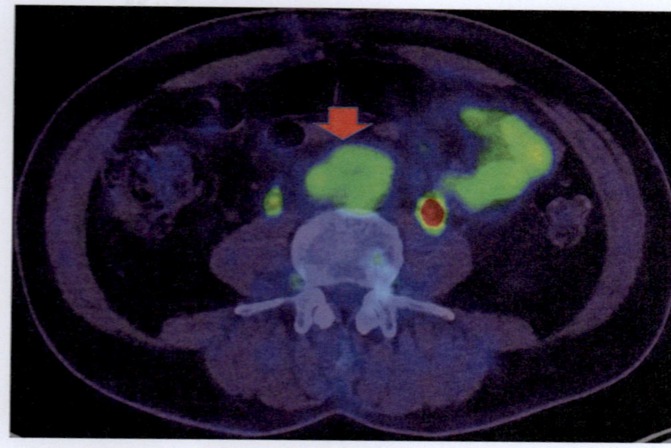

Fig. 5.12 Base line FDG-PET/CT axial image

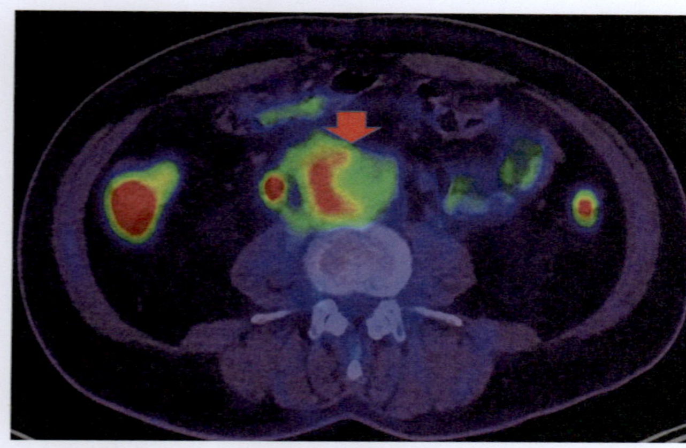

Fig. 5.13 FDG-PET/CT axial image during follow-up

5.5.3 Technique

- Patient preparation: patient should not take anything except water without sugar for more than 6 h before administration of FDG.
- 5 MBq per kg (Body weight) of FDG administered intravenously using automatic injector.
- Imaging device: Whole body PET/CT camera (Siemens Biograph mCT Flow64) with a 780 mm field of view, continuous bed motion of 1.3 cm/min for body stem and 2.0 cm/min for head. Image reconstruction with matrix size of 200, iterations 2, subsets 21, Gaussian filter and CT condition of slice thickness of 2 mm, 120 kV, 70mAs, CARE Dose 4D.

5.5.4 Image Interpretation

Initial axial image of abdominal aortic wall (Fig. 5.12), just above the bifurcation to common iliac arteries, showed slightly increased FDG uptake (SUV_{max}: 2.9). Follow-up FDG PET (Figs. 5.13 and 5.14) showed increased FDG uptake (SUV_{max}: 6.6) in the right abdominal aortic wall, suggesting reactivated abdominal aortitis.

5.5.5 Differential Diagnosis

- Inflammatory abdominal aortic aneurysm
- Bacterial aneurysm
- Atherosclerosis

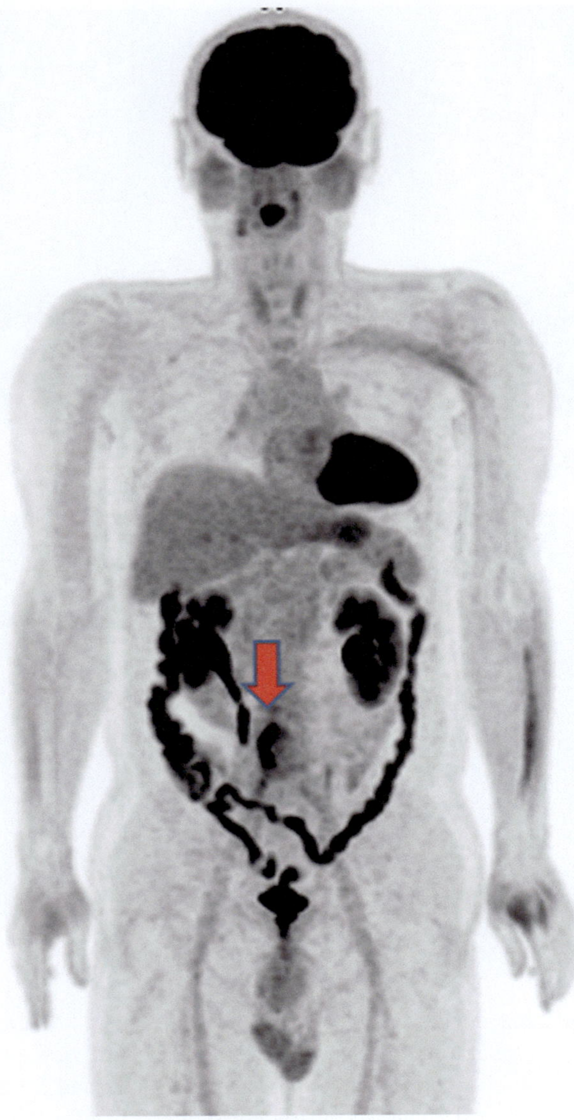

Fig. 5.14 FDG-PET MIP image

5.5.6 Diagnosis and Clinical Follow-ups

Follow-up FDG-PET/CT (Figs. 5.13 and 5.14) showed the severely increased FDG uptake in the abdominal aorta (arrow). Enhanced CT image (Fig. 5.15) showed progressively enlarged abdominal aortic lumen and high density component in the right adjacent tissue (arrow), suggesting imminent rupture of abdominal aortic aneurysm.

5.5.7 Discussion

Reactivation of Takayasu disease can induce severe complication like rupture of aortic aneurysm shown in this case. Monitoring of inflammatory activity by CRP or clinical symptom is sometimes inaccurate during steroid treatment.

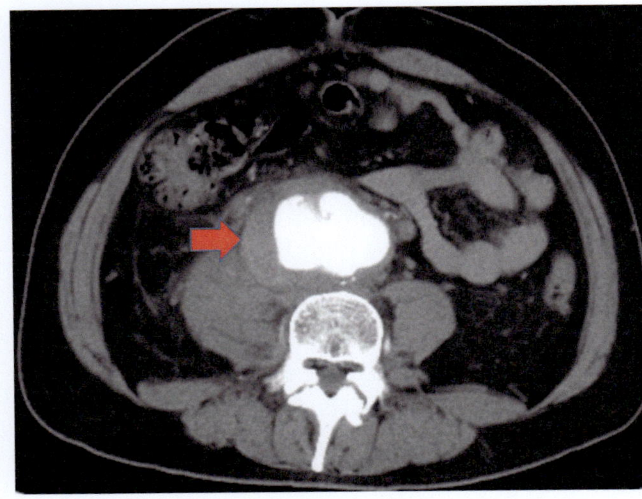

Fig. 5.15 Enhanced abdominal CT image

Additional finding in FDG-PET/CT can be used as a useful monitoring tool for early detection of severe complication.

5.6 Takayasu Arteritis 5

Shinro Matsuo

Abstract Aortitis syndrome (Takayasu arteritis) is a chronic nonspecific panarteritis involving the aorta and its main branches. Flureine-18-labeled 2-denxy-2-fluoro-D-glucose (FDG) positron emission computed tomography combined with computed tomography (PET/CT) has been proven to be useful in diagnosing and monitoring disease activity in Takayasu syndrome. A FDG-PET scan of a 43-year-old woman could make a direct assessment of the locality of the disease activity of her ascending aorta. The FDG-PET/CT scan demonstrated a vascular inflammation of the patient, confirming a diagnosis of Takayasu aortitis. It is fast becoming a reliable tool for the evaluation of patients with Takayasu vasculitis.

Keywords: FDG, Takayasu disease, CPR, Ascending aorta, PET

5.6.1 Clinical Presentation

The patient was a 43-year-old woman admitted with fever and a cool sensation in her right upper limb. She had also noticed a general fatigue over the previous 3 months and described weakness and decreased energy levels. Laboratory examination indicated that anemia was present (hemoglobin 8.5 g/dL). The serum level of C-reactive protein (CRP) was elevated (1.9 mg/dL; normal range: up to 0.3 mg/d). The ESR was prolonged (ESR; 102 mm/h; normal: 15 mm/h).

5.6.2 Key Images

5.6.3 Technique

- A FDG PET/CT was conducted. 185 MBq of FDG was administered intravenously.
- Patient preparation: patient was advised not to swallow anything for 6 h before administration of the radiopharmaceutical.
- Imaging device: whole body PET/CT camera (GE) with resolution of 5.0 mm FWHM.

5.6.4 Image Interpretation

The FDG-PET/CT demonstrated high-level radiolabel uptake along the arterial wall of the ascending aorta (Fig. 5.16). The images showed an accumulation of the tracer along the wall of the ascending aorta (SUV_{max}: 3.1) in a patient with Takayasu disease.

5.6.5 Differential Diagnosis

- Giant-cell arteritis.
- Polyarteritis nodosa.
- Buerger's disease.
- Syphilic aortitis.

5.6.6 Diagnosis and Clinical Follow-ups

The FDG-PET scan demonstrated a vascular inflammation of the patient confirming a diagnosis of Takayasu aortitis. The patient was treated with prednisone (20 mg/day). The fever subsided several days after the steroid administration. Then all symptoms improved after the treatment.

5.6.7 Discussion

FDG-PET/CT is a sensitive, noninvasive technique for the diagnosis of Takayasu disease [80]. CRP concentration only moderately reflects the FDG PET vascular positivity in Takayasu syndrome [81]. FDG-PET could make a direct assessment of the locality of the disease activity and displays increased FDG uptake in the inflamed artery wall. It is fast becoming a reliable tool for the evaluation of patients with Takayasu vasculitis [82].

5.7 Giant Cell Arteritis 1

Chao Cheng

Abstract Giant-cell arteritis (GCA) is the most frequent systemic vasculitis in patients over 50. Arteritis of the temporal arteries, which are one of the preferential sites in GCA, results in headache, jaw claudication, scalp tenderness, and

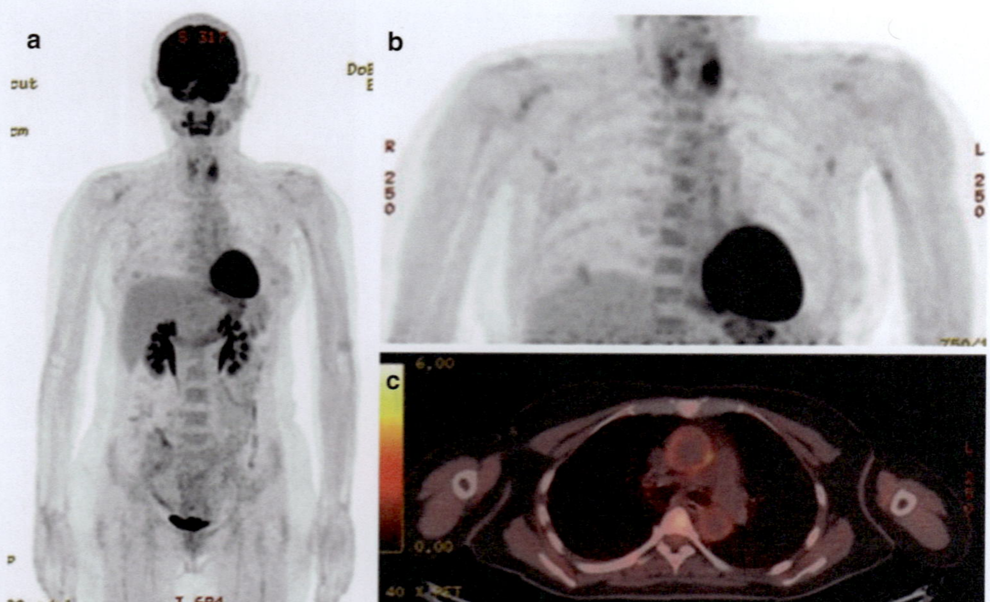

Fig. 5.16 FDG-PET/CT scan in a delayed phase. FDG uptake in the ascending aorta is observed. (**a**), early image; (**b**) delayed image; (**c**) PET/CT

visual impairment. Involvement of the aorta is rarely symptomatic, but its diagnosis could help lead to GCA diagnosis. Aortic CT angiography (CTA) was the first and most frequently used procedure to demonstrate large-vessel involvement. In recent years, 18F-fluorodeoxyglucose (FDG) positron emission tomography (FDG-PET/CT) has also shown the ability to demonstrate large-vessel vasculitis. Recent studies have demonstrated the value of PET for the diagnosis of aortitis in GCA patients, and this method seems to be very sensitive (Hommada M, et al. Autoimmun Rev. 2017;16(11):1131–1137; de Boysson H, et al. Eur J Nucl Med Mol Imaging. 2017;44(13):2274–2279).

Keywords: Giant-cell arteritis, FDG, PET/CT

5.7.1 Clinical Presentation

A 51-year-old female known with weakness for more than 10 months, fever for more than 2 months. The body temperature rises more regularly, about 38–38.5 °C. Laboratory examination found: ESR, 140 mm/H; CRP, 94.80 mg/L; WBC, 7.74 × 10^9/L; Hb, 64 g/L; PLT, 677 × 10^9/L.

5.7.2 Key Images

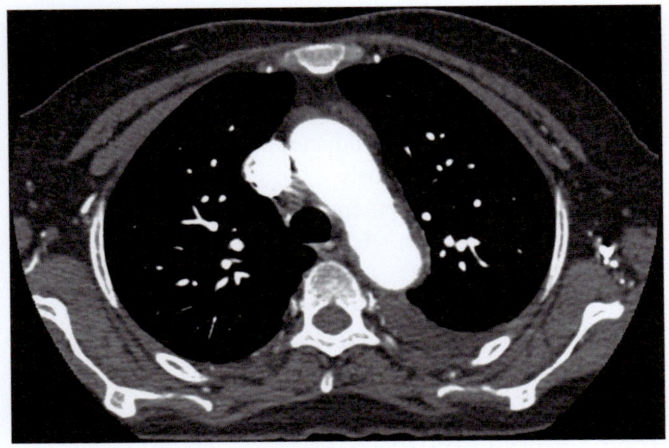

Fig. 5.18 Contrast-enhanced CT image

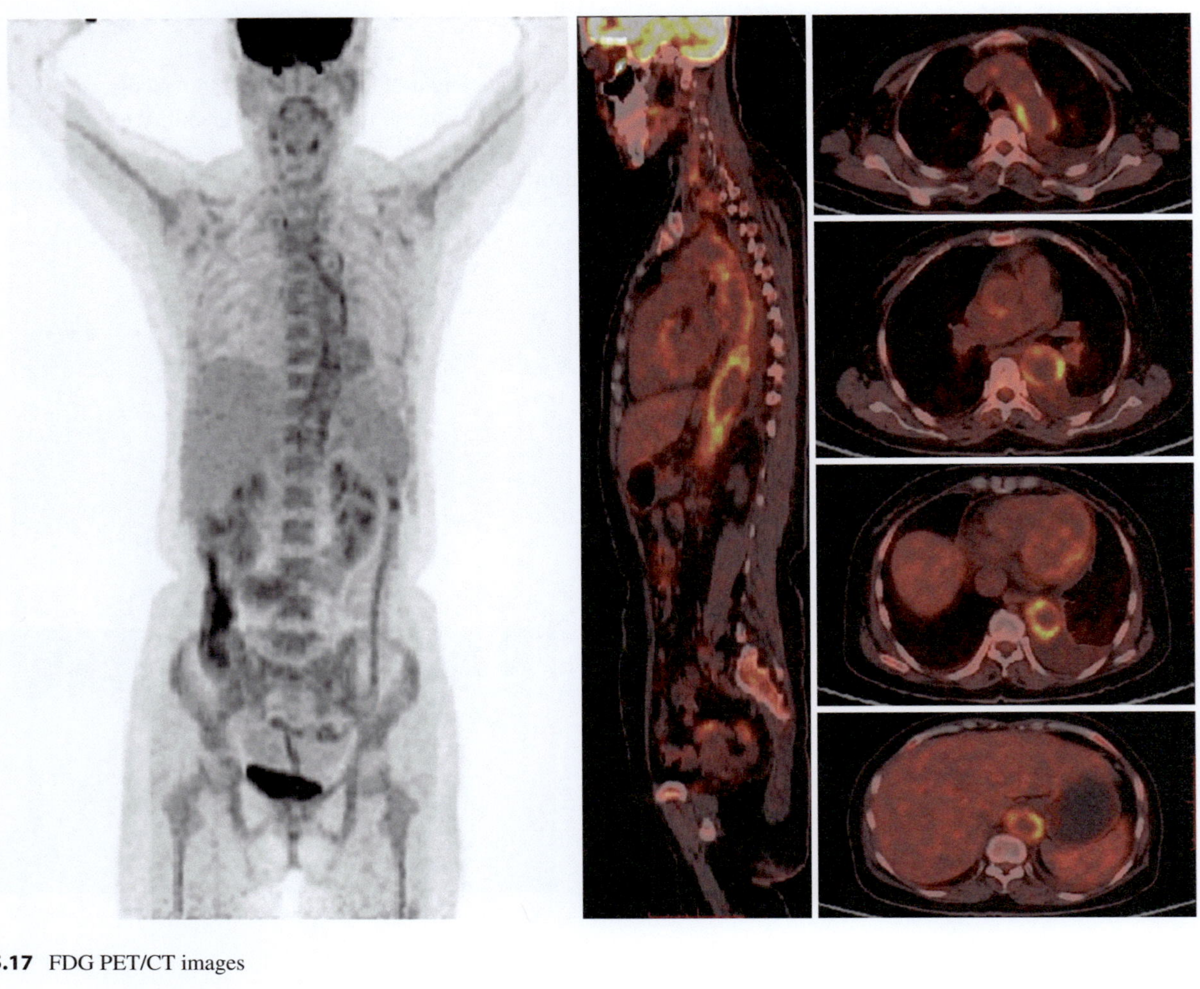

Fig. 5.17 FDG PET/CT images

5.7.3 Technique

- Patient preparation: patient should not take anything by mouth for 6 h before administration of radiopharmaceutical.
- 320 MBq of 18FDG administered intravenously (Body Weight = 53Kg).
- Imaging device: whole body PET/CT camera (Siemens biograph 64) with resolution of 4.0 mm FWHM,

5.7.4 Image Interpretation

18F-FDG PET/CT images (Fig. 5.17) demonstrate the aortic arch, thoracic aorta, and abdominal aortic wall increased uptake of FDG (SUV_{max} = 4.7). Thoracic aorta CT enhancement angiography (Fig. 5.18) show aortic arch vessel wall is uneven.

5.7.5 Differential Diagnosis

- Henoch-Schonlein.
- Takayasu arteritis.

5.7.6 Diagnosis and Clinical Follow-ups

Supplementary medical history suggested the patient had an intermittent headache and mandibular joint pain about 10 months ago. The patient received prednisone and hydroxychloroquine therapy and recovered promptly.

5.7.7 Discussion

Imaging tools are mainly helpful in the diagnosis of incomplete clinical forms of the disease, especially when temporal artery biopsy (TAB) fails to demonstrate vasculitis. Aortic CTA can demonstrate changes in the morphology of large vessels, such as wall thickening, vessel stenosis or thrombosis, or aortic dilation or dissection. FDG PET/CT identifies morphological and metabolic changes in large vessels, and vascular inflammation can appear as homogeneous and linear vascular FDG uptakes [9, 83, 84].

5.8 Giant Cell Arteritis 2

Jingping Zhang

Abstract A 65-year-old woman had fever 2 years ago, presenting persistent low fever, accompanied by headache and temporomandibular joint pain. The diagnosis was giant-cell arteritis. Two months ago she found that tumor markers elevated. Reexamination every half a month indicated that CA724 gradually increased. PET/CT showed increasing metabolism shadow of right brachiocephalic vein, left subclavian artery and abdominal aortic wall and hepatic cyst.

Keywords: ^{18}F-FDG PET/CT, Giant-cell arteritis, Fever

5.8.1 Clinical Presentation

A 65-year-old women had fever 2 years ago, accompanied by headache and temporomandibular joint pain, anti-infective therapy was not effected. Then she had a diagnosis of "giant-cell arteritis" at Union Medical College Hospital. Two months ago, due to fever and pneumonia, she was found CA724 rising in the hospital. Reexamination every half a month indicated that CA724 gradually increased. Loss of weight, no fever, no other symptoms were observed.

5.8.2 Key Images

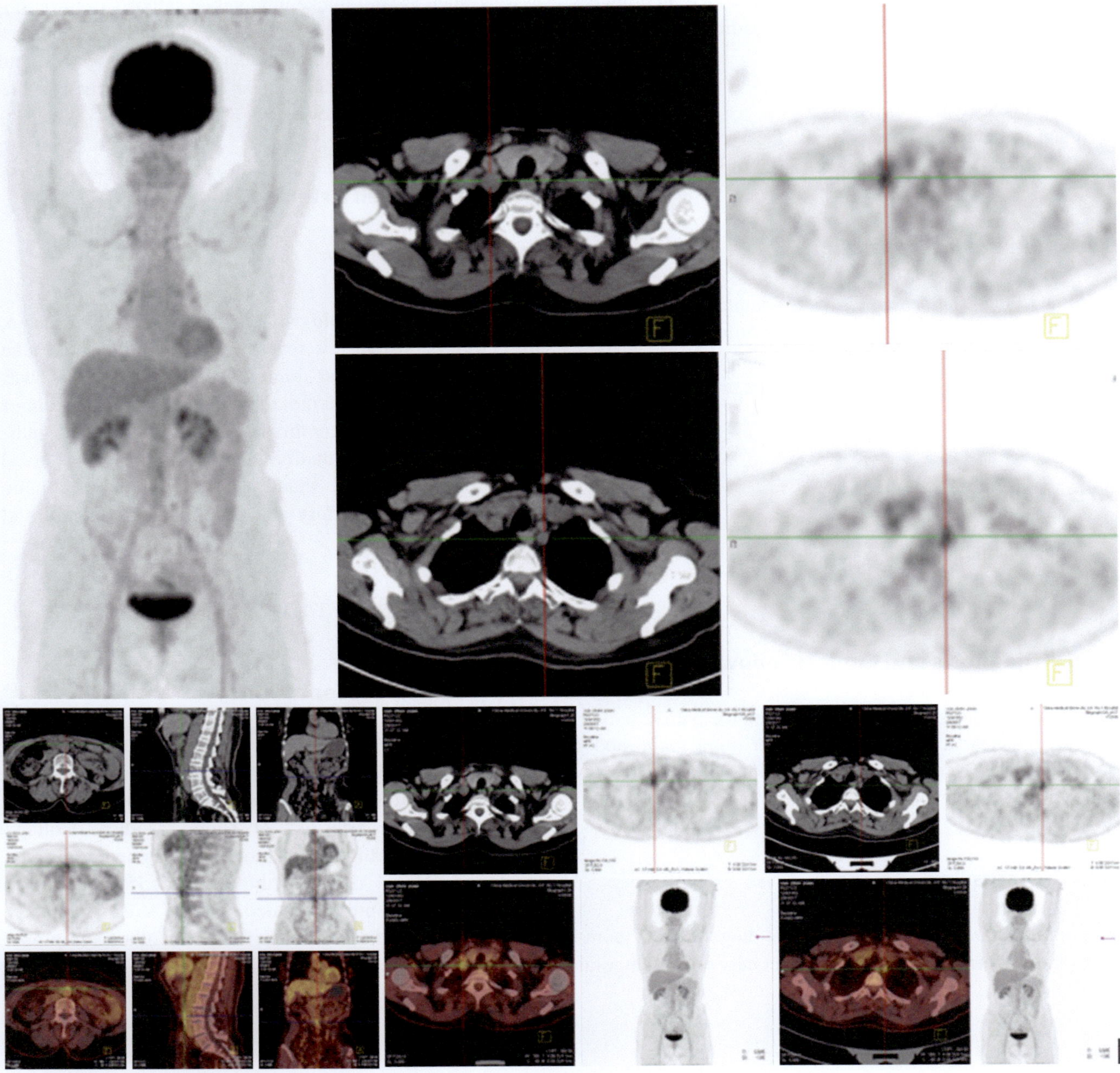

Fig. 5.19 Increased metabolism shadow of right brachiocephalic vein, left subclavian artery, and abdominal aortic wall

Fig. 5.20 Middle lobe of right lung has linear shadows, nodules in upper lobe of left lung, no metabolism increase. Increasing metabolism of double hilar lymph node

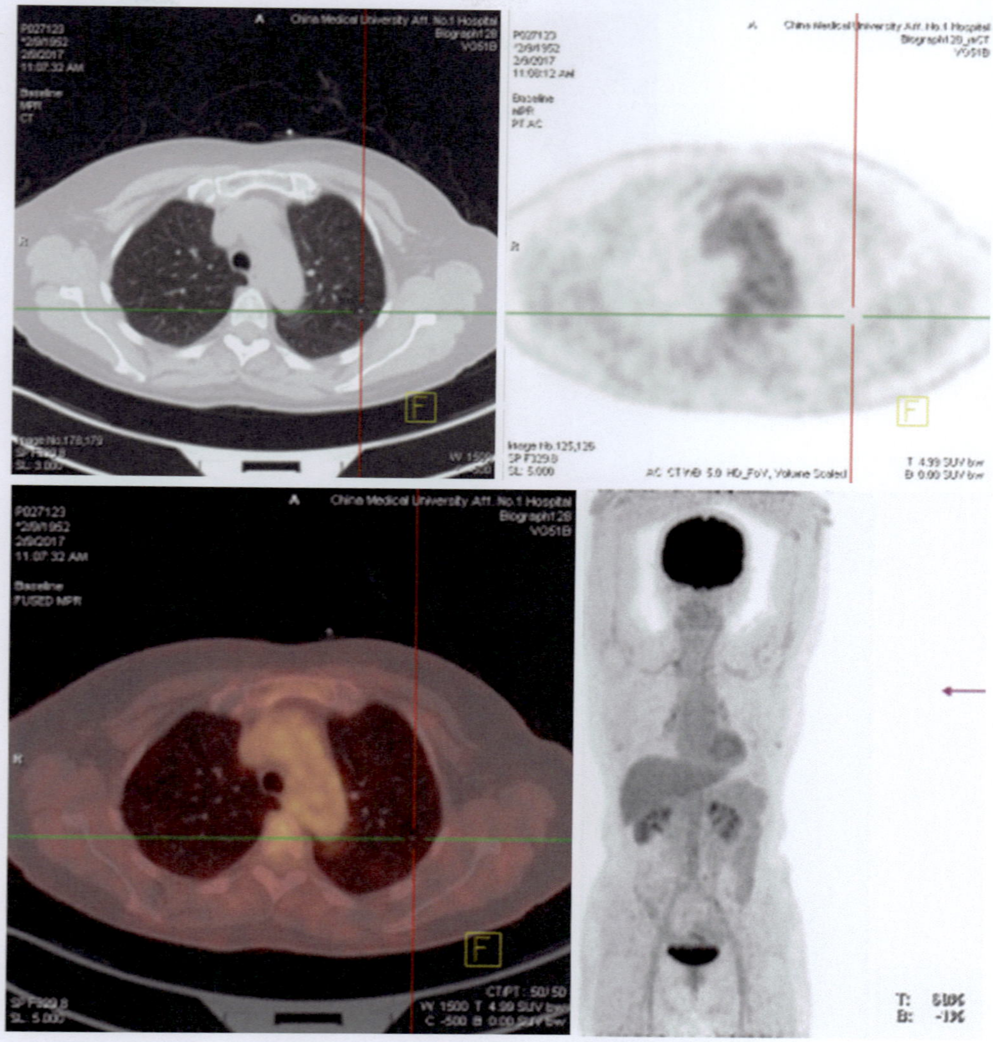

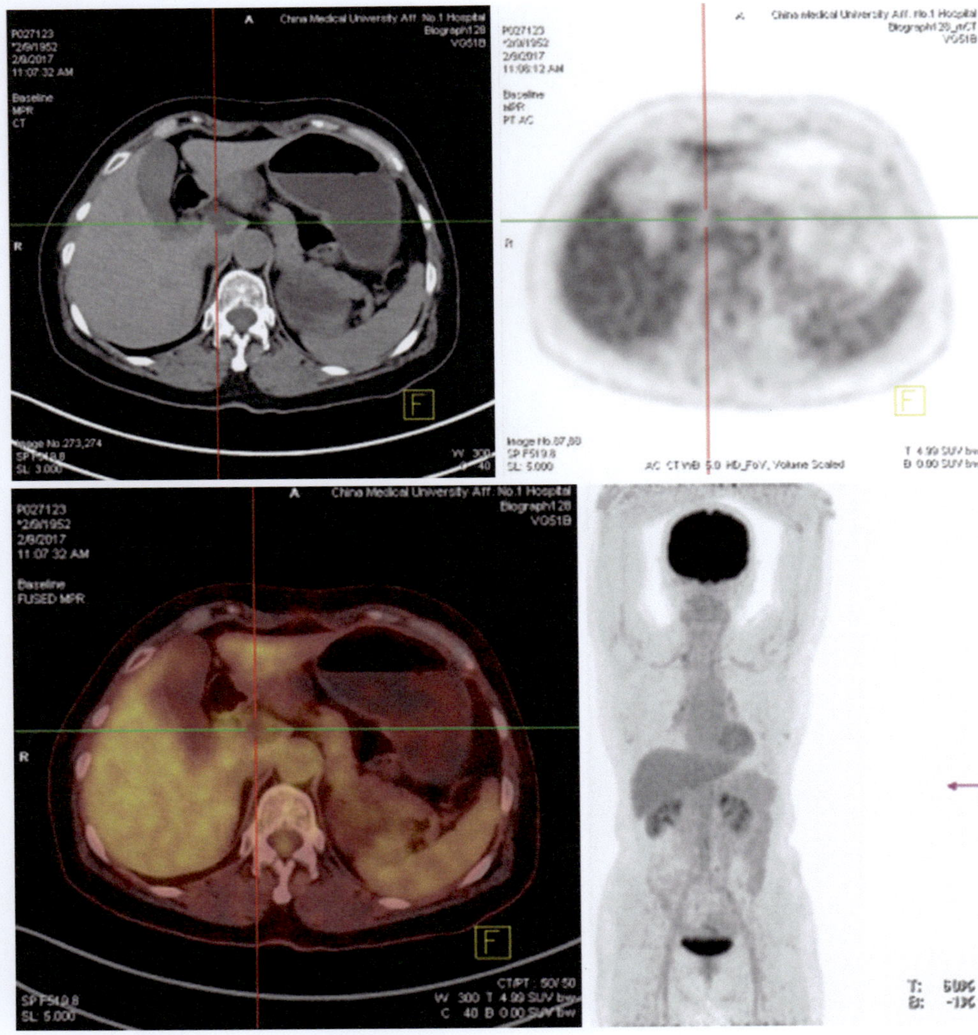

Fig. 5.21 Hepatic cyst

5.8.3 Technique

- Patient preparation: patient should not take anything by mouth for 6 h before administration of radiopharmaceutical.
- 185 MBq of ^{18}F-FDG administered intravenously.
- Imaging device: Whole-body PET/CT scanning was performed using Siemens biograph mCT scanner with resolution of 5.0 mm FWHM.

5.8.4 Differential Diagnosis

- Polyarteritis nodosa,
- Wegener granuloma,
- Hypersensitivity vasculitis.

5.8.5 Diagnosis and Clinical Follow-ups

Diagnosis of "giant-cell arteritis" at Union Medical College Hospital was performed using Hormone and Tripterygium wilfordii. Two months ago the patient was hospitalized for fever and found CA724 increased. PETCT was performed to determine the cause of increasing tumor markers. PET/CT showed the increasing metabolism shadow of right brachiocephalic vein, left subclavian artery and abdominal aortic wall and hepatic cyst.

5.8.6 Discussion

The advantage of 18FDG PET/CT scan of giant-cell arteritis is that it can comprehensively detect the lesions, accurately locate and judge the benign and malignant lesions, so it can detect the lesions early, quickly, accurately, and comprehensively.

5.9 Giant Cell Arteritis 3

Jun Hashimoto, Yuri Yamada, Toshiki Kazama, Takakiyo Nomura, and Yutaka Imai

Abstract We present a case of giant-cell arteritis (GCA) associated with polymyalgia rheumatica (PMR) who underwent ^{18}F-FDG-PET/CT twice before and after steroid therapy. The case is a female in her 60s. Her symptoms were fever, joint pain, and mandibular pain during chewing. Values of CRP and ESR increased. Temporal artery biopsy revealed GCA. ^{18}F-FDG-PET/CT was performed twice before and after steroid therapy. First PET showed increased FDG uptake in the walls of arteries, joints, and vertebrae, which disappeared after steroid administration. FDG-PET/CT is useful to assess the sites and activities of inflammation and therapeutic effects.

Keywords: FDG, PET/CT, Giant-cell arteritis, Polymyalgia rheumatica, Therapeutic effect

5.9.1 Clinical Presentation

The case is a female in her 60s. She suffered from common cold, and after that she felt pain in shoulder and knee joints. Subsequent symptoms comprised fever and mandibular pain during chewing. Increased values of CRP and ESR were also observed. She underwent steroid therapy.

5.9.2 Key Images

5.9.3 Technique

- Patient preparation: patient should not take anything by mouth except water for 5 h before administration of radiopharmaceutical.
- 185 MBq of ^{18}F-FDG administered intravenously.
- Imaging device: whole body PET/CT camera (TruePoint Biograph 16 (Siemens Medical Solutions, Knoxville, TN)) with resolution of 5 mm FWHM.

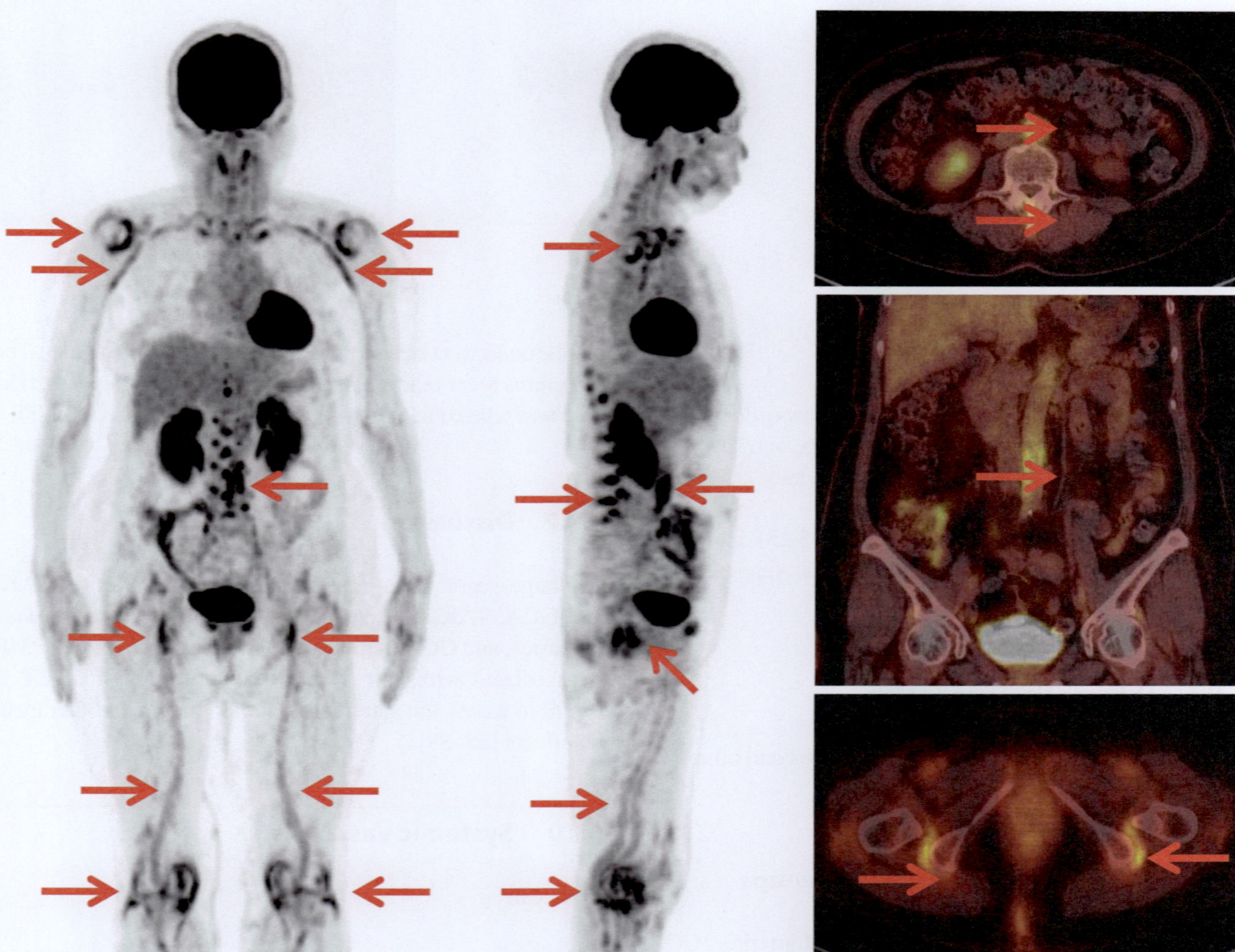

Fig. 5.22 ^{18}F-FDG-PET/CT images before therapy

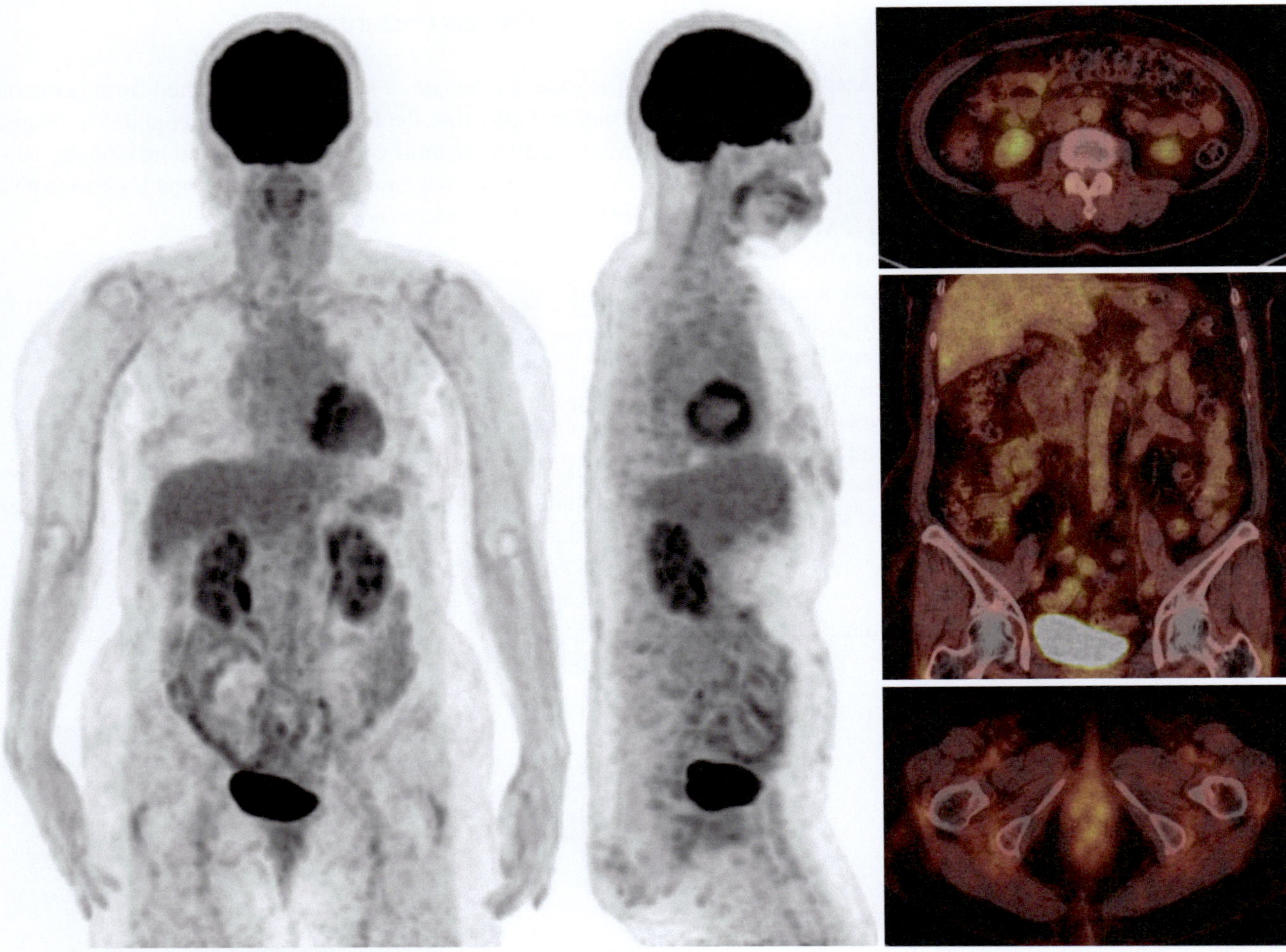

Fig. 5.23 ^{18}F-FDG-PET/CT images after therapy

5.9.4 Image Interpretation

Images before therapy (Fig. 5.22, red arrows) demonstrate increased tracer uptake in the walls of aorta, subclavian and femoral arteries, joints (shoulder, hip and knee), vertebrae, and ischiogluteal bursa.

The second PET after therapy (Fig. 5.23) manifested decreased FDG uptake in the above sites, suggesting the therapeutic effect.

5.9.5 Differential Diagnosis

- Large-vessel vasculitis (giant-cell arteritis and others).
- Collagen diseases.

5.9.6 Diagnosis and Clinical Follow-ups

Temporal artery biopsy revealed giant-cell arteritis (GCA). The symptoms and laboratory findings also met the criteria of polymyalgia rheumatica (PMR).

She underwent steroid therapy with a dose of 60 mg/day. The symptoms were relieved soon after initiating the therapy. The dose was tapered to 6 mg/day just before the second PET/CT.

5.9.7 Discussion

The large-vessel vasculitis includes Takayasu arteritis (TAK) and GCA. TAK is often seen in younger females in Asian countries, and GCA in the elderly in western countries. PMR is associated with half of GCA patients. FDG-PET/CT is useful to assess the activities of inflammation and therapeutic effects [85–88].

5.10 Systemic Vasculitis 1

Chao Cheng

Abstract Systemic vasculitis generally refers to a group of autoimmune diseases in which vascular inflammation and destruction are major pathological changes. Inflammatory cells infiltrate around the vessel wall and blood vessels, accompanied by vascular damage, including cellulose deposition, collagen fibrosis, and endothelial cells. And myocyte necrosis. Can be divided into large vasculitis, vasculitis, and small vasculitis. Patients with primary systemic vasculitis may present with organ-specific or frequently with nonspecific symptoms such as fever, malaise, arthralgia, myalgia, weight loss, and so on. These patients tend to have elevated inflammatory markers, but there are no specific blood tests which can confirm the diagnosis. MRI can overestimate the degree of severity of stenosis by up to 15%. Conventional angiography, considered the gold standard to assess vasculitis, is invasive and associated with morbidity, radiation exposure, and risk of contrast toxicity. FDG-PET is very useful in early diagnosis of TAK and also in the serial assessment of disease activity in stable, relapsing, as well as untreated patients.

Keywords: Takayasu arteritis, FDG, PET/CT

5.10.1 Clinical Presentation

A 61-year-old man known with repeated fever, fatigue, and microscopic hematuria for more than 1 month, and left eye congestion for more than 1 month. The body temperature rises more regularly, about 37.5 °C in the morning, about 38.0 °C in the afternoon, and 39.0 °C in the night. When the fever is accompanied by body aches and weakness, the consciousness is obviously weight loss. Laboratory examination found: ESR, 65 mm/H; CRP, >180 mg/L; WBC, 10.1 × 10^9/L, Hb 98 g/L, ANA(negative), ANCA(negative), Anti-ku antibody (positive).

5.10.2 Key Images

The left side of Figs. 5.24 and 5.25 are the MIP (maximum intensity projection) view of early phase and delay phase images of FDG PET. The right side of Figs. 5.24 and 5.25 are the fusion images of the different transverse section, which

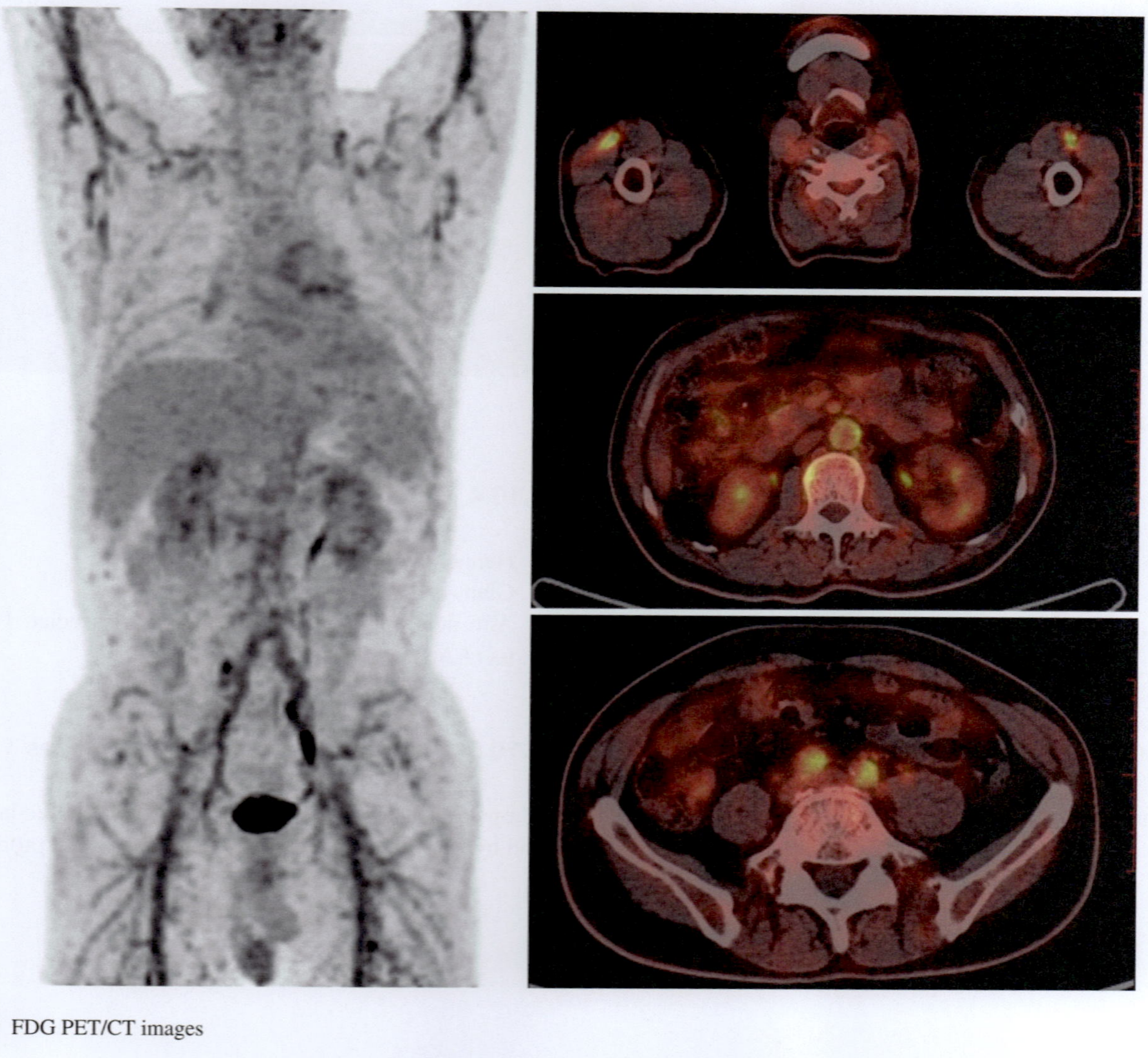

Fig. 5.24 FDG PET/CT images

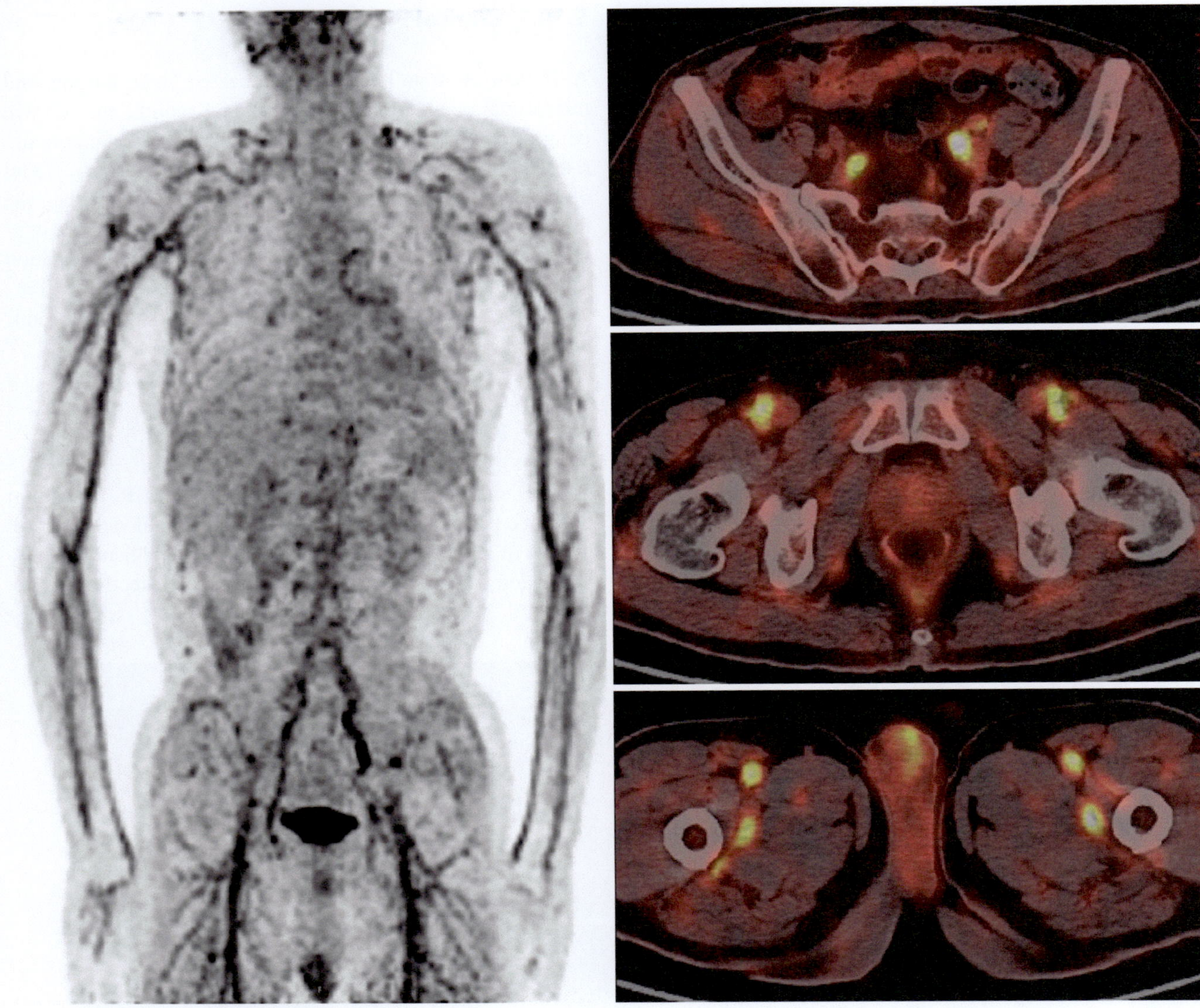

Fig. 5.25 FDG PET/CT images

demonstrate multiple arterial ingestion FDG, SUV_{max} = 16.7 (early phase of left radial artery).

5.10.3 Technique

- Patient preparation: patient should not take anything by mouth for 6 h before administration of radiopharmaceutical.
- 380 MBq of 18FDG administered intravenously (Body Weight = 72 kg).
- Imaging device: whole body PET/CT camera (Siemens biograph 64) with resolution of 4.0 mm FWHM.

5.10.4 Differential Diagnosis

- Henoch-Schonlein.
- Giant-cell arteritis.
- Anti-neutrophil cytoplasmic antibody-associated vasculitis (AAS).

5.10.5 Diagnosis and Clinical Follow-ups

The patient received cyclophosphamide, Methylprednisolone, and hydroxychloroquine therapy and recovered promptly.

5.10.6 Discussion

A primary systemic vasculitis is a group of heterogeneous disorders, characterized by inflammation of blood vessels causing end-organ damage from ischemia, aneurysm formation, or dissection. Delay in the early diagnosis owing to nonspecific symptoms, lack of definitive serological tests, limited availability of biopsy, and standard imaging tests pose a significant challenge in the management of these diseases. FDG-PET can be useful for early diagnosis and probably for serial assessment of disease activity [89–92].

5.11 Systemic Vasculitis 2

Xuena Li

Abstract ANCA-associated vasculitis is a group of systemic vasculitis characterized by inflammatory infiltration or fibrinoid necrosis of capillary, micro arterial, and micro venous wall, which can accumulate multiple systems. The lungs are the main organs involved. A 72-year-old female presented dyspnea and fever a month ago, and had no significant remission after 10 days of anti-inflammatory treatment. Laboratory reports showed positive anti-neutrophil cytoplasmic antibody. The patient underwent ^{18}F-FDG PET/CT imaging. The imaging showed multiple patches and nodules shadows with increased metabolism involving both lungs. The patient was diagnosed with ANCA-associated vasculitis. The symptoms relieved after treatment with cyclophosphamide.

Keywords: Antineutrophil cytoplasmic antibodies-associated vasculitis, FDG, PET

5.11.1 Clinical Presentation

A 72-year-old female presented dyspnea and fever a month ago, and had no significant remission after 10 days of anti-inflammatory treatment. Laboratory reports showed positive anti-neutrophil cytoplasmic antibody.

5.11.2 Key Images

5.11.3 Technique

– Patient preparation: patient should not take anything by mouth for 6 h before administration of radiopharmaceutical.
– 185 MBq of 18F-FDG administered intravenously.
– Imaging device: whole body of PET/CT camera (Siemens biograph) with resolution of 5.0 mm FWHM.

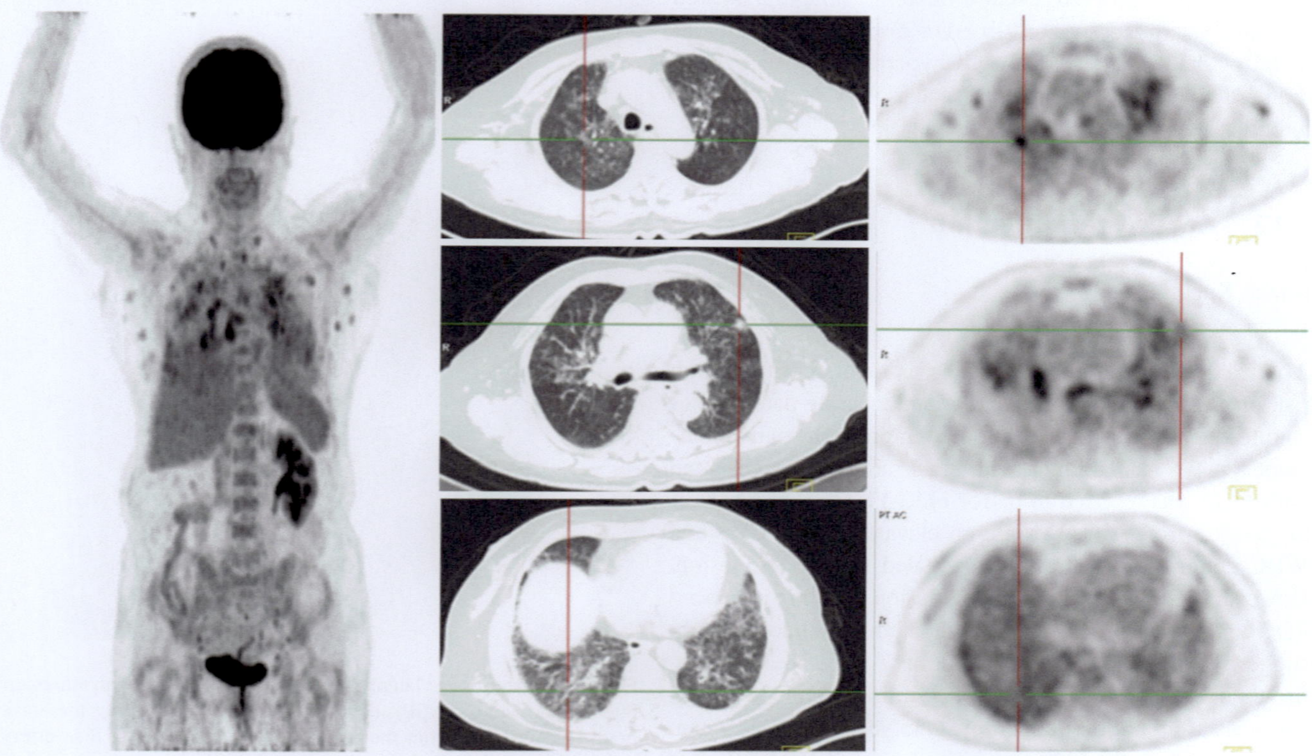

Fig. 5.26 ^{18}F-FDG PET/CT image

5.11.4 Image Interpretation

PET/CT imaging showed multiple patches and nodules shadows with increased FDG uptakes involving both lungs (SUV_{max} = 5.0, delayed imaging SUV_{max} = 6.4) and multiple lymph node enlargement with increased FDG uptakes in the mediastinum, bilateral hilum, bilateral axilla, and below bilateral pectoralis minor muscle (SUV_{max} = 6.4, delayed imaging SUV_{max} = 8.3).

5.11.5 Differential Diagnosis

- Pneumonia
- Lung cancer

5.11.6 Diagnosis and Clinical Follow-ups

The patient was diagnosed with ANCA-associated vasculitis. The symptoms relieved after treatment with cyclophosphamide.

5.11.7 Discussion

ANCA-associated vasculitis involves small blood vessels, encroaching upon small arteries, arterioles, capillaries, and venules of the viscera such as lung. Pulmonary capillaries are commonly involved, usually bilateral. Imaging showed irregular-patchy, spotty-cord-like dense impact and scattered-nodular shadow. PET showed hypermetabolism, which required laboratory examination such as ANCA to make differential diagnosis.

5.12 Aortic Graft Infection

Kazuo Kubota

Abstract Aortic graft infection is associated with a high risk of mortality. Therefore, early and accurate detection of an infected aortic graft is essential to improve the patient outcomes. A 50-year-old man with renal failure who presented with FUO was referred to us for FDG-PET/CT as a part of the workup for FUO. Despite an elevated serum CRP and WBC count, non-contrast CT revealed no specific lesion. However, FDGPET/CT revealed a lesion showing enhanced FDG uptake (SUV 11.2) around the abdominal aortic graft, suggestive of prosthetic graft infection. A blood culture confirmed infection with *Staphylococcus aureus*, and the patient was started on antibiotic therapy. One year later, significant decrease of both the FDG uptake and serum CRP level were observed. FDGPET/CT successfully detected aortic prosthetic graft infection.

Keywords: Prosthetic aortic graft, Infection, FUO, Antibiotic therapy

5.12.1 Clinical Presentation

A 50-year-old man with end-stage renal disease caused by polycystic kidneys who presented with FUO was referred to us for an FDG-PET examination as part of the workup for FUO. An elevated CRP level (5.44) and WBC count (11540) were observed. He gave a history of having undergone surgery for aortic aneurysm with placement of a prosthetic graft 2 years earlier, and of having had no significant postoperative complications.

5.12.2 Key Images

Anterior and lateral maximum-intensity projection images (Figure 5.27). Axial images of PET, CT, and fusion images (Figure 5.28). All the images show a lesion with enhanced FDG uptake along the prosthetic aortic graft in the abdomen.

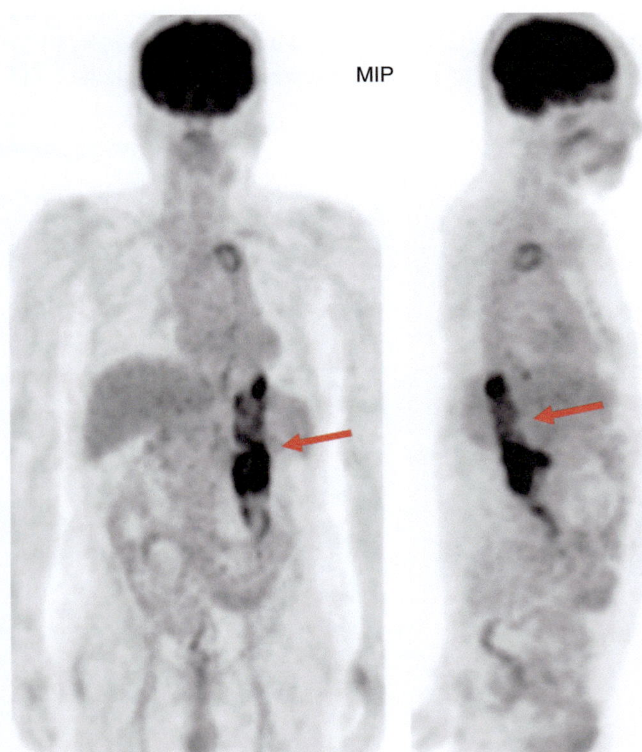

Fig. 5.27 Anterior and lateral images of FDG-PET/CT with maximum intensity projection (MIP). High FDG uptake surrounding the aortic graft was observed from the diaphragm to the common iliac artery. Arrows indicated the lesion

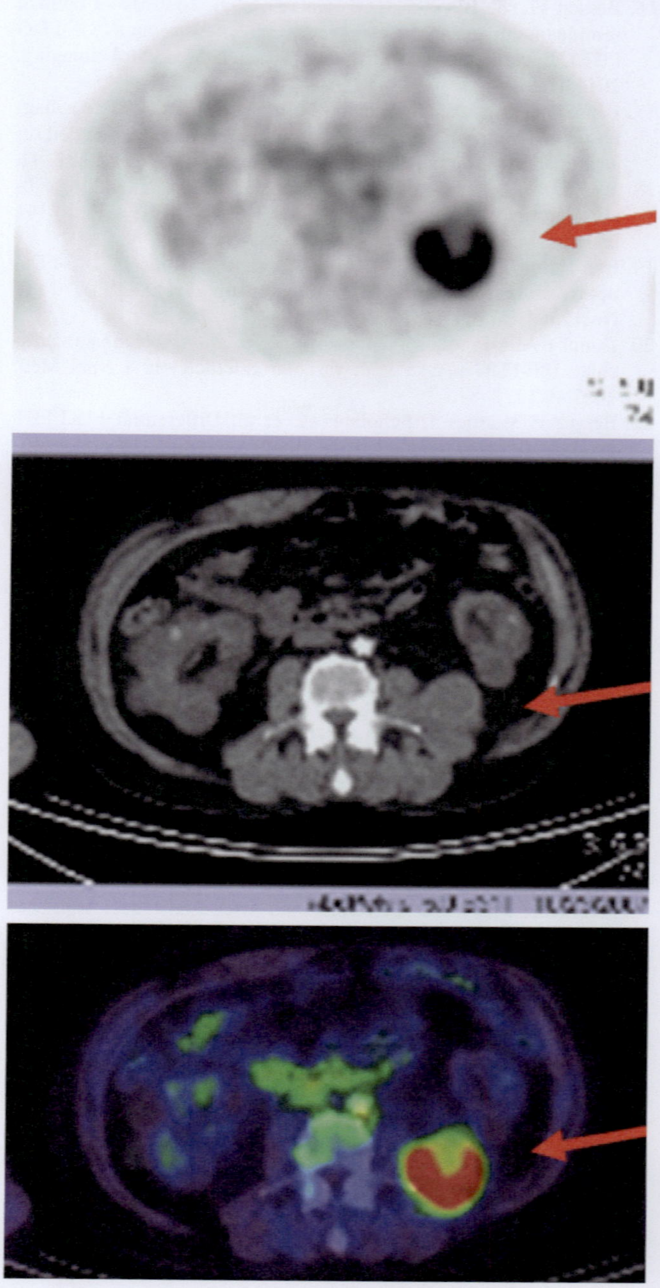

Fig. 5.28 Axial images of PET, CT and fusion images of PET/CT from top to bottom. Please note the left kidney locating anterior to the FDG avid aortic graft, having no FDG uptake due to the renal failure. Arrows indicated the lesion

5.12.3 Technique

- Patient preparation: The patient was instructed to take nothing by mouth for 5 h before administration of the radiopharmaceutical.
- 300 MBq of 18FDG is administered by intravenous injection.
- Imaging device: Whole-body PET/CT camera (Siemens biograph 16) with a resolution of 5.0 mm FWHM.

5.12.4 Image Interpretation

A CT scan without contrast enhancement performed before the FDG-PET/CT revealed the presence of fibrosis around the aortic graft. FDG-PET/CT showed a high FDG uptake (SUV 11.2) in the region around the aortic graft, extending from the diaphragm to the common iliac artery. These findings were consistent with graft infection.

5.12.5 Differential Diagnosis

- Noninfected inflammatory uptake by a vascular graft.
- Large-vessel vasculitis.

5.12.6 Diagnosis and Clinical Follow-ups

A blood culture performed after the FDGPET/CT imaging confirmed infection with *Staphylococcus aureus*, and the patient was started on antibiotic therapy. One year later, significant decrease of both the FDG uptake and serum CRP level was observed (SUV, 4.2; CRP, 0.05). FDGPET/CT images after the therapy are shown in Fig. 5.29. (Note: the case was from our previous publication [93]).

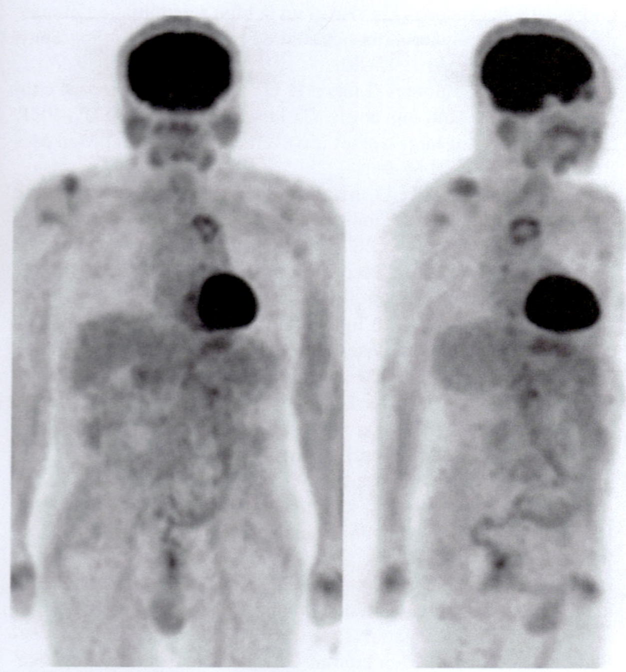

Fig. 5.29 Anterior and lateral MIP images of FDG-PET/CT after antibiotics therapy. FDG uptake by aortic graft was decreased significantly

5.12.7 Discussion

FDGPET/CT successfully detected aortic prosthetic graft infection that could not be detected by CT. Several reports have shown very good results of FDGPET/CT for the diagnosis of prosthetic aortic graft infection, especially for lesions that show high FDG uptake [94, 95]. As inflammatory FDG uptake by noninfected grafts has been reported to mimic the findings of infected grafts [96, 97], careful evaluation of not only FDGPET and CT images, but also of the markers of inflammation, is mandatory.

References

1. Jennette JC, Falk RJ, Bacon PA, et al. 2012 revised International Chapel Hill Consensus Conference Nomenclature of Vasculitides. Arthritis Rheum. 2013;65:1–11.
2. Gross WL, Trabandt A, Reinhold-Keller E. Diagnosis and evaluation of vasculitis. Rheumatology (Oxford). 2000;39:245–52.
3. Kermani TA, Warrington KJ, Crowson CS, et al. Large-vessel involvement in giant cell arteritis: a population-based cohort study of the incidence-trends and prognosis. Ann Rheum Dis. 2013;72:1989–94.
4. Ernst D, Baerlecken NT, Schmidt RE, et al. Large vessel vasculitis and spondyloarthritis: coincidence or associated diseases? Scand J Rheumatol. 2014;43:246–8.
5. Blockmans D, Stroobants S, Maes A, et al. Positron emission tomography in giant cell arteritis and polymyalgia rheumatica: evidence for inflammation of the aortic arch. Am J Med. 2000;108:246–9.
6. Hotchi M. Pathological studies on Takayasu arteritis. Heart Vessels Suppl. 1992;7:11–7.
7. Gornik HL, Creager MA. Aortitis. Circulation. 2008;117:3039–51.
8. Kubota R, Yamada S, Kubota K, et al. Intratumoral distribution of fluorine-18-fluorodeoxyglucose in vivo: high accumulation in macrophages and granulation tissues studied by microautoradiography. J Nucl Med. 1992;33:1972–80.
9. de Boysson H, Dumont A, Liozon E, et al. Giant-cell arteritis: concordance study between aortic CT angiography and FDG-PET/CT in detection of large-vessel involvement. Eur J Nucl Med Mol Imaging. 2017;44:2274–9.
10. Slart R. FDG-PET/CT(A) imaging in large vessel vasculitis and polymyalgia rheumatica: joint procedural recommendation of the EANM, SNMMI, and the PET Interest Group (PIG), and endorsed by the ASNC. Eur J Nucl Med Mol Imaging. 2018;45:1250–69.
11. Bucerius J, Mani V, Moncrieff C, et al. Optimizing 18F-FDG PET/CT imaging of vessel wall inflammation: the impact of 18F-FDG circulation time, injected dose, uptake parameters, and fasting blood glucose levels. Eur J Nucl Med Mol Imaging. 2014;41:369–83.
12. Stellingwerff MD, Brouwer E, Lensen KJ, et al. Different scoring methods of FDG PET/CT in giant cell arteritis: need for standardization. Medicine (Baltimore). 2015;94:e1542.
13. Martinez-Rodriguez I, Martinez-Amador N, Banzo I, et al. Assessment of aortitis by semiquantitative analysis of 180-min 18F-FDG PET/CT acquisition images. Eur J Nucl Med Mol Imaging. 2014;41:2319–24.
14. Lensen KD, Comans EF, Voskuyl AE, et al. Large-vessel vasculitis: interobserver agreement and diagnostic accuracy of 18F-FDG-PET/CT. Biomed Res Int. 2015;2015:914692.
15. Soussan M, Nicolas P, Schramm C, et al. Management of large-vessel vasculitis with FDG-PET. Medicine. 2015;94:e622.
16. Besson FL, de Boysson H, Parienti JJ, et al. Towards an optimal semiquantitative approach in giant cell arteritis: an (18)F-FDG PET/CT case-control study. Eur J Nucl Med Mol Imaging. 2014;41:155–66.
17. Lehmann P, Buchtala S, Achajew N, et al. 18F-FDG PET as a diagnostic procedure in large vessel vasculitis-a controlled, blinded re-examination of routine PET scans. Clin Rheumatol. 2011;30:37–42.
18. Wasselius JA, Larsson SA, Jacobsson H. FDG-accumulating atherosclerotic plaques identified with 18F-FDG-PET/CT in 141 patients. Mol Imaging Biol. 2009;11:455–9.
19. Ben-Haim S, Kupzov E, Tamir A, et al. Evaluation of 18F-FDG uptake and arterial wall calcifications using 18F-FDG PET/CT. J Nucl Med. 2004;45:1816–21.
20. Dunphy MP, Freiman A, Larson SM, et al. Association of vascular 18F-FDG uptake with vascular calcification. J Nucl Med. 2005;46:1278–84.
21. Berger P, Vaartjes I, Scholtens A, et al. Differential FDG-PET uptake patterns in uninfected and infected central prosthetic vascular grafts. Eur J Vasc Endovasc Surg. 2015;50:376–83.
22. Cimmino MA, Camellino D, Paparo F, et al. High frequency of capsular knee involvement in polymyalgia rheumatica/giant cell arteritis patients studied by positron emission tomography. Rheumatology (Oxford). 2013;52:1865–72.
23. Rehak Z, Szturz P. Comment on: FDG PET in the early diagnosis of large-vessel vasculitis. Eur J Nucl Med Mol Imaging. 2014;41:579–80.
24. de Boysson H, Liozon E, Lambert M, et al. 18F-fluorodeoxyglucose positron emission tomography and the risk of subsequent aortic complications in giant-cell arteritis: a multicenter cohort of 130 patients. Medicine (Baltimore). 2016;95:e3851.
25. Besson FL, Parienti JJ, Bienvenu B, et al. Diagnostic performance of (18)F-fluorodeoxyglucose positron emission tomography in giant cell arteritis: a systematic review and meta-analysis. Eur J Nucl Med Mol Imaging. 2011;38:1764–72.
26. Meller J, Strutz F, Siefker U, et al. Early diagnosis and follow-up of aortitis with [(18)F]FDG PET and MRI. Eur J Nucl Med Mol Imaging. 2003;30:730–6.
27. Nielsen BD, Gormsen LC, Hansen IT, et al. Three days of high-dose glucocorticoid treatment attenuates large-vessel 18F-FDG uptake in large-vessel giant cell arteritis but with a limited impact on diagnostic accuracy. Eur J Nucl Med Mol Imaging. 2018;45:1119–28.
28. Palard-Novello X, Querellou S, Gouillou M, et al. Value of (18) F-FDG PET/CT for therapeutic assessment of patients with polymyalgia rheumatica receiving tocilizumab as first-line treatment. Eur J Nucl Med Mol Imaging. 2016;43:773–9.
29. Yoshifuji H. Pathophysiology of large vessel vasculitis and utility of interleukin-6 inhibition therapy. Mod Rheumatol. 2019;29:287–93.
30. Watanabe Y, Miyata T, Tanemoto K. Current clinical features of new patients with Takayasu Arteritis observed from Cross-Country Research in Japan: age and sex specificity. Circulation. 2015;132:1701–9.
31. Kobayashi Y, Ishii K, Oda K, et al. Aortic wall inflammation due to Takayasu arteritis imaged with 18F-FDG PET coregistered with enhanced CT. J Nucl Med. 2005;46:917–22.
32. Pagnoux C, Seror R, Henegar C, et al. Clinical features and outcomes in 348 patients with polyarteritis nodosa: a systematic retrospective study of patients diagnosed between 1963 and 2005 and entered into the French Vasculitis Study Group Database. Arthritis Rheum. 2010;62:616–26.
33. Maksimowicz-McKinnon K, Clark TM, Hoffman GS. Takayasu arteritis and giant cell arteritis: a spectrum within the same disease? Medicine. 2009;88:221–6.
34. Grayson PC, Maksimowicz-McKinnon K, Clark TM, et al. Distribution of arterial lesions in Takayasu's arteritis and giant cell arteritis. Ann Rheum Dis. 2012;71:1329–34.

35. Kermani TA, Crowson CS, Muratore F, Schmidt J, Matteson EL, Warrington KJ. Extra-cranial giant cell arteritis and Takayasu arteritis: how similar are they? Semin Arthritis Rheum. 2015;44:724–8.
36. Yoshida M, Watanabe R, Ishii T, et al. Retrospective analysis of 95 patients with large vessel vasculitis: a single center experience. Int J Rheum Dis. 2016;19:87–94.
37. Maksimowicz-McKinnon K, Clark TM, Hoffman GS. Limitations of therapy and a guarded prognosis in an American cohort of Takayasu arteritis patients. Arthritis Rheum. 2007;56:1000–9.
38. Hoffman GS, Merkel PA, Brasington RD, Lenschow DJ, Liang P. Anti-tumor necrosis factor therapy in patients with difficult to treat Takayasu arteritis. Arthritis Rheum. 2004;50:2296–304.
39. Molloy ES, Langford CA, Clark TM, Gota CE, Hoffman GS. Anti-tumour necrosis factor therapy in patients with refractory Takayasu arteritis: long-term follow-up. Ann Rheum Dis. 2008;67:1567–9.
40. Schmidt J, Kermani TA, Bacani AK, Crowson CS, Matteson EL, Warrington KJ. Tumor necrosis factor inhibitors in patients with Takayasu arteritis: experience from a referral center with long-term followup. Arthritis Care Res. 2012;64:1079–83.
41. Comarmond C, Plaisier E, Dahan K, et al. Anti TNF-alpha in refractory Takayasu's arteritis: cases series and review of the literature. Autoimmun Rev. 2012;11:678–84.
42. Mekinian A, Neel A, Sibilia J, et al. Efficacy and tolerance of infliximab in refractory Takayasu arteritis: French multicentre study. Rheumatology (Oxford). 2012;51:882–6.
43. Gudbrandsson B, Molberg O, Palm O. TNF inhibitors appear to inhibit disease progression and improve outcome in Takayasu arteritis; an observational, population-based time trend study. Arthritis Res Ther. 2017;19:99.
44. Novikov PI, Smitienko IO, Sokolova MV, et al. Certolizumab pegol in the treatment of Takayasu arteritis. Rheumatology (Oxford). 2018;57:2101–5.
45. Nakaoka Y, Higuchi K, Arita Y, et al. Tocilizumab for the treatment of patients with refractory Takayasu arteritis. Int Heart J. 2013;54:405–11.
46. Mekinian A, Resche-Rigon M, Comarmond C, et al. Efficacy of tocilizumab in Takayasu arteritis: Multicenter retrospective study of 46 patients. J Autoimmun. 2018;91:55–60.
47. Nakaoka Y, Isobe M, Takei S, et al. Efficacy and safety of tocilizumab in patients with refractory Takayasu arteritis: results from a randomised, double-blind, placebo-controlled, phase 3 trial in Japan (the TAKT study). Ann Rheum Dis. 2018;77:348–54.
48. Terao C, Yoshifuji H, Nakajima T, Yukawa N, Matsuda F, Mimori T. Ustekinumab as a therapeutic option for Takayasu arteritis: from genetic findings to clinical application. Scand J Rheumatol. 2016;45:80–2.
49. Langford CA, Cuthbertson D, Ytterberg SR, et al. A randomized, double-blind trial of Abatacept (CTLA-4Ig) for the treatment of Takayasu arteritis. Arthritis Rheumatol (Hoboken NJ). 2017;69:846–53.
50. Azak A, Huddam B, Kocak G, Kilic F, Kocak E, Duranay M. Takayasu arteritis and ulcerative colitis; coexistence or misdiagnosis? Sarcoidosis Vasc Diffuse Lung Dis. 2012;29:53–4.
51. Watanabe R, Ishii T, Nakamura K, et al. Ulcerative colitis is not a rare complication of Takayasu arteritis. Mod Rheumatol. 2014;24:372–3.
52. Terao C, Matsumura T, Yoshifuji H, et al. Takayasu arteritis and ulcerative colitis: high rate of co-occurrence and genetic overlap. Arthritis Rheum (Hoboken NJ). 2015;67:2226–32.
53. Lande A. Abdominal Takayasu's aortitis, the middle aortic syndrome and atherosclerosis. A critical review. Int Angiol. 1998;17:1–9.
54. Agard C, Barrier JH, Dupas B, et al. Aortic involvement in recent-onset giant cell (temporal) arteritis: a case-control prospective study using helical aortic computed tomodensitometric scan. Arthritis Rheum. 2008;59:670–6.
55. Espinoza JL, Ai S, Matsumura I. New insights on the pathogenesis of Takayasu arteritis: revisiting the microbial theory. Pathogens. 2018;7:73. https://doi.org/10.3390/pathogens7030073.
56. Jennete JC, Falk RJ, Bacon PA, et al. Revised international Chapel Hill consensus conference nomenclature of Vasculitides. Arthritis Rheum. 2013;65:1–11.
57. Fuchs M, Briel M, Daikeler T, et al. The impact of 18F-FDG PET on the management of patients with suspected large vessel vasculitis. Eur J Nucl Med Mol Imaging. 2012;39:344–53.
58. Papathanasiou ND, Du Y, Menezes LJ, et al. 18F-Fludeoxyglucose PET/CT in the evaluation of large-vessel vasculitis: diagnostic performance and correlation with clinical and laboratory parameters. Br J Radiol. 2012;85:e188–94.
59. Jamar F, Buscombe J, Chiti A, et al. EANM/SNMMI guideline for 18F-FDG use in inflammation and infection. J Nucl Med. 2013;54:647–58.
60. Signore A, Glaudemans AWJM. The molecular imaging approach to image infections and inflammation by nuclear medicine techniques. Ann Nucl Med. 2011;25:681–700.
61. Schollhammer R, Schwartz P, Jullie ML, et al. 18F-FDG PET/CT imaging of popliteal vasculitis associated with polyarteritis nodosa. Clin Nucl Med. 2017;42:e385–7.
62. De Geeter F, Gykiere P. (18)F-FDG PET imaging of granulomatosis with polyangiitis-Wegener's syndrome. Hell J Nucl Med. 2016;19:53–6.
63. Morita H, Yokoyama I, Yamada N, et al. Usefulness of 18FDG/13N-ammonia PET imaging for evaluation of the cardiac damage in Churg-Strauss syndrome. Eur J Nucl Med Mol Imaging. 2004;31:1218.
64. Elourimi G, Soussan M, Warzocha U, et al. Efficacy of tocilizumab highlighted by FDG-PET/CT in a patient with relapsing polychondritis-associated aortitis. Rheumatol Int. 2017;37:1931–5.
65. Ishikawa K. Diagnostic approach and proposed criteria for the clinical diagnosis of Takayasu's arteriopathy. J Am Coll Cardiol. 1988;12:964–72.
66. Ohigashi H, Haraguchi G, Konishi M, et al. Improved prognosis of Takayasu arteritis over the past decade: comprehensive analysis of 106 patients. Circ J. 2012;76:1004–11.
67. Comarmond C, Cluzel P, Toledano D, et al. Findings of cardiac magnetic resonance imaging in asymptomatic myocardial ischemic disease in Takayasu arteritis. Am J Cardiol. 2014;113:881–7.
68. Mukhtyar C, Guillevin L, Cid MC, Dasgupta B, de Groot K, Gross W, et al. EULAR recommendations for the management of large vessel vasculitis. Ann Rheum Dis. 2009;68:318–23.
69. Mirouse A, Biard L, Comarmond C, et al. Overall survival and mortality risk factors in Takayasu's arteritis: a multicenter study of 318 patients. J Autoimmun. 2019;96:35–9.
70. Arend WP, Michel BA, Bloch DA, et al. The American College of Rheumatology 1990 criteria for the classification of Takayasu arteritis. Arthritis Rheum. 1990;33:1129–34.
71. Tezuka D, Haraguchi G, Ishihara T, et al. Role of FDG PET-CT in Takayasu arteritis. sensitive detection of recurrences. J Am Coll Cardiol Img. 2012;5:422–9.
72. Santhosh S, Mittal BR, Gayana S, et al. F-18 FDG PET/CT in the evaluation of Takayasu arteritis: an experience from the tropics. J Nucl Cardiol. 2014;21:993–1000.
73. Kerr GS, Ha llahan CW, Giordano J, et al. Takayasu arteritis. Ann Intern Med. 1994;120:919–29.
74. Han Q, Liang Q, Kang F, et al. An increased major vessel uptake by 18F-FDG-PET/CT in NIH criteria inactive patients with Takayasu's arteritis. Clin Exp Rheumatol. 2018;36(Suppl 111(2)):88–92.
75. Terao C, Matsumura T, Yoshifuji H, et al. Takayasu arteritis and ulcerative colitis: high rate of co- occurrence and genetic overlap. Arthritis Rheumatol. 2015;67:2226–32.

76. Soriano A, Pazzola G, Boiardi L, Casali M, Muratore F, Pipitone N, et al. Distribution patterns of 18F-fluorodeoxyglucose in large vessels of Takayasu's and giant cell arteritis using positron emission tomography. Clin Exp Rheumatol. 2018;36(Suppl 111(2)):99–106.
77. Grayson PC, Maksimowicz-McKinnon K, Clark TM, Tomasson G, Cuthbertson D, Carette S, et al. Distribution of arterial lesions in Takayasu's arteritis and giant cell arteritis. Ann Rheum Dis. 2012;71(8):1329–34. https://doi.org/10.1136/annrheumdis-2011-200795.
78. Kerr GS, et al. Takayasu arteritis. Ann Intern Med. 1994;120:919–29.
79. Kobayashi Y, et al. Aortic wall inflammation due to Takayasu arteritis imaged with 18F-FDG PET coregistered with enhanced CT. J Nucl Med. 2005;46(6):917–22.
80. Isobe M. Takayasu. Arteritis revisited: current diagnosis and treatment. Int J Cardiol. 2013;168(1):3–10.
81. Gomez L, et al. Effect of CRP value on ^{18}F–FDG PET vascular positivity in Takayasu arteritis: a systematic review and per-patient based meta-analysis. Eur J Nucl Med Mol Imaging. 2018;45(4):575–81.
82. Tezuka D, et al. Role of FDG PET-CT in Takayasu arteritis: sensitive detection of recurrences. JACC Cardiovasc Imaging. 2012;5:422–9.
83. Hommada M, Mekinian A, Brillet PY, et al. Aortitis in giant cell arteritis: diagnosis with FDG PET/CT and agreement with CT angiography. Autoimmun Rev. 2017;16(11):1131–7.
84. Hay B, Mariano-Goulart D, Bourdon A, et al. Diagnostic performance of 18F-FDG PET-CT for large vessel involvement assessment in patients with suspected giant cell arteritis and negative temporal artery biopsy. Ann Nucl Med. 2019;33(7):512–20.
85. Blockmans D, et al. Positron emission tomography in giant cell arteritis and polymyalgia rheumatica: evidence for inflammation of the aortic arch. Am J Med. 2000;108:246–9.
86. Treglia G, et al. Usefulness of whole-body fluorine-18-fluorodeoxyglucose positron emission tomography in patients with large-vessel vasculitis: a systematic review. Clin Rheumatol. 2011;30:1265–75.
87. Lee KH, et al. The role of ^{18}F-fluorodeoxyglucose-positron emission tomography in the assessment of disease activity in patients with takayasu arteritis. Arthritis Rheum. 2012;64:866–75.
88. Grayson PC, et al. ^{18} F-Fluorodeoxyglucose-positron emission tomography as an imaging biomarker in a prospective, longitudinal cohort of patients with large vessel vasculitis. Arthritis Rheum. 2018;70:439–49.
89. Danve A, O'DELL J. The role of 18F Fluorodeoxyglucose positron emission tomography scanning in the diagnosis and Management of Systemic Vasculitis. Int J Rheum Dis. 2015;18:714–24.
90. Kim J, Song H-C. Role of PET/CT in the evaluation of aortic disease. Chonnam Med J. 2018;54:143–52.
91. Schmidta WA, Blockmansb D, et al. Investigations in systemic vasculitis e the role ofimaging. Best Pract Res Clin Rheumatol. 2018;32:63–82.
92. Martínez-Rodríguez I, Jiménez-Alonso M, Quirce R, et al. 18F-FDG PET/CT in the follow-up of large-vessel vasculitis: a study of 37 consecutive patients. Semin Arthritis Rheum. 2018;47(4):530–7.
93. Kubota K, Nakamoto Y, Tamaki N, et al. FDG-PET for the diagnosis of fever of unknown origin: a Japanese multi-center study. Ann Nucl Med. 2011;25:355–64.
94. Tokuda Y, Oshima H, Araki Y, et al. Detection of thoracic aortic prosthetic graft infection with 18F-Fluorodeoxyglucose positron emission tomography/computed tomography. Eur J Cardiothorac Surg. 2013;43:1183–7.
95. Mitra A, Pencharz D, Davis M, Wagner T. Determining the diagnostic value of 18F-Fluorodeoxyglucose positron emission/computed tomography in detecting prosthetic aortic graft infection. Ann Vasc Surg. 2018;53:78–85.
96. Keidar Z, Pirmisashvili N, Leiderman M, et al. 18F-FDG uptake in noninfected prosthetic vascular grafts: incidence, patterns, and changes over time. J Nucl Med. 2014;55:392–5.
97. Lee M, Ryu JS, Suh CH, et al. Intense 18F-FDG activity in aortoiliac bypass graft mimicking infection. Medicine. 2018;97(7):e9876.

Suggested Reading

Frary EC, Hess S, Gerke O, et al. ^{18}F-fluoro-deoxy-glucose positron emission tomography combined with computed tomography can reliably rule-out infection and cancer in patients with anti-neutrophil cytoplasmic antibody-associated vasculitis suspected of disease relapse. Medicine. 2017;96(30):e7613.

Hofheinz K, Bertz S, Wacker J, Schett G, Manger B. Fever of unknown origin, giant cell arteritis, and aortic dissection. Z Rheumatol. 2017;76(1):83–6. https://doi.org/10.1007/s00393-016-0245-5.

Kemna MJ, Vanderheynst F, Vöö S, Blocklet D, et al. Positron emission tomography scanning in anti-neutrophil cytoplasmic antibodies-associatedvasculitis. Medicine. 2015;94(20):e747.

Smith JH, Swanson JW. Giant cell arteritis. Headache. 2014;54(8):1273–89. https://doi.org/10.1111/head.12425.

Soussan M, Abisror N, Abad S, et al. FDG-PET/CT in patients with ANCA-associated vasculitis: case-series and literature review. Autoimmun Rev. 2014;13:125–31.

Watanabe S, Gono T, Nishina K, et al. Rheumatoid factor is correlated with disease activity and inflammatory markers in antineutrophil cytoplasmic antibody-associated vasculitis. BMC Immunol. 2017;18(1):53.

FDG PET/CT for Rheumatic Diseases (Collagen Diseases)

6

Hiroyuki Yamashita, Chao Cheng, Xuena Li, Azusa Tokue, Kimiteru Ito, Kazuhiro Oguchi, Masatoyo Nakajo, and Noriko Oyama-Manabe

6.1 Role of FDG PET/CT in the Diagnosis of Rheumatic Diseases

Hiroyuki Yamashita

Abstract Advanced imaging techniques may enable early diagnosis and monitoring of therapy in various rheumatic diseases. To prevent irreversible tissue damage, inflammatory rheumatic disease must be diagnosed and treated in preclinical stages, requiring highly sensitive detection techniques. PET provides highly sensitive, quantitative imaging at a molecular level, revealing the important pathophysiological processes underlying inflammation. This section provides an overview of the current utility of FDG-PET/CT in patients with active rheumatic diseases such as rheumatoid arthritis (RA), polymyalgia rheumatica (PMR), spondyloarthritis (SpA), relapsing polychondritis (RPC), adult-onset Still's disease (AOSD), large vessel vasculitis (LVV), immunoglobulin G4-related disease (IgG4-RD), polymyositis/dermatomyositis (PM/DM), and Granulomatosis with polyangitis (GPA). We also discuss the role of FDG-PET/CT in the diagnosis and monitoring of these diseases.

H. Yamashita (✉)
Division of Rheumatic Diseases, National Center for Global Health and Medicine, Tokyo, Japan
e-mail: hiroyuki_yjp2005@yahoo.co.jp

C. Cheng
Shanghai Changhai Hospital, Shanghai, China
e-mail: chao_cheng_1999@163.com

X. Li
Department of Nuclear Medicine, The First Hospital of China Medical University, Shenyang, Liaoning Province, China
e-mail: lixuenacmunm@163.com

A. Tokue
Department of Diagnostic Radiology and Nuclear Medicine, Gunma University Hospital, Maebashi, Gunma, Japan
e-mail: azut@gunma-u.ac.jp

K. Ito
Department of Diagnostic Radiology, National Cancer Center Hospital, Tokyo, Japan
e-mail: kimito@ncc.go.jp

K. Oguchi
Positron Imaging Center, Aizawa Hospital, Matsumoto, Nagano, Japan
e-mail: pet-dr@ai-hosp.or.jp

M. Nakajo
Department of Radiology, Graduate School of Medical and Dental Sciences, Kagoshima University, Kagoshima, Japan
e-mail: toyo.nakajo@dolphin.ocn.ne.jp

N. Oyama-Manabe
Department of Diagnostic and Interventional Radiology, Hokkaido University Hospital, Sapporo, Hokkaido, Japan
e-mail: norikooyama@med.hokudai.ac.jp

Keywords: Rheumatoid arthritis (RA), Polymyalgia rheumatica (PMR), Spondyloarthritis (SpA), Relapsing polychondritis (RPC), Adult-onset Still's disease (AOSD), Large vessel vasculitis (LVV), Immunoglobulin G4-related disease (IgG4-RD), Polymyositis/dermatomyositis (PM/DM), Granulomatosis with polyangitis (GPA), FDG-PET/CT

6.1.1 Introduction

Timely diagnosis and early effective treatment can improve the outcome of various inflammatory rheumatic diseases [1]. To enable early diagnosis and individualized therapeutic protocols, sensitive monitoring tools such as advanced imaging techniques are needed. Promising results have already been obtained using anatomical imaging modalities, such as MRI and ultrasound (US), which allow highly sensitive detection of synovitis and bone marrow edema in inflammatory arthropathies and vascular thickening in systemic vasculitis [2–5]. Each technique, however, has drawbacks and limitations; MRI usually produces images within a limited field of view, and US is limited by variability and labor intensity. In addition, in the presence of inflammation, both techniques can visualize indirect inflammatory signs such as increased tissue water content and hyperperfusion. Because diagnosis and assessment of disease activity at subclinical stages is

H. Toyama et al. (eds.), *PET/CT for Inflammatory Diseases*, https://doi.org/10.1007/978-981-15-0810-3_6

increasingly important, nuclear imaging techniques are becoming more widely used.

FDG is used to trace glucose metabolism. Many cancer cells showed elevated expression of glucose transporters and hexokinase. Most cancer cells are FDG avid, and a fusion imaging technique combining PET/CT, which provides information on both anatomy and glucose metabolism, has improved the diagnostic accuracy and is now widely used in oncology. FDG uptake is not limited to cancer cells; uptake may also occur in various inflammatory cells. Elevated FDG uptake by activated macrophages and by newly formed granulation tissue was demonstrated by Kubota et al. in the early 1990s [6, 7]. The uptake of FDG by cancer cells is postulated to involve the same mechanism as in inflammatory cells. Cramer et al. reported that HIF1α activation is essential for myeloid cell (granulocytes and monocytes/macrophages) infiltration and activation an in vivo inflammation model [8]. More recently, Matsui et al. reported FDG uptake in the area in which inflammatory cell infiltration and synovial cell hyperplasia were visible in an arthritis model. Based on in vitro experiments, Matsui et al. suggested that the cell types responsible for FDG uptake are activated macrophages and proliferating fibroblasts in the presence of cytokine stimulation and under hypoxic circumstances within a joint [9]. The FDG uptake by inflammatory tissue, such as arthritis lesions, seems to reflect the inflammatory activity accurately.

Such studies have strongly encouraged the clinical application of FDGPET/CT for rheumatic diseases.

6.1.2 Rheumatoid Arthritis (RA)

RA is a symmetric, inflammatory, peripheral polyarthritis of unknown etiology. It typically leads to deformity through the stretching of tendons and ligaments and destruction of joints through the erosion of cartilage and bone. If it is untreated or unresponsive to therapy, inflammation and joint destruction lead to loss of physical function, inability to carry out daily tasks of living, and difficulties in maintaining employment. Therefore, early diagnosis of RA and evaluation of latent activity are important, and FDG-PET/CT may be useful for this purpose.

In 1995, the first FDG-PET studies in active RA patients revealed increased ^{18}F-FDG uptake in clinically inflamed wrist joints. Further, standardized uptake values (SUVs) for ^{18}F-FDG were correlated with clinical indicators such as tenderness and swelling [10]; these findings were confirmed in other studies [11, 12]. ^{18}F-FDG SUV data in arthritis is also correlated with disease activity score 28 (DAS28) and simple disease activity index (SDAI) values. The number of FDG-positive joints is also strongly correlated with their cumulative SUV and disease duration [11]. However, Kubota et al. [12] and Goerres et al. [13] found that simple visual semiquantitative scoring from 0 to 4 based on ^{18}F-FDG joint uptake [12] also reflected clinical evidence of inflammation in joints. This approach eliminates the need to quantify tracer uptake and makes the technique more accessible to routine clinical practice.

Beckers et al. [11] reported sensitivities of up to 90% in a study evaluating 356 joints of 21 established RA patients using ^{18}F-FDG PET. In this study, visually identified FDG positivity was clearly associated, according to odds ratios, with both joint swelling and tenderness. Regarding specificity, ^{18}F-FDG PET allows excellent differentiation between inflamed and healthy joints, both among RA patients and between patients and healthy controls; healthy joints do not take up the tracer at all [11, 14]. However, despite a greater number of FDG-positive joints in RA than in osteoarthritis patients, absolute values for tracer uptake do not differ between these two conditions [15]. Nonetheless, whole-body PET may aid in differentiation between RA and other inflammatory joint diseases, as differences in bio-distribution patterns have allowed distinction between some forms of arthritis associated with connective tissue disease [16].

Although clinical treatment response is not correlated with semiquantitative PET measures, ^{18}F-FDG PET images do detect reductions in metabolism and treatment-related changes in the volume of pannus that are not detectable with conventional imaging [10]. In 2006, Beckers et al. [17] used ^{18}F-FDG PET to image joints before and after anti-TNF therapy and found that that PET-positivity was correlated with higher SUVs. In contrast, ^{18}F-FDG PET revealed no significant metabolic changes following acupuncture treatment of affected knees in six chronic RA patients [18].

Several studies have indicated that subclinical disease is present during clinical remission and may be related to progression of joint damage [19]. Due to its high sensitivity and ability to scan multiple joints in one session, PET may allow detection of such subclinical disease activity. Whole-body PET scanning in 18 RA patients, four of whom were in remission [10], showed significant differences between those with active arthritis and those in clinical remission [12]. ^{18}F-FDG uptake by large joints, total visual PET scores for involved joints, SUV_{max}, and the mean number of joints per patient with high FDG uptake were all significantly lower for patients in clinical remission. In all patients in remission, however, increased ^{18}F-FDG uptake was still observed in one or more joints, suggesting subclinical disease activity.

Besides its ability to detect and monitor subclinical disease, PET may also have prognostic power. Recently, ^{18}F-FDG changes in inflamed hand joints after 2 weeks of infliximab treatment were correlated with DAS28 joint scores at 14–22 weeks of treatment [20]. In contrast, erythrocyte sedimentation rate (ESR), C-reactive protein (CRP), and DAS28 scores had no such predictive value after 2 weeks of therapy.

A number of studies have examined the ability of PET to accurately indicate treatment outcomes compared to MRI. Before and during treatment with nonsteroidal anti-inflammatory drugs (NSAIDs), prednisone, or methotrexate, changes in joint uptake of ^{18}F-FDG, as revealed by PET, were strongly correlated with synovial volume upon MRI in RA patients [10, 21]. Comparison of semiquantitative PET data with US data and clinical findings [11] revealed a significant linear correlation between SUVs and synovial thickness, as measured by US, for nearly all joints. This relationship was stronger for larger joints, as these are more accurately evaluated by semiquantitative scoring [22]. Moreover, some small joints in the hand cannot easily be evaluated in three dimensions by US for anatomical reasons [23]. The first study simultaneously investigating PET, MRI, and US in RA patients showed that enhanced FDG uptake was associated with positive findings obtained by the other two imaging techniques. In addition, the study also revealed correlations among SUVs from PET, relative contrast enhancement from MRI, and synovial thickness from US. Changes in SUVs in RA-affected knees after initiation of anti-TNF therapy were also correlated with changes in MRI parameters and serum CRP and metalloproteinase-3 (MMP-3) levels, but not with changes in synovial thickness as measured via US [17].

Hybrid PET-CT and PET-MRI have become available. Combining PET with CT has helped place pathophysiologic PET information in its anatomic context [24]. Thus, hybrid imaging should allow more precise localization of PET signals and PET-MRI should limit radiation exposure [25].

Recent reports have demonstrated that a higher baseline SUV for joints correlate with a higher risk for subsequent joint damage [26, 27].

6.1.3 Polymyalgia Rheumatica

PMR is an inflammatory rheumatic disease characterized by aches and morning stiffness in the shoulders, hip girdle, and neck in patients over 50 years of age. PMR is diagnosed by the exclusion of other disorders causing similar complaints and by its rapid response to low-dose corticosteroid therapy [28, 29]. Although its pathology is unknown, synovitis and bursitis are common features of this disease. MRI and US frequently reveal inflammation of the tenosynovial sheaths of patients' hands or feet [30–32].

Moosig et al. [33] quantified FDG accumulation in large vessels in 13 untreated patients with PMR by PET, and compared these data with serological markers of inflammation. By visual evaluation, FDG uptake by the aorta or its major branches increased in 12 of 13 patients. In active PMR, the mean region of interest (ROI) index for all vascular regions exceeded that of controls by 70%. Among the eight patients who underwent follow-up PET, this index declined substantially. In active PMR, FDG uptake was significantly correlated with CRP, ESR, and platelet counts. The observed FDG accumulation in the aorta and its branches and the strong correlation between tracer uptake and markers of inflammation suggests that large vessel arteritis is characteristic of active PMR.

Brockmans et al. [34] investigated whether FDG deposition in various vascular lesions and large joints of patients with isolated PMR predicts relapse. All patients underwent an FDG-PET scan before steroid treatment and at 3 and 6 months; seven vascular areas were scored and a total vascular score (TVS) was calculated, ranging from 0 to 21. At diagnosis, vascular FDG uptake was noted in 31% of patients, predominantly at the subclavian arteries. FDG uptake in the shoulders was noted in 94% of patients, in the hips in 89%, and in the spinous processes of the vertebrae in 51%. FDG uptake intensity was not correlated with the risk of relapse in either the large vessels or large joints.

While Brockmans et al. [34] analyzed FDG-PET changes in patients with PMR, we analyzed the precise distribution of lesions via PET/CT and evaluated differences in FDG accumulation between PMR and similar diseases. In PMR patients, FDG uptake was increased in ischial tuberosities, greater trochanters, and lumbar spinous processes [35]. Positive results at two or more of these sites were highly sensitive (85.7%) and specific (88.2%) for the diagnosis of PMR, and shoulder or hip joint involvement were not disease-specific. High FDG accumulation was found in the aortas and subclavian arteries of two PMR patients in whom FDG uptake did not identify temporal arteritis or scanty synovium and perisynovium. PET/CT images of the 12 PMR patients without apparent vascular involvement revealed synovitis and/or perisynovitis.

Furthermore, we compared PET/CT findings in a large number of PMR cases with those in patients with elderly-onset RA (EORA), which is extremely difficult to distinguish from PMR. We observed no significant difference in FDG uptake in the shoulders or hips. However, specific uptake patterns were observed in each group: circular and linear uptake patterns around the humeral head in EORA, and focal and nonlinear uptake patterns in PMR. Moreover, focal uptake at the front of the hip joint, indicating iliopectineal bursitis, tended to be limited to the PMR group. The sensitivity and specificity for PMR diagnosis were very high at 92.6% and 90.0%, respectively, when at least three of the five items, including findings characteristic of shoulder and iliopectineal bursitis, FDG uptake in ischial tuberosities and spinal spinous processes, and lack of FDG uptake in the wrists, were satisfied. FDG-PET/CT may be useful for the detection of PMR lesions, which are difficult to identify using other methods [36].

Subsequently, several papers on PET findings in PMR were published. Based on a detailed analysis of PET findings in knee joints with PMR, Cimmino et al. hypothesized that capsulitis is the source of inflammation [37]. Wakura et al. hypothesized that not only bursitis but also enthesitis may be the main cause of lesions and that these conditions may have developed from synovitis and inflammation of the surrounding area [38]. Owen et al. demonstrated that hamstring peritendonitis is a typical manifestation of PMR on PET/CT [39]. Rehak et al. comprehensively examined PET results from the affected site of PMR and roughly divided the sites into large arteries (V), proximal joints (A), and extraarticular synovial structures (E). The authors also demonstrated that PMR can be classified into six types: A (alone), E (alone), A + E, A + V, E + V, and A + E + V [40]. Furthermore, an increase in praepubic FDG uptake was also shown to be typical in PMR [41]. Praepubic inflammation is probably related to enthesitis and tenosynovitis at the origin of pectineus and adductor longus muscles ventrally from the pubis. Camellino et al. compared the PET findings and clinical symptoms of PMR and demonstrated that the clinical symptoms do not always correlate with the findings of cervical and lumbar interspinous bursitis [42]. Palard–Novello et al. compared the PET findings in PMR before and after treatment with Tocilizumab and demonstrated its usefulness in evaluating disease activity [43].。 .

6.1.4 Spondyloarthritis (SpA)

SpA includes ankylosing spondylitis (AS), psoriatic arthritis (PsA), reactive arthritis (ReA), enteropathic arthritis, and undifferentiated spondyloarthritis (uSpA) [44]. SpA often involves enthesitis, sacroiliitis, and inflammatory spondylitis [45].

Taniguchi et al. [46] evaluated the accuracy of FDG-PET/CT in detecting enthesitis in patients with SpA. PET/CT scans of the shoulder, hip, and knee joints revealed that FDG accumulates at the entheses in SpA and in the synovium in RA patients. SUV_{max} was significantly higher at the entheses of the lumbar spinous process, pubic symphysis, and ischial tuberosity in SpA patients than in RA patients. Lumbar spinous processes and ischial tuberosities appeared more frequently via PET/CT than MRI in SpA patients. They concluded that PET/CT represents an alternative modality to identifying enthesitis, and will likely contribute to the early diagnosis of SpA.

Strobel et al. [47] evaluated the performance of FDG-PET/CT for the diagnosis of sacroiliac joint (SIJ) arthritis in patients with active AS using patients with mechanical low back pain (MLBP) as a control. The mean ratio of FDG uptake in the SIJ to that in the sacrum in AS patients was 1.66, while that in MLBP patients was 1.12. With plain radiography as the gold standard and using an SIJ/S ratio of 1.3 as the threshold, the sensitivity and specificity of FDG-PET/CT for arthritis were 80% and 77%, respectively. On a per-SIJ basis, the greatest sensitivity (94%) was found in grade 3 sacroiliitis. These results suggest that quantitative FDG-PET/CT may be useful to diagnose sacroiliitis in active AS, providing an alternative to conventional bone scintigraphy in times of molybdenum shortage.

We used FDG-PET/CT to compare SUVs in various joints in 53 patients with SpA, PMR, and RA [48]. In PMR patients, the SUV_{max} for ischial tuberosities was significantly higher than in SpA or RA patients, and those in the greater trochanter and spinous processes were also significantly higher than in RA patients. In SpA patients, SUV_{max} in the SIJ was greater than in PMR or RA patients. No significant difference in vertebral scores was observed among groups. PET/CT findings can thus distinguish SpA from RA and PMR and are useful for the early diagnosis of sacroiliitis.

Vijayant et al. [49] evaluated the potential of FDG-PET in the early assessment of treatment response in various rheumatic diseases, including 11 newly diagnosed SpA patients and one patient with PsA. In the SpA group, FDG uptake in the affected joint was heterogeneous, low grade, and non-symmetrical, with intense tendon and muscular uptake in symptomatic joints. In contrast, FDG uptake in the PsA patient was intense in the joints and soft tissue. If larger studies corroborate these findings, FDG-PET could be useful to distinguish RA from SpA. FDG-PET also appears to be a sensitive tool in the early assessment of treatment response, especially when using quantitative information.

Subsequently, several papers on SpA and PET were published. Bruijnen et al. argued that unlike for RA, PET/CT is not as useful for AS from the perspective of evaluating activity. The authors argued that the activity of AS is reflected by ossification rather than inflammation in PET/CT [50]. Meanwhile, Lee et al. argued that not only syndesmophyte in the spine of patients with AS but also inflammatory lesions are associated with active bone synthesis, as evaluated by FDG uptake [51]. Based on a study concerning active AS using hybrid PET/MRI, Buchbender et al. hypothesized that bone marrow edema rather than chronic changes is more closely associated with osteoblastic activity. The authors reported that the accumulation of FDG was due to bone marrow edema and fat deposition [52]. Takata et al. discovered that asymptomatic enthesitis can be identified in PsA patients based on PET/CT images; further, they indicated that there are more cases of asymptomatic PsA than previously expected [53]. Chaudhari et al. evaluated PsA-affected hands and wrist joints using high-resolution FDG–PET/CT and reported that the technique is useful in the quantitative evaluation of disease activity (synovitis, enthesitis, edema, and bone fracture) [54]. Idolazzi et al. performed PET/CT in patients with AS and confirmed a correlation between the number of FDG-positive sites and disease activity. They also argued that PET/CT may be a useful tool for follow-up evaluations of AS [55]. Based on their results, Park et al. stated that FDG-PET may be useful in identifying patients with AS at a higher risk for future syndesmophyte formation [56]. Based on dual-phase PET/MRI findings of sacroiliac joints in patients with AS, Sawicki et al. reported a possibility that regional hyperemia and osteoblast activity, and not chronic AS lesions, are associated with inflammation [57].

6.1.5 Relapsing Polycondritis (RPC)

Relapsing polychondritis (RPC) is an immune-mediated condition associated with inflammation in cartilaginous structures and other tissues throughout the body, particularly the ears, nose, eyes, joints, and respiratory tract. The clinical features and course of RPC vary considerably from patient to patient. Subtle, early manifestations often remain unrecognized for prolonged periods. As a result, the diagnosis is frequently obtained only after the emergence of classic features such as auricular inflammation, saddle-nose deformity, or other features of cartilage destruction.

We first investigated the utility of FDG-PET/CT for the diagnosis and evaluation of disease activity in five RPC patients undergoing FDG-PET/CT in our hospital and eight cases in the literature [58]. Typical FDG accumulation was noted in tracheobronchial trees, costal cartilage, joints, larynx, nasal cavity/paranasal sinuses, auricles, lymph nodes, and the aorta. In one patient, PET revealed nasal chondritis despite an absence of nasal changes upon physical examination. Of five patients with costochondritis, four remained asymptomatic. Of the nine patients with airway FDG accumulation, eight developed respiratory symptoms and all had CT abnormalities. In the remaining patient, airway FDG accumulation was evident despite the absence of airway symptoms and a lack of abnormalities in the respiratory function test or CT. PET also revealed bronchial chondritis in asymptomatic patients. In the five patients examined by PET posttreatment, FDG accumulation diminished as symptoms improved and inflammation decreased. We conclude that FDG-PET/CT is a potentially powerful tool for the early diagnosis of RPC, especially in patients with affected organs that are difficult to biopsy. This modality also facilitates the evaluation of the extent of disease and disease activity during treatment.

Subsequently, Lei et al. conducted a similar study and reported similar findings [59].

6.1.6 Adult Onset of Still Disease (AOSD)

Adult-onset Still's disease (AOSD) is a systemic inflammatory disease of unknown etiology and pathogenesis. It is characterized by fever, skin eruptions, systemic organ involvement, and arthralgias. Arthralgias and arthritis occur in the majority of patients with AOSD, with incidences ranging from 69 to 96%. Hepatosplenomegaly is also often seen in this disease. Frequency of hepatomegaly and splenomegaly has been reported to be 18.2–50.0% and 18.2–57.0%, respectively, and the frequency of increased liver enzyme was 63.6–84.0%. The diagnosis of AOSD remains a clinical diagnosis. It is difficult to diagnose because of its low prevalence, heterogeneous clinical manifestations, and absence of pathognomic clinical features. The disease also lacks a specific diagnostic test. Before the final diagnosis of AOSD is made in suspected subjects, it is important to rule out a wide range of other diseases including infectious diseases, malignancies, and rheumatic diseases.

We first evaluated FDG-PET/CT for diagnosis and disease evaluation of AOSD by investigating FDG uptake for characteristic findings in seven patients with AOSD and reviewing the literature on seven previous reports of PET/CT in AOSD patients [60]. FDG accumulation was positive mainly in the bone marrow (100%), spleen (90.9%), lymph nodes (80.0%), and joints (75.0%). In addition, FDG uptake was positive in the pericardium, pleura, salivary glands, eyelids, muscle, and major blood vessels. Follow-up PET/CT showed diminished FDG accumulation, as measured by SUV_{max}, in the bone marrow, spleen, and lymph nodes. The only correlation with laboratory data was between lactate dehydrogenase (LDH) and spleen SUV. In conclusion, FDG-PET/CT is useful for long-term assessment of AOSD activity in individual patients. However, PET/CT findings alone are not sufficient to make a differential diagnosis of AOSD versus malignant lymphoma.

Subsequently, Dong et al. conducted a similar study and reported somewhat similar findings [61].

6.1.7 Large-Vessel Vasculitis (LVV)

Large-vessel vasculitis (LVV) can be clinically diagnosed and classified according to specific criteria. During the Chapel Hill Conference in 2012, two forms of primary LVV were distinguished: giant cell arteritis (GCA) and Takayasu arteritis (TAK). Early diagnosis and assessment of the extent of LVV are crucial factors for adequate therapeutic management. LVV diagnosis is often difficult because of the absence of specific symptoms and signs and the limited specificity of the available biochemical tests. Morphological imaging techniques such as angiography, CT, MRI, and US cannot detect the early phase of inflammation of the vessel wall because of slight anatomical changes at this time. It is also difficult to distinguish active inflammatory lesions from the residual anatomical changes of scarring.

From a systematic review on FDG-PET/CT in patients with LVV, Treglia et al. [62] drew several conclusions. First, FDG-PET/CT appears to be useful in early diagnosis and in the assessment of disease activity and extent. Second, the correlation between FDG-PET findings and serological inflammatory markers, as well as the usefulness of FDG-PET/CT in evaluating treatment response, require further investigation. Additionally, FDG-PET/CT appears to be superior to conventional imaging methods, such as US or MRI, in the diagnosis of LVV, but not in assessing response to immunosuppressive treatment, predicting relapse, or evaluating vascular complications. Lastly, PET analysis and diagnostic criteria should be standardized to allow reproducible, directly comparable results.

We also studied the usefulness of FDG-PET/CT and contrast-enhanced CT in early diagnosis and treatment follow-up of patients with LVV presenting as elderly-onset inflammation of unknown origin (IUO) [63]. For quantitative comparison, we evaluated SUV_{max} and PET scores of the aortic wall, as well as aortic wall thickness (W) and its ratio with respect to aortic radius (W/R) by contrast-enhanced CT, and compared pretreatment and posttreatment values. Of 124 patients who were hospitalized due to advanced age and IUO, 10.5% had LVV, and more than half had nonspecific symptoms. Compared to control subjects, patients with LVV showed significantly higher aortic wall SUV_{max}, higher PET scores as revealed by FDG-PET/CT, and increased aortic wall thicknesses as revealed by contrast-enhanced CT. PET scores and contrast-enhanced CT revealed significant reductions in aortic wall thickness following treatment. In conclusion, LVV is an important cause of IUO with nonspecific symptoms in elderly patients. Combined contrast-enhanced CT and FDG-PET/CT is useful for early diagnosis and early treatment evaluation of LVV, as it detects amelioration of aortic wall thickening.

Notably, FDG-PET/CT may be negative for old lesions even if the arterial stricture is severe. Lesions in which the inflammatory activity has already subsided may not be appropriate for evaluation by FDG-PET; in such cases, morphological imaging such as MRI or contrast-enhanced CT may be used. Again, LVV should be diagnosed in the early phase with FDG-PET/CT to prevent stricture formation.

6.1.8 Immunoglobulin G4-Related Disease (IgG4-RD)

IgG4-RD is a systemic disorder associated with lesions characterized by mass formation in multiple specific organs. This disorder comprises Mikulicz's disease (MD), autoimmune pancreatitis (AIP), hypophysitis, Riedel thyroiditis, interstitial pneumonitis, interstitial nephritis, lymphadenopathy, retroperitoneal fibrosis, and inflammatory pseudotumor [64]. The combination of such lesions on FDG-PET/CT may strongly suggest or support the diagnosis of IgG-4RD.

Shigekawa et al. noted that the FDG-PET pattern at baseline, including extra-abdominal lymph nodes and/or salivary glands and the involvement of the eyes and biliary ducts, can be useful for discriminating between AIP and pancreatic cancer [65]. Ozaki et al. also found that FDG uptake by hilar lymph nodes was significantly more frequent in AIP than in pancreatic cancer and reported that uptake by the lacrimal gland, salivary gland, biliary duct, retroperitoneal space, and prostate were seen only in AIP [3]. They reported that a longitudinal pattern, heterogeneous accumulation, and multiple localizations in the pancreas indicated AIP rather than pancreatic cancer [66].

Ebbo et al. [67] evaluated FDG-PET/CT for disease staging and treatment evaluation in 46 FDG-PET/CT images from 21 IgG4-RD patients. At diagnosis or relapse, all patients presented abnormal FDG uptake at sites typically affected by IgG4-RD. In most cases, FDG-PET/CT was more sensitive than conventional imaging to detect organ involvement, especially in the arteries, salivary glands, and lymph nodes. In a few cases, FDG-PET/CT failed to identify small or contiguous lesions in the brain or kidneys. Evaluation before and after treatment showed that FDG-PET/CT results were generally correlated with treatment response and disease activity. This retrospective study shows that FDG-PET/CT imaging is useful for staging IgG4-RD and assessing treatment response.

In addition, we evaluated the utility of FDG-PET/CT in eight IgG4-RD patients [68]. Although nearly all patients were negative for CRP, various organs took up significant amounts of FDG. In conclusion, FDG accumulation in organs characteristically affected by IgG4-RD allows diagnosis without evidence of an associated inflammatory reaction.

Subsequently, several similar reports showed the utility of FDG–PET/CT in IgG4-RD [69–73]. Berti et al. examined the relationship between IgG4-RD disease activity and FDG uptake and reported that FDG accumulation in IgG4-RD reflects perturbations in the B-cell compartment. The authors concluded that PET is a reliable method for evaluating IgG4-RD disease activity [74]. Takano et al. compared the PET findings of patients with and those suspected of having IgG4-related sclerosing sialadenitis (IgG4-SS) and argued that IgG4-SS may be noninvasively diagnosed by reviewing the PET findings in addition to serum IgG4 level and clinical findings [75].

6.1.9 Polymyositis/Dermatomyositis (PM/DM)

Polymyositis (PM) and dermatomyositis (DM) are idiopathic inflammatory myopathies, characterized by the shared features of proximal skeletal muscle weakness and evidence of muscle inflammation. DM, unlike PM, is associated with a variety of characteristic skin manifestations. The association between malignancy and inflammatory myopathy has been supported by numerous epidemiologic studies, with the strongest association occurring in those with DM.

Owada et al. [76] examined whether FDG-PET can detect myositis or extramuscular lesions in patients with PM and DM, and observed increased FDG uptake in muscle in 33% of patients. The sensitivity of FDG-PET to detect myositis was lower than that of electromyography (EMG), MRI, and muscle biopsy, and patients with and without increased FDG uptake in muscle did not differ clinically, although those with FDG muscle uptake had a tendency toward extended myositis with endomysial cell infiltration. In contrast, FDG-PET did detect neoplasms in patients with associated malignancy, which accounted for 38.9% of patients with interstitial lung disease. Thus, FDG-PET imaging appears to have limited usefulness for the evaluation of myositis in patients with PM and DM because of its low sensitivity.

On the other hand, Tanaka et al. [77] also conducted a retrospective study to determine whether FDG-PET/CT discriminates PM and DM from nonmuscular diseases and whether FDG uptake in proximal muscles reflects severity of muscular inflammation. Mean proximal muscle SUVs were significantly greater in PM and DM patients than in controls and were correlated with mean proximal manual muscle test scores and serum creatine kinase and aldolase levels. Furthermore, SUVs in proximal muscles from which biopsy specimens were obtained were significantly correlated with histological grade for inflammatory cell infiltration. These results suggest that FDG-PET/CT is useful in the diagnosis of PM and DM when inflammation in proximal muscles is also quantitatively assessed by other means. These results also indicate that local FDG uptake reflects inflammatory activity in proximal muscle and can help guide biopsy site selection.

Several studies concerning PET findings in inflammatory myositis have been reported, and all of their results suggest a correlation between myositis disease activity and the FDG accumulation degree [78–81]. In particular, Matuszak et al. reported that screening for malignant tumors was useful [78], whereas Motegi et al. noted that FDG-PET was useful in evaluating the activity of interstitial pneumonia with myositis [79].

6.1.10 Granulomatosis with Polyangitis (GPA)

Wegener's granulomatosis (WG), namely granulomatosis with polyangiitis (GPA), is a relatively rare disease characterized by granulomatous necrotising vasculitis. In the first evaluation of FDG-PET/CT imaging for the diagnosis and monitoring of WG [80], we retrospectively analyzed 13 FDG-PET/CT images obtained from eight patients. WG lesions of the upper respiratory tract and lung were more clearly detected by FDG-PET/CT fusion imaging than by nonenhanced CT alone, and all active lesions showed decreased FDG uptake after treatment. In addition, FDG-PET/CT can be combined with other imaging methods to inform selection of biopsy sites. In conclusion, FDG PET/CT is a feasible modality for evaluating lesion activity and therapeutic efficacy in WG.

Several research studies on PET findings in GPA have been published. Similar to the aforementioned reports, FDG–PET/CT was indicated as useful in identifying lesions and biopsy sites as well as evaluating disease activity [81–83]. Some reports also stated that the FDG-PET was useful in evaluating inflammation in aortitis as a complication of GPA [84].

6.1.11 Conclusion

FDG-PET/CT can provide information on active inflammatory lesions. It is a very sensitive but nonspecific imaging modality. The distribution patterns of inflammatory foci sometimes suggest specific disease. In general, if FDG-PET/CT imaging is used appropriately, it may provide very helpful information for accurate diagnosis, particularly for identification of biopsy sites. In addition, FDG-PET/CT is very sensitive for monitoring disease activity. It could be applied to the prediction of therapeutic response, but further studies are required. FDG-PET/CT is a promising imaging modality for rheumatic diseases.

6.2 Adult-Onset Still's Disease

Chao Cheng

Abstract The diagnosis of adult-onset Still's disease (AOSD) is nonspecific and requires the exclusion of other diseases including infectious, inflammatory and malignant diseases. AOSD has been referred to as the archetypal febrile autoinflammatory illness. It typically causes a diurnal fever, highest in the evening accompanied by a salmon-pink rash and arthralgia, with both the fever and rash subsiding completely within hours. Currently, the diagnosis is largely clinical due to low prevalence, vague symptoms and the absence of any diagnostic test. AOSD is the archetypal febrile autoimmune disease.

Keywords: Adult-onset Still's disease, FDG, PET/CT, Lymph nodes

6.2.1 Clinical Presentation

A 33-year-old female known with intermittent fever (T_{max} of 39 °C) for more than 10 days without obvious incentives. The rash was widely located in the skin of hip and arm, with obvious pharynx and body sore. The patient had no chills, no cough. Laboratory examination found: WBC, 10.6 × 10^9/L; NEUT, 10.08 × 10^9/L; ESR, 44 mm/H; CRP, 129 mg/L; PCT,0.228 ng/mL; ANA (negative); ALT, 1004 U/L; AST,893 U/L; IgE, 255.00 IU/mL.

6.2.2 Key Images

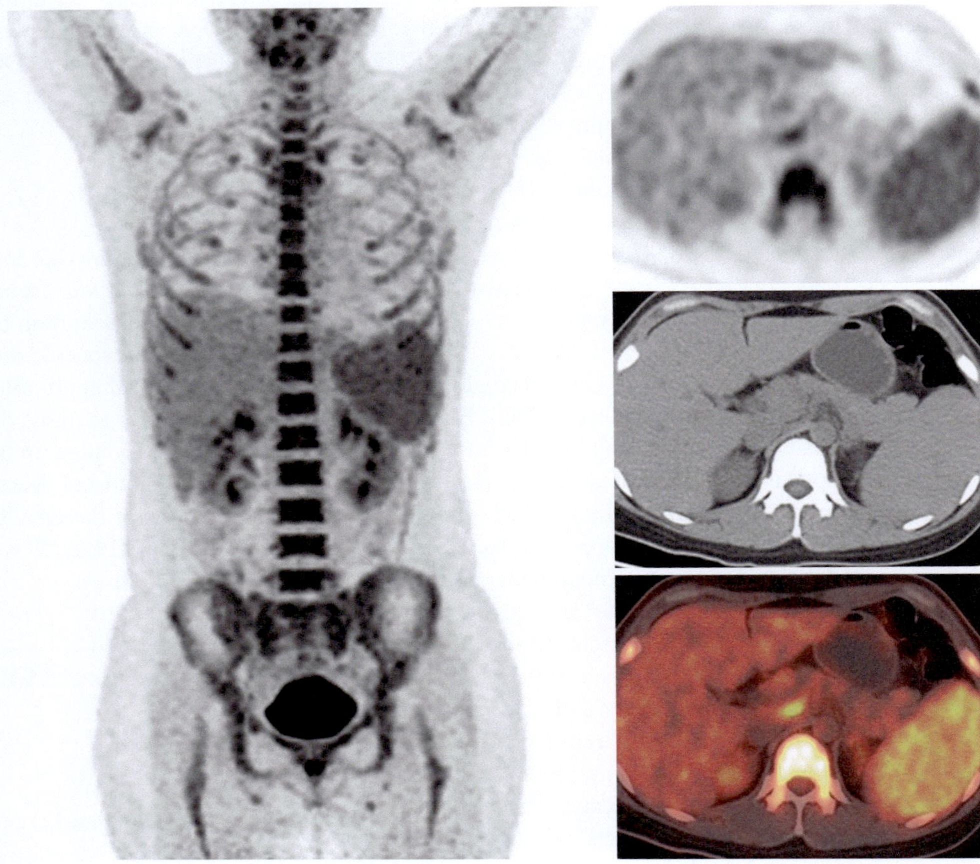

Fig. 6.1 Demonstrate increased FDG uptake for ^{18}F-FDG PET/CT images in the bone (SUV_{max} = 7.7), spleen (SUV_{max} = 4.0) and multiple lymph nodes (SUV_{max} = 4.5)

6.2.3 Technique

- Patient preparation: patient should not take anything by mouth for 6 h before administration of radiopharmaceutical.
- 344 MBq of F18-FDG administered intravenously (body weight = 65 Kg).
- Imaging device: whole body PET/CT camera (Siemens biograph 64) with resolution of 4.0 mm FWHM.

6.2.4 Differential Diagnosis

- Malignant lymphoma,
- Tuberculosis,
- Metastatic tumor.

6.2.5 Diagnosis and Clinical Follow-Ups

The patient received anti-inflammatory therapy (Methylprednisolone, Hydroxychloroquine, Human Immumoglobulin) and recovered promptly.

6.2.6 Discussion

AOSD is a chronic systemic inflammatory disease. Due to the nonspecific features in clinical performance, laboratory tests, and imaging modalities, AOSD remains difficult to diagnose. FDG-PET/CT has been suggested to be useful for AOSD diagnosis and evaluation of disease activity [60, 85]. Especially grossly 18F-FDG accumulation in the bone marrow and spleen is considered to be a characteristic of AOSD. Although the definitive diagnosis cannot be made based only on FDG-PET/CT findings in a case with suspected AOSD, these findings are extremely useful as support for the diagnosis [86].

6.3 Polymyositis/Dermatomyositis

Chao Cheng

Abstract Idiopathic inflammatory myopathies are a heterogeneous group of disorders clinically characterized by progressive proximal muscle weakness and pathologically by mononuclear cell infiltration and fiber necrosis in muscles. Polymyositis (PM), dermatomyositis (DM) and inclusion body myositis are representative phenotypes. PM/DM can present with prominent truncal muscle weakness or preferential involvement of respiratory muscles. We can visually evaluate the extent and pattern of muscle lesions systemically by F-18 FDG PET/CT.

Keywords: Polymyositis, Dermatomyositis, FDG, PET/CT

6.3.1 Clinical Presentation

A 41-year-old man known with Intermittent limb muscle soreness for more than 1 year, increased in the past week and accompanied by limb weakness. Electromyogram examination suggests myogenic damage. Laboratory examination found: CK, 5537 U/L; CKMB 61.0 U/L, LDH 226 U/L, K^+, 1.9 mmol/L. The levels of tumor markers were normal.

6.3.2 Key Images

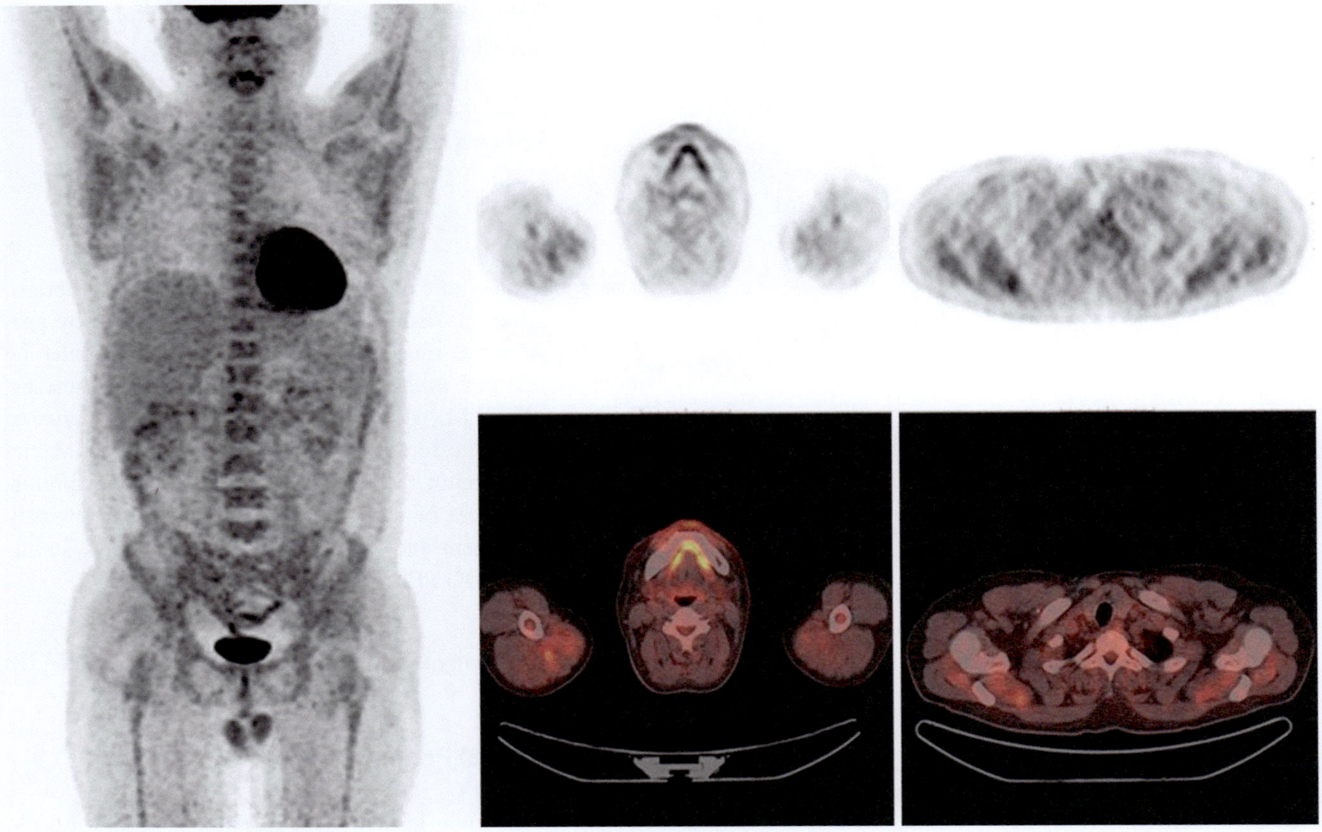

Fig. 6.2 Demonstrates moderate increased FDG uptake in PET/CT images in the whole body muscle, especially the bilateral upper limb muscles. In addition, systemic bone radioactivity uptake was significantly increased

6.3.3 Technique

- Patient preparation: the patient should not take anything by mouth for 6 h before administration of radiopharmaceutical.
- 460 MBq of 18FDG administered intravenously (body weight = 87 kg).
- Imaging device: whole body PET/CT camera (Siemens Biograph 64) with resolution of 4.0 mm FWHM.

6.3.4 Differential Diagnosis

- Infectious myopathy
- Metabolic myopathy
- Polymyalgia rheumatica
- Muscular dystrophy
- Tumor-associated myopathy

6.3.5 Diagnosis and Clinical Follow-Ups

This patient developed muscle aches and limb weakness in the limbs, and simultaneous hypokalemia. After receiving hormone combined with methotrexate therapy, the condition of the patient tended to be stable and is discharged from hospital.

6.3.6 Discussion

PM (polymyositis) and DM (dermatomyositis) are chronic inflammatory diseases that affect systemic skeletal muscles and extramuscular organs including the lungs [87, 88]. F18-FDG PET/CT has practicality and convenience in the clinical characterization of PM/DM [89, 90]. The biggest advantage of FDG PET is the fact that it can screen the entire body in one scan [91, 92].

6.4 Polymyositis

Xuena Li

Abstract Polymyositis is a disease with characteristic rash dominated by inflammation of skin and striated muscles. Skin and muscle damage can disappear or be mitigated after removal of tumors. An 18-year-old female developed lower limb weakness without inducement 6 months ago. Symptoms gradually worsened. The patient had difficulty swallowing in the past half-month, and occasionally coughed when drinking water. To exclude malignant tumors, the patient underwent PET/CT. Imaging showed multiple, symmetrical, and diffuse increased FDG uptake in head, neck, psoas major, and limb muscles, the viscera showed no lesion of increased metabolism. Muscle biopsy suggested myositis. Symptoms improved after hormone therapy.

Keywords: Polymyositis, FDG, PET

6.4.1 Clinical Presentation

An 18-year-old female developed lower limb weakness without obvious inducement 6 months ago, and her symptoms gradually worsened. The patient had difficulty swallowing in the past half-month, and occasionally had a cough when drinking water. Normal limb muscle tension. Head MRI prompted normal.

6.4.2 **Key Images** (Fig. 6.3)

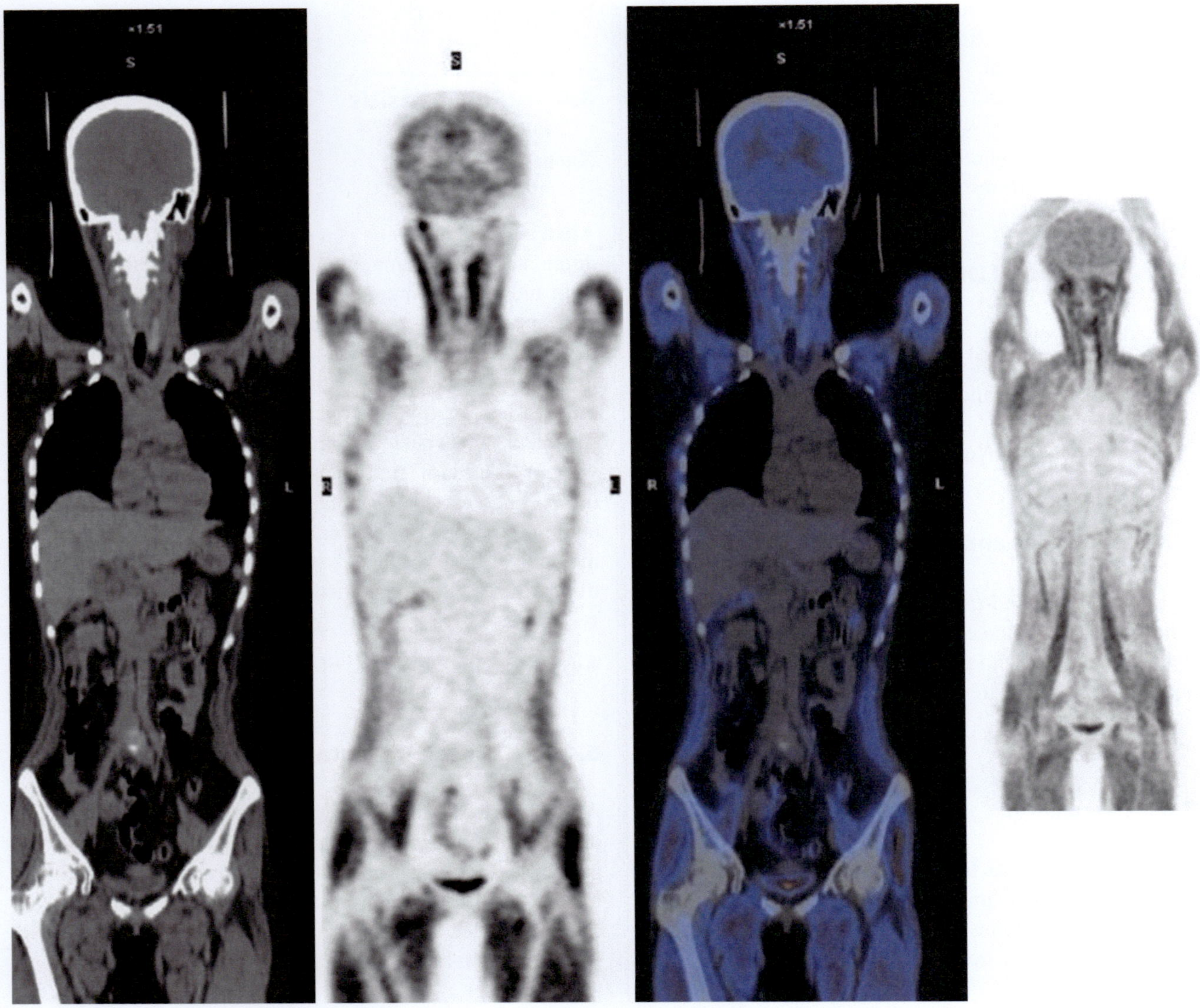

Fig. 6.3 ^{18}F-FDG PET/CT image

PET/CT imaging shows multiple, symmetrical, and diffuse increased FDG uptake in head, neck, psoas major, and limb muscles (SUV_{max} = 7.3), the viscera shows no lesions of increased metabolism

6.4.3 Technique

- Patient preparation: patient should not take anything by mouth for 6 h before administration of radiopharmaceutical.
- 185 MBq of 18F-FDG administered intravenously.
- Imaging device: whole body PET/CT camera (Siemens biograph) with resolution of 5.0 mm FWHM,

6.4.4 Differential Diagnosis

- Primary muscle tumor.
- Sarcoidosis.

6.4.5 Diagnosis and Clinical Follow-Ups

Muscle biopsy suggested myositis. The symptoms improved after the hormone therapy.

6.4.6 Discussion

Polymyositis is a disease with characteristic rash dominated by inflammation of skin and striated muscles. Inflammatory myopathy is a group of heterogeneous diseases. Malignant tumors are associated with polymyositis. Imaging contributes to exclude tumor-associated polymyositis [93, 94]. As a whole-body imaging, it shows lesions' distribution throughout the body and provides information for diagnosis [95, 96].

6.5 Dermatomyositis 1

Xuena Li

Abstract Polymyositis (PM) and dermatomyositis (DM) are idiopathic inflammatory myopathies that mainly involve skeletal muscles and other organs. Patients with DM present with characteristic skin lesions. A 65-year-old male was diagnosed with "systemic lupus erythematosus" 9 years ago, and his symptoms did not significantly improve after treatment with externally used drug. One month ago, the patient suffered from fatigue, facial edema, and rashes. Laboratory tests showed raisedd NSE. PET/CT imaging showed multiple elevated FDG uptake in the muscle with no primary tumors observed. The skin biopsy indicated DM.

Keywords: Dermatomyositis, FDG, PET

6.5.1 Clinical Presentation

A 65-year-old man was diagnosed with "systemic lupus erythematosus"9 years ago, and his symptoms did not significantly improved after external medication therapy. One month ago, the patient suffered from fatigue, facial edema, and rashes. Laboratory tests showed elevated NSE (30.47), serum levels of CK (128 U/L) and LDH (206 U/L).

6.5.2 Key Images

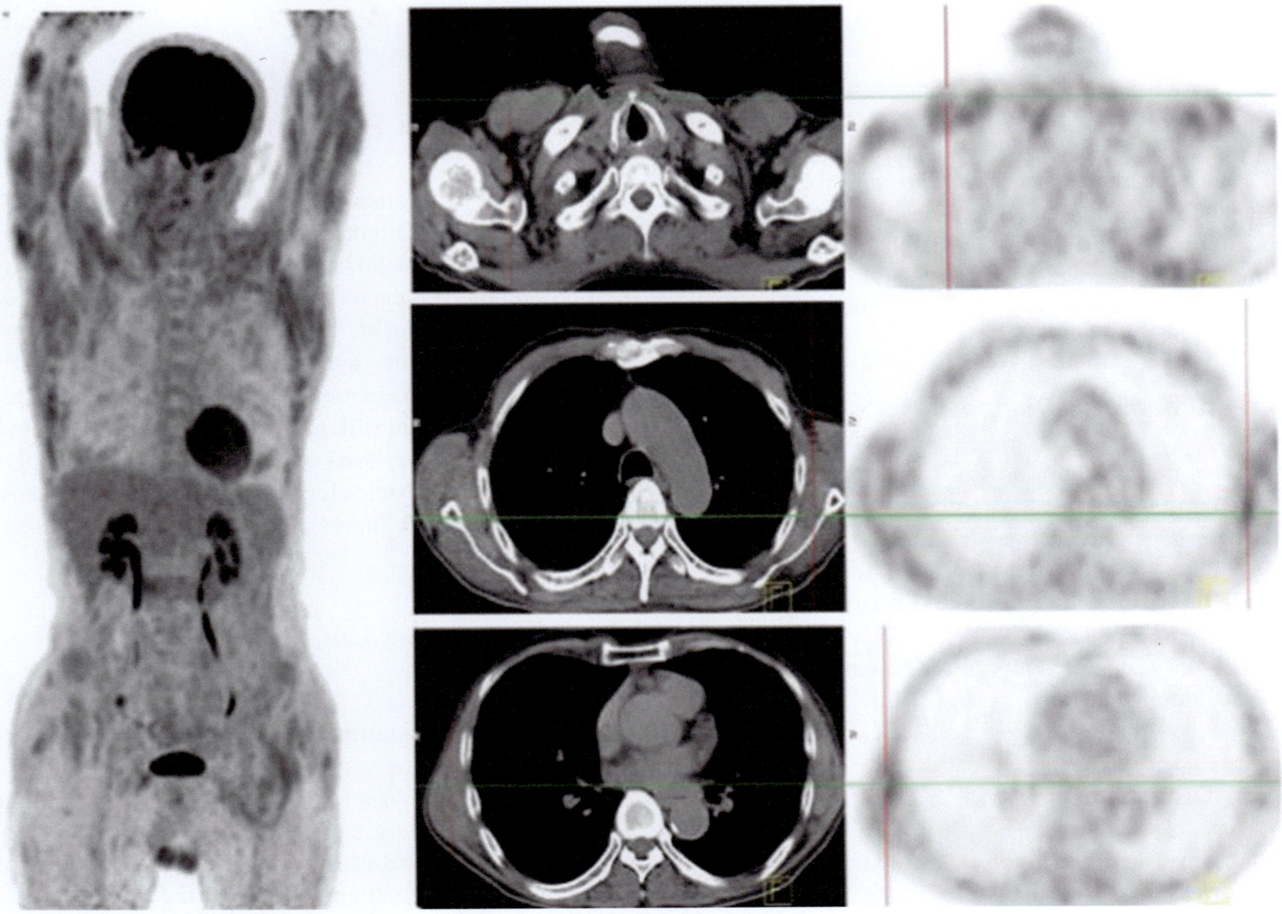

Fig. 6.4 ^{18}F-FDG PET/CT image

PET/CT imaging shows multiple elevated FDG uptake in the muscles without primary tumors

6.5.3 Technique

- Patient preparation: patient should not take anything by mouth for 6 h before administration of radiopharmaceutical.
- 185 MBq of 18F-FDG administered intravenously.
- Imaging device: whole body PET/CT camera (Siemens biograph) with resolution of 5.0 mm FWHM.

6.5.4 Differential Diagnosis

- Primary muscle tumor.
- Sarcoidosis.

6.5.5 Diagnosis and Clinical Follow-Ups

The skin pathology indicated dermatitis. The symptoms improved after specialist treatment.

6.5.6 Discussion

The diagnosis of DM is mainly based on the diagnostic and revised criteria proposed by Bohan and Peter in 1975. Some patients have no objective evidence of muscle inflammation. PET imaging has diagnostic value for DM and reflects disease activity by evaluating the metabolic activity of proximal band muscles [97–100].

6.6 Dermatomyositis 2

Azusa Tokue

Abstract Dermatomyositis (DM) is an idiopathic inflammatory myopathy characterized by skin rash and symmetric weakness of proximal muscles. We present a case of DM with FDG uptake in muscles assessed by PET/CT. The inflammatory lesions with increased FDG uptake were consistent with those of myositis detected by MRI. DM is often associated with malignancy and interstitial lung disease (ILD). FDG PET/CT may be useful for detection of malignancy and evaluation of active muscle inflammation, interstitial pneumonia in patients with DM.

Keywords: Dermatomyositis, FDG-PET/CT, Malignancy, Interstitial lung disease

6.6.1 Clinical Presentation

A 38-year-old woman presented with high fever, joint pain, and muscle pain for 2 months. She had heliotrope rash, Gottron's signs, mechanic's hands, and the weakness of proximal muscles. Muscle strength was evaluated by manual muscle test (MMT). Serum creatine kinase level was normal.

6.6.2 Key Images

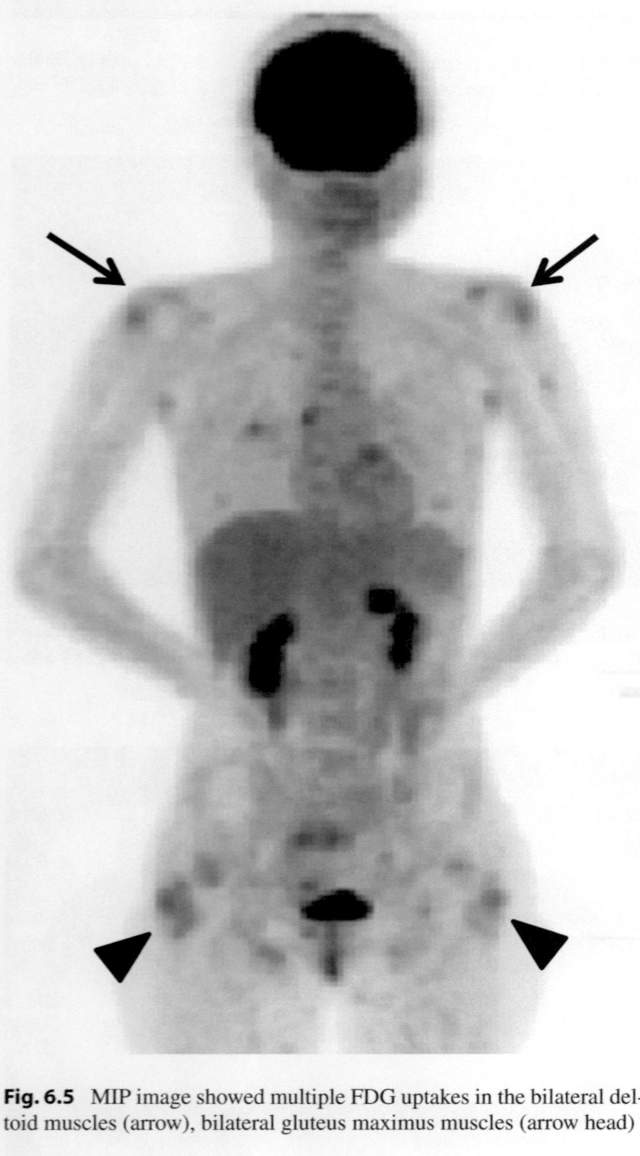

Fig. 6.5 MIP image showed multiple FDG uptakes in the bilateral deltoid muscles (arrow), bilateral gluteus maximus muscles (arrow head)

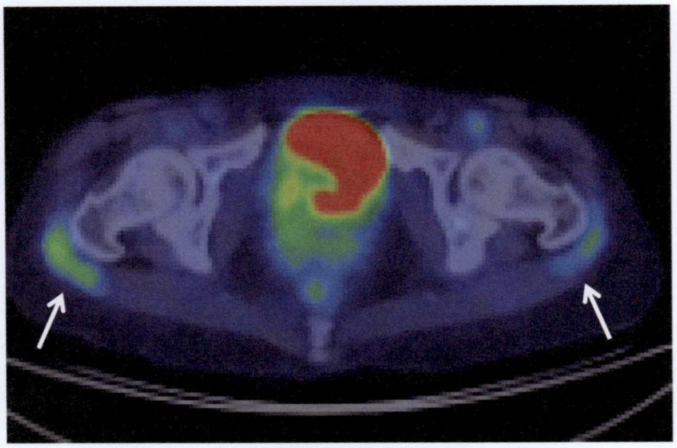

Fig. 6.6 PET/CT fusion image showed increased FDG uptakes in the bilateral gluteus maximus muscles (SUV_{max}: 2.1–2.8) (arrow)

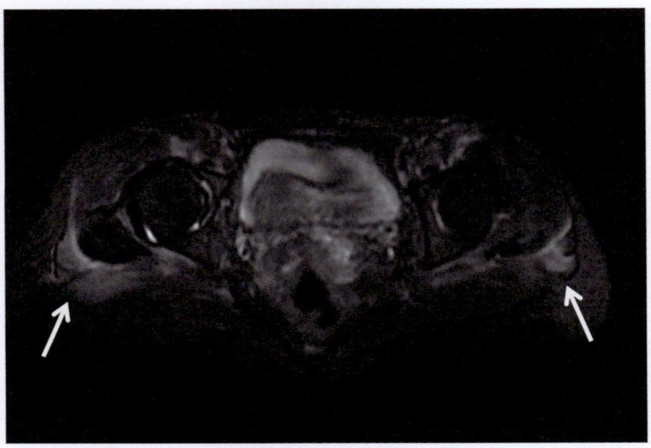

Fig. 6.7 Clinical diagnosis was DM. MRI scan demonstrated enhancement of bilateral gluteus maximus muscles consistent with FDG accumulation (arrow)

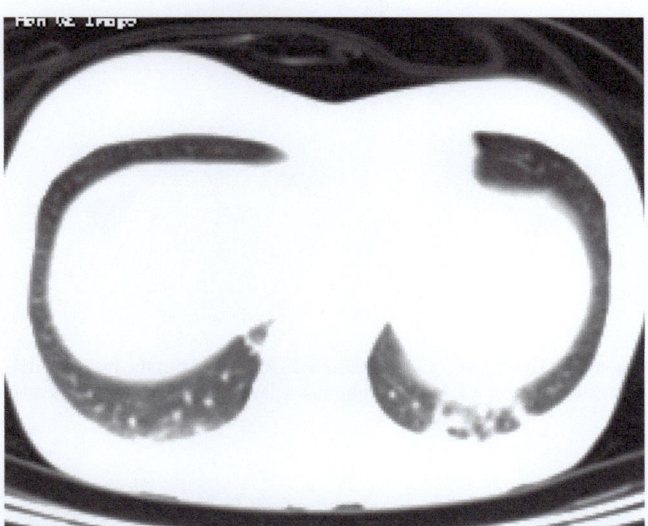

Fig. 6.8 CT showed reticular opacity in both lower lung and the complication of ILD was observed. She was treated with prednisolone, cyclophosphamide, and tacrolimus

6.6.3 Technique

- After fasting for at least 6 h, the patient was injected with FDG (5 MBq/kg) intravenously.
- PET/CT imaging was acquired 1 h after injection on a whole body PET/CT camera (Biograph 16, Siemens Medical Solutions) with resolution of 5.0 mm FWHM.
- MRI scan (Signa 1.5 T, GE) with a body total imaging matrix array coil was acquired.

6.6.4 Differential Diagnosis

- muscle strain,
- sarcoidosis.

6.6.5 Discussion

DM is a systemic autoimmune inflammatory myopathy with characteristic skin lesions and skeletal muscle inflammation [101]. Since DM patient often presents with malignancy and ILD [102], it is necessary to evaluate the distribution of whole body lesions before treatment. FDG PET/CT is useful for screening for malignancy, detecting inflammatory lesion of muscle and evaluating lung inflammation [103–105].

6.7 Rheumatoid Arthritis 1

Hiroyuki Yamashita

Abstract The main pathological manifestations of rheumatoid arthritis (RA) include synovitis, pannus formation and bone erosion. These pathological changes are usually assessed by plain X-ray, US, CT, and contrast-enhanced, fat-suppressed MRI. PET with 18F-FDG can be used to evaluate the metabolic activity of synovitis and measure the disease activity in RA patients by whole-body imaging. Imaging studies using 18F-FDG-PET have been performed to assess the metabolic activity of synovitis in patients with RA and to evaluate the disease activity of RA. Several reports have indicated that there was a significant correlation between the visual assessment of FDG uptake and clinical evaluation of disease activity.

Keywords: Rheumatoid arthritis, 18F-FDG-PET/CT, Disease activity

6.7.1 Clinical Presentation

An 86-year-old woman presented with polyarthritis. She had symmetrical polyarthritis that continued for more than 19 weeks with a severe inflammatory reaction (CRP, 12.72 mg/dL) and MRI findings that showed synovitis and tendinitis.

6.7.2 Key Images

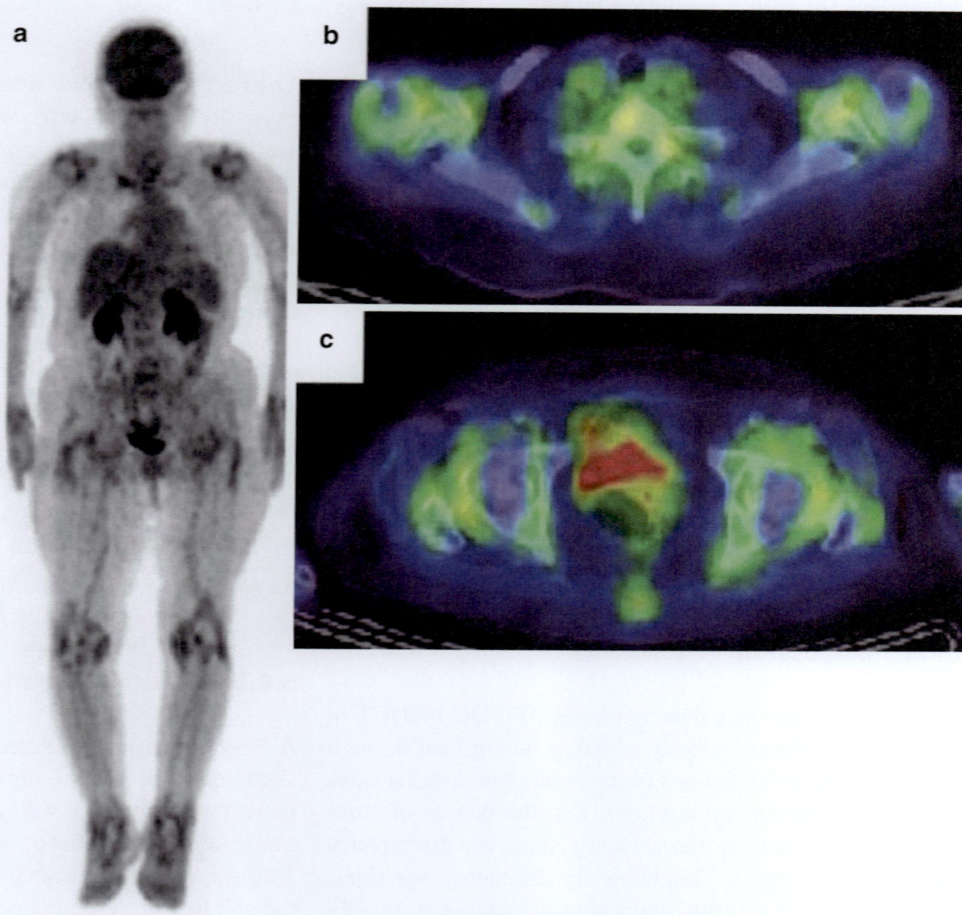

Fig. 6.9 (**a**–**c**) shows (**a**) MIP and (**b**, **c**) axial FDG-PET/CT findings. FDG-PET/CT showed (**a**) symmetrical arthritis and remarkable circular FDG uptake due to synovitis around the (**b**) shoulders and (**c**) hips.

6.7.3 Technique

- Patient preparation: The patient should not take anything orally up to 4 h before the administration of ^{18}FDG.
- 4–6 MBq/kg of ^{18}F-FDG was intravenously administered.
- Imaging device: Whole body PET/CT camera (Siemens biograph 16) with a resolution of 3.75 mm FWHM was used.

6.7.4 Differential Diagnosis

- Polymyalgia rheumatica (PMR)
- Spondyloarthritis (SpA)

6.7.5 Diagnosis and Clinical Follow-Ups

For this patient, clear synovitis was confirmed on MRI. Because polyarthritis in >11 sites and inflammatory reaction were observed, and the symptoms lasted for >6 weeks in spite of negative RF and anti-CCP antibody results, a diagnosis of RA was made based on the 2010 ACR/EULAR RA classification criteria.

6.7.6 Discussion

Active RA lesions were detected using ^{18}F-FDG PET/CT in our case. The disease activity of RA is determined through comprehensive examinations of the number of arthritis sites, degree of inflammatory reactions, and the degree of complaints from the patient. Occasionally, there is a discrepancy between the patient's complaints, inflammatory reactions, and the degree of arthritis upon physical examination. ^{18}F-FDG PET/CT is useful when comprehensively screening for latent arthritis and performing differential diagnoses of similar diseases, such as PMR and SpA [106–109].

6.8 Rheumatoid Arthritis 2

Xuena Li

Abstract Rheumatoid arthritis (RA) is a chronic autoimmune disorder with unknown etiology. The major clinical manifestations are chronic, symmetrical arthritis and extraarticular lesions. A 75-year-old male suffered from swelling and pain of the shoulders, knees, and hips without obvious inducement, accompanied by elevated blood NSE, underwent ^{18}F-FDG PET/CT for cancer screening. PET images showed increased FDG uptake of the bilateral shoulder joints, bilateral hip joints, gall bladder, and right cervical lymph nodes. Laboratory reports showed elevated C-reactive protein, erythrocyte sedimentation rate, and rheumatoid factor. The patient was diagnosed with rheumatoid arthritis and cholecystitis. After specialist treatment, his symptoms markedly improved.

Keywords: Rheumatoid arthritis, FDG, PET

6.8.1 Clinical Presentation

A 75-year-old man suffered from swelling and pain of the shoulders, knees, and hips with no apparent cause. The patient was diagnosed with gout by local hospital. The symptoms did not relieve after corresponding treatment. Ultrasonography indicated slightly higher echogenicity in the gall bladder. Laboratory reports showed elevated NSE.

6.8.2 Key Images

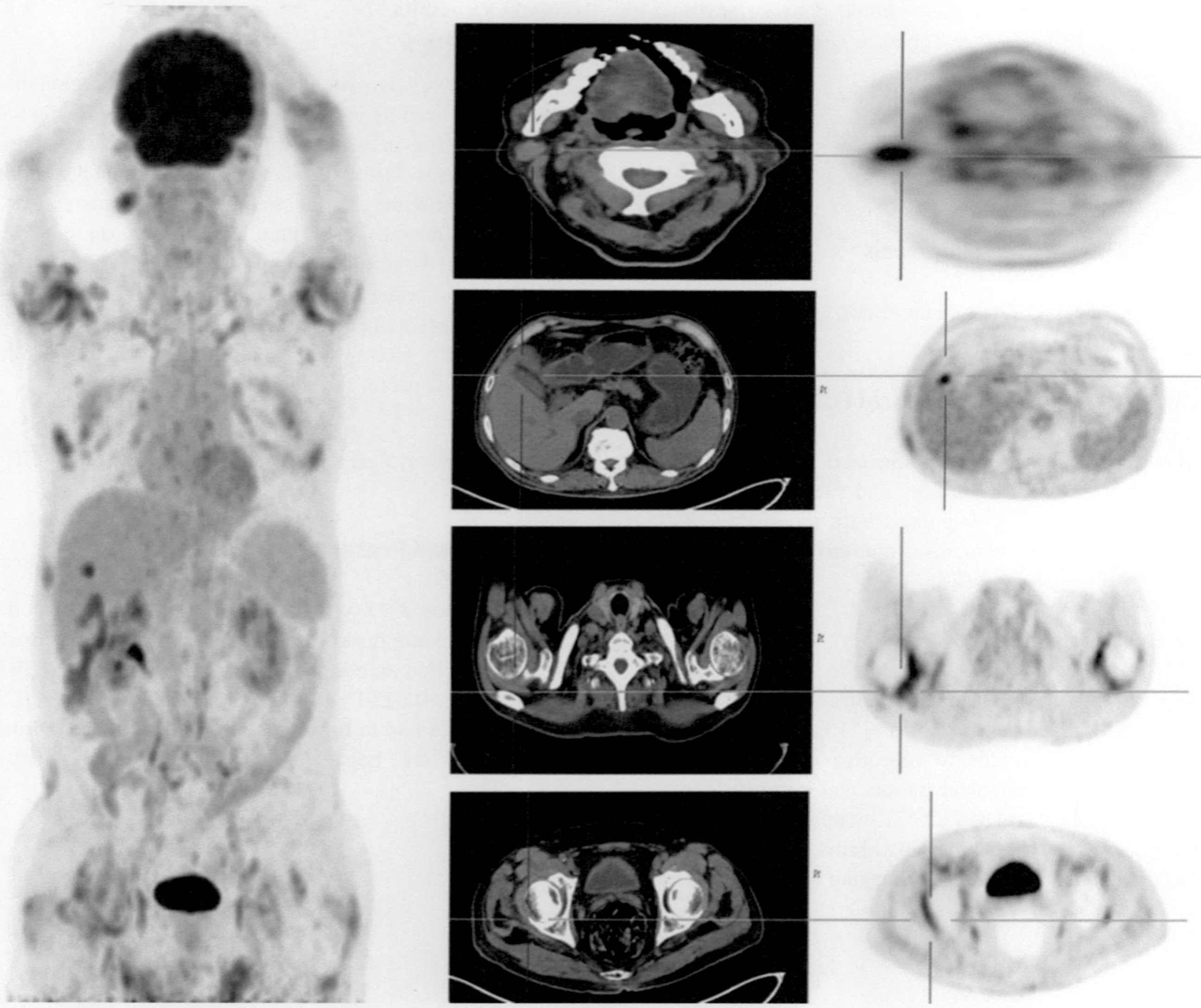

Fig. 6.10 ^{18}F-FDG PET/CT image

MIP image (Fig. 6.10) demonstrates increased tracer uptake in the bilateral shoulder joints, bilateral hip joints, gall bladder, and right cervical lymph nodes. Transverse image shows soft tissue in the bilateral shoulder joints and bilateral hip joints with increased FDG uptake

6.8.3 Technique

- Patient preparation: patient should not take anything by mouth for 6 h before administration of radiopharmaceutical.
- 185 MBq of 18F-FDG administered intravenously.
- Imaging device: whole body PET/CT camera (Siemens biograph) with resolution of 5.0 mm FWHM.

6.8.4 Differential Diagnosis

- Bone metastasis of malignant tumor.

6.8.5 Diagnosis and Clinical Follow-Ups

Laboratory reports showed elevated C-reactive protein, erythrocyte sedimentation rate, and rheumatoid factor. The patient was clinically diagnosed with rheumatoid arthritis. After specialist treatment, his symptoms markedly improved.

6.8.6 Discussion

FDG PET/CT has contributed to diagnosis and differential diagnosis of rheumatoid arthritis [110, 111]. This imaging always provides relatively objective overall information, helps to exclude malignant tumors and improves diagnostic accuracy [112]. ^{18}F-FDG PET/CT imaging can reflect activity and impact scope of rheumatoid arthritis, show more valuable information than conventional imaging modalities [113].

6.9 Polymyalgia Rheumatica

Hiroyuki Yamashita

Abstract Polymyalgia rheumatica (PMR) is a common disorder characterized by inflammatory pain and stiffness in the shoulder as well as in the pelvic girdle and neck. The diagnosis requires the exclusion of other conditions causing similar symptoms. Sometimes the complaints of PMR patients are vague and the diagnosis is difficult, based only on the chief complaints and the physical findings. FDG-PET/CT is useful for covering the entire body and identifying bursitis, a characteristic of PMR, which has vague symptoms and is difficult to identify from other imaging tests. As a result, FDG-PET/CT is useful for diagnosing PMR.

Keywords: Polymyalgia rheumatic, Bursitis, FDG-PET/CT

6.9.1 Clinical Presentation

The patient was a 58-year-old female whose chief complaint was an acute onset of neck pain and proximal myalgia. She exhibited an elevated inflammatory reaction (CRP level, 7.52 mg/dL; ESR, 104 mm/h), and an FDG-PET/CT scan was performed to investigate the cause. Blood culture test results were negative, and bacteremia was also negative.

6.9.2 Key Images (Fig. 6.11)

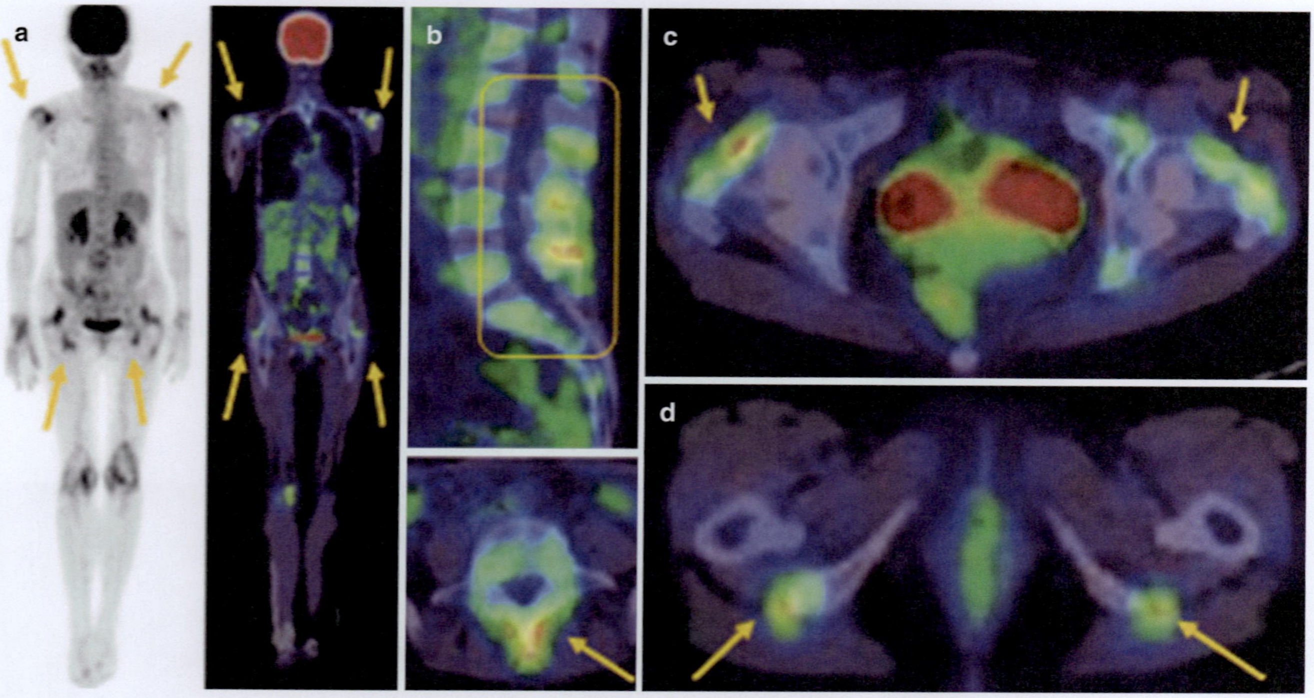

Fig. 6.11 (**a**, **b**) FDG-PET shows inflammatory FDG uptake in the shoulders and hips (arrows). Axial and sagittal FDG-PET/CT fusion images clearly show high FDG uptake in the intervertebral joints, interspinal ligaments, and surrounding muscles of the lumbar region (arrows) (**b**), and bursae in the greater trochanter (arrows) (**c**) and ischial tuberosity (arrows) (**d**)

6.9.3 Technique

- Patient preparation: patient should not take anything by mouth for 6 h before administration of radiopharmaceutical.
- -185 MBq of 18FDG administered intravenously.
- Imaging device: whole body PET/CT camera (Siemens biograph) with resolution of 5.0 mm FWHM.

6.9.4 Differential Diagnosis

- Rheumatoid arthritis (RA).
- Spondyloarthritis (SpA).

6.9.5 Diagnosis and Clinical Follow-Ups (Fig. 6.12)

6.9.6 Discussion

Active RA lesions were detected using ^{18}F-FDG PET/CT in our case. PMR patients showed increased FDG uptake in ischial tuberosities, greater trochanters, and lumbar spinous processes [114]. Positive results at two or more of these sites showed high sensitivity and specificity for the diagnosis of PMR. Moreover, the pattern of accumulation in the shoulder (focal and nonlinear uptake patterns) and the identification of iliopectineal bursitis are useful in diagnosing PMR, which is at times difficult to differentiate from elderly-onsetRA [109, 115].

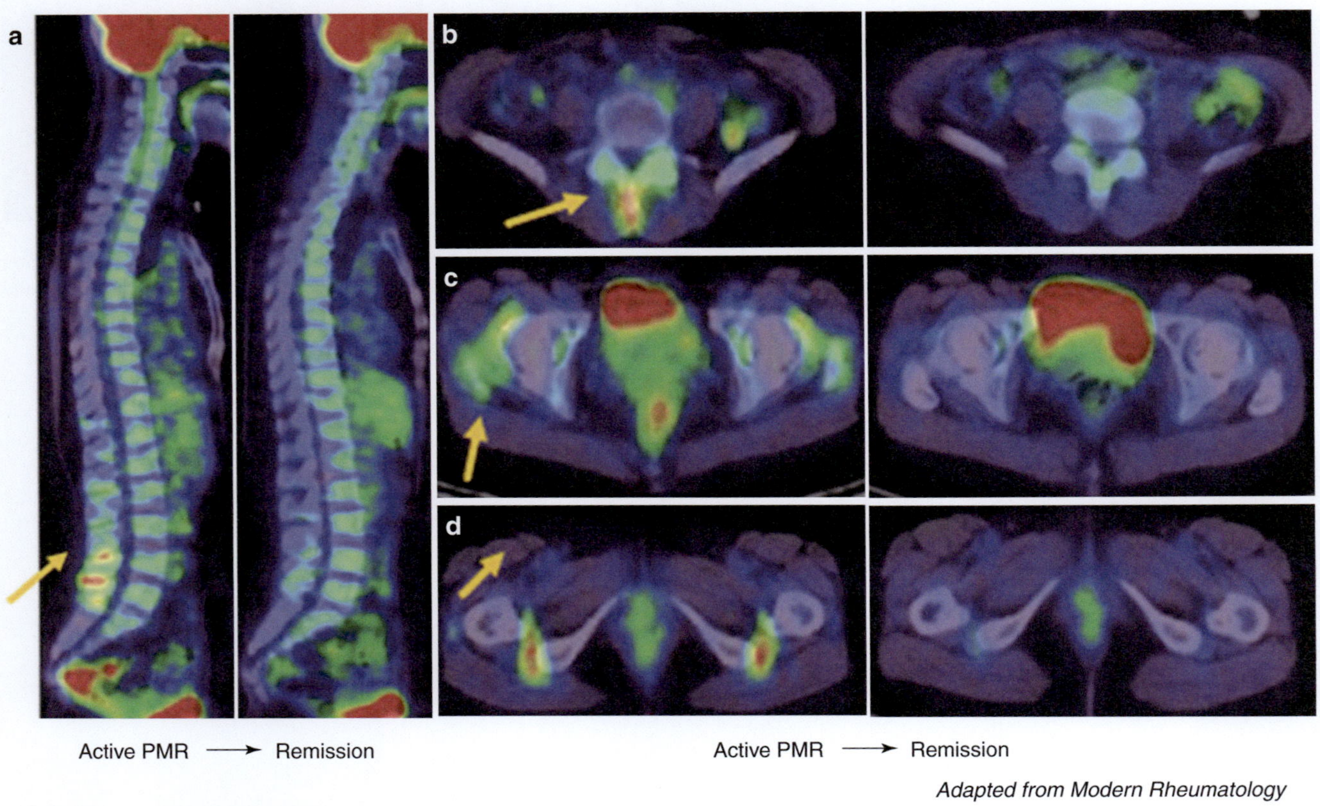

Fig. 6.12 Because the patient was ≥50 years, her ESR was ≥40 mm/h; further, she had proximal myalgia and experienced a prompt therapeutic reaction to steroids. She was evaluated as having met the Chuang et al. and Healy criteria, which led to a diagnosis of PMR. A follow-up FDG-PET/CT shows that FDG uptake in the spinous processes of the lower lumbar vertebrae (**a**, **b**, arrows), greater trochanter (**c**, arrows), and ischial tuberosity (**d**, arrows) normalized after therapy (**a**–**d**, right panels)

6.10 Relapsing Polycondritis

Hiroyuki Yamashita

Abstract Relapsing polychondritis (RPC) is a rare multisystemic disease characterized by recurrent inflammation of the cartilaginous structures of the external ear, nose, peripheral joints, larynx, and tracheobronchial tree. Much remains unknown about the epidemiology of RPC. Diagnosis is made according to the empirically defined clinical criteria of McAdam et al. No specific histological finding is considered pathognomonic for this disease. FDG-PET/CT may be a powerful tool for the early diagnosis of relapsing polychondritis, especially when patients have no involvement of organs that are easily biopsied such as the ears or nose. It is also useful for determining the extent of disease and monitoring disease activity during treatment.

Keywords: Relapsing polychondritis, FDG-PET/CT

6.10.1 Clinical Presentation

A 74-year-old female presented with nasal symptoms. She was positive for type II anti-collagen antibody, and nasal cartilage biopsy findings were consistent with RPC.

6.10.2 Key Images (Fig. 6.13)

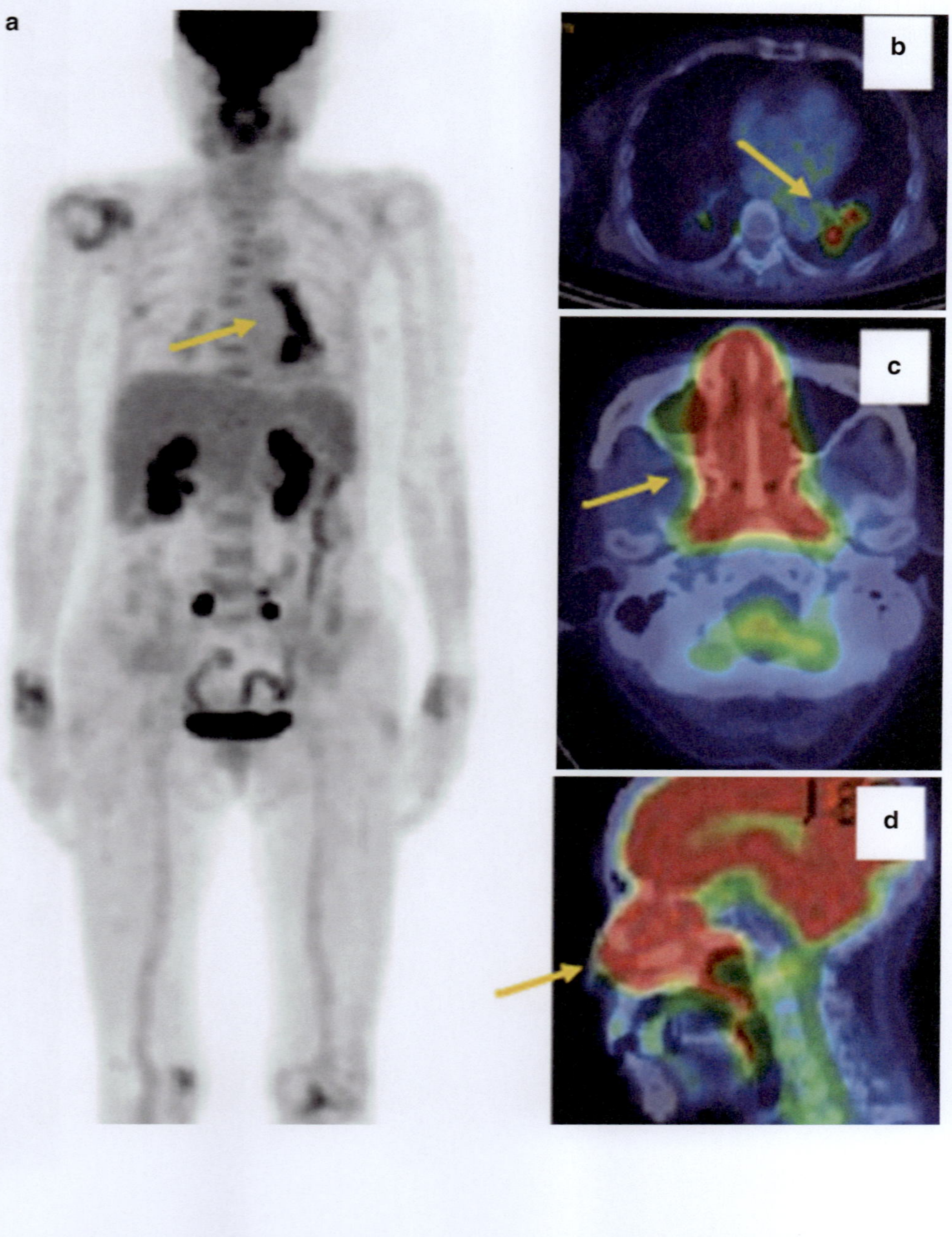

Fig. 6.13 Well-defined FDG accumulations (SUV_{max}: 13.03) in the area extending from the infrahilar region of the left inferior lobe to the pulmonary hilus are noted (**a**, **b**, *arrow*). There was no radiographic evidence of bronchial wall thickening or bronchial stricture. Conspicuous FDG accumulation (SUV_{max}: 9.50) was also noted in the nasal cavity (**c**, **d**, *arrow*)

6.10.3 Technique

- Patient preparation: patient should not take anything by mouth for 6 h before administration of radiopharmaceutical.
- 185 MBq of 18FDG administered intravenously.
- Imaging device: whole body PET/CT camera (Siemens biograph) with resolution of 5.0 mm FWHM.

6.10.4 Differential Diagnosis

- Infection or malignancy
- Chondrodermatitis nodularis helicis
- Red ear syndrome Epiglottitis Rhinoscleroma Pemphigus vulgaris
- Mediastinal lesions affecting the tracheal wall
- Granulomatosis with polyangiitis
- Systemic inflammatory polyarthritis
- Aortitis and aortic aneurysms

6.10.5 Diagnosis and Clinical Follow-Ups (Fig. 6.14)

Based on the diagnostic criteria established by Damiani et al., the definitive diagnosis was RPC, because nasal chondritis and associated histological findings were confirmed.

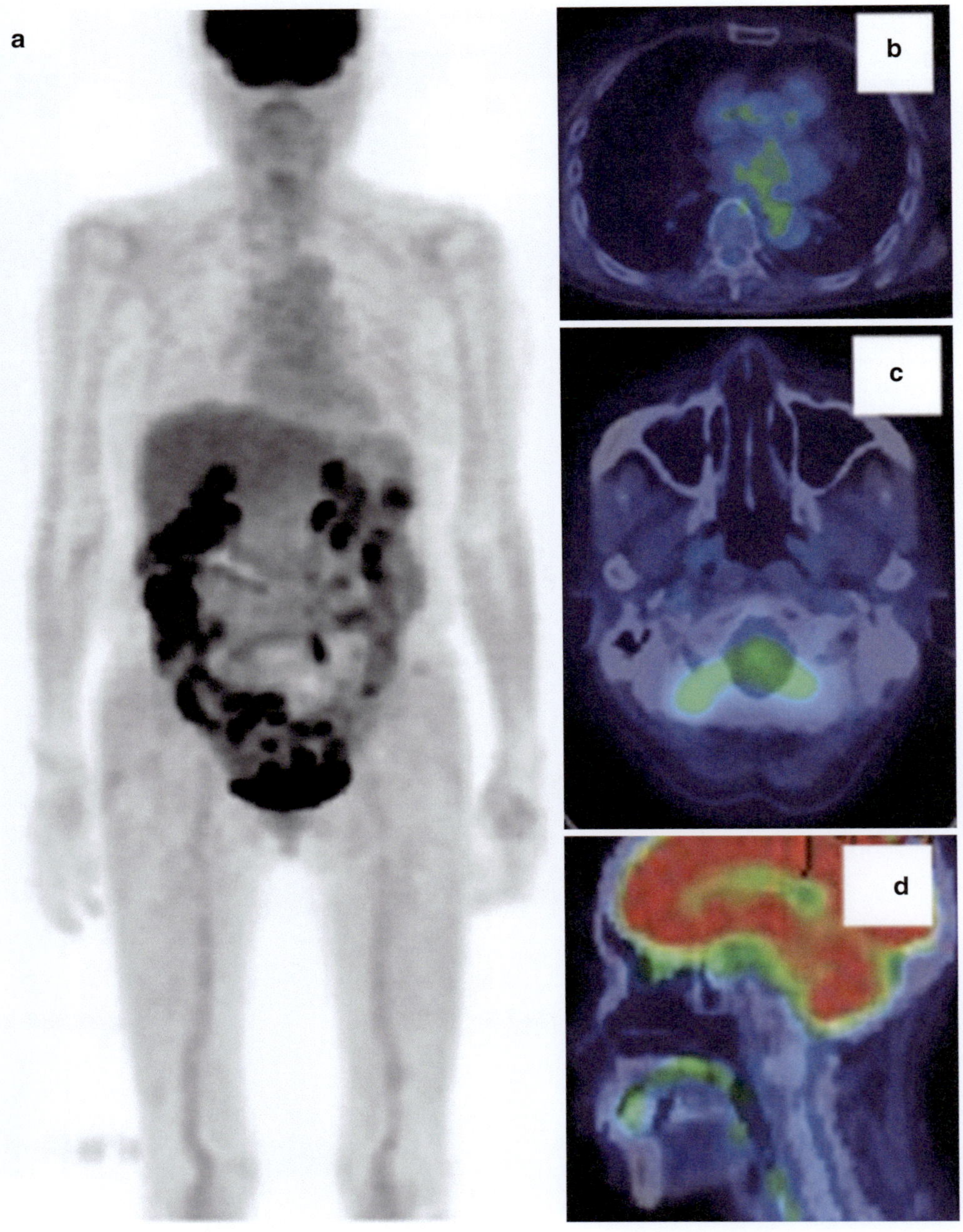

Fig. 6.14 (**a**, **b**) Posttreatment FDG PET/CT images showed complete lack of FDG accumulation in the area extending from the infrahilar region of the left inferior lobe to the pulmonary hilus. (**c**, **d**) Conspicuous FDG accumulation in the nasal cavity disappeared completely after treatment

6.10.6 Discussion

FDG-PET/CT is a potentially powerful tool for the early diagnosis of RPC, especially in patients without easily biopsied organ involvement [109, 116, 117]. This modality also facilitates the evaluation of extent of disease and disease activity during treatment. In addition, FDG-PET/CT guides biopsy site by identifying the active inflammation of asymptomatic lesions in relapsing polychondritis.

6.11 Granulomatosis with Polyangiitis 1

Xuena Li

Abstract Granulomatosis with polyangiitis (GPA) is complex, various and lack of specificity in clinical manifestations. The most commonly involved organs and systems are ears, nose, throat, lungs, and kidneys. A 56-year-old male appeared with epistaxis, discharging pus, and smelly secretions 6 months ago. It was considered sinusitis. In the past 2 months, instep skin and the sacrococcygeal region ulcerated and formed scabs. PET imaging was used to exclude malignant tumors. PET/CT showed soft tissue density shadow in bilateral maxillary sinus and nasal cavity, FDG uptake increased uneven. Metabolism in spleen and bone marrow increased diffusely. Laboratory tests showed positive ANCA. Symptoms relieved after hormone therapy.

Keywords: Granulomatosis with polyangiitis, FDG, PET

6.11.1 Clinical Presentation

A 56-year-old male appeared with epistaxis, discharging pus, and smelly secretions 6 months ago. It was considered sinusitis. Anti-inflammatory treatment is not effective. In the past 2 months, instep skin and sacrococcygeal region ulcerated and formed scabs. He had pain in lower limbs with swelling feet and difficulty in walking. CA12-5 and CRP increased (Fig. 6.15).

Key Images PET/CT imaging shows soft tissue density shadow in the bilateral maxillary sinus and nasal cavity, the FDG uptake increases uneven (SUV_{max} = 8.7), the metabolism in the spleen and bone marrow in visual field increases diffusely (SUV_{max} = 5.1)

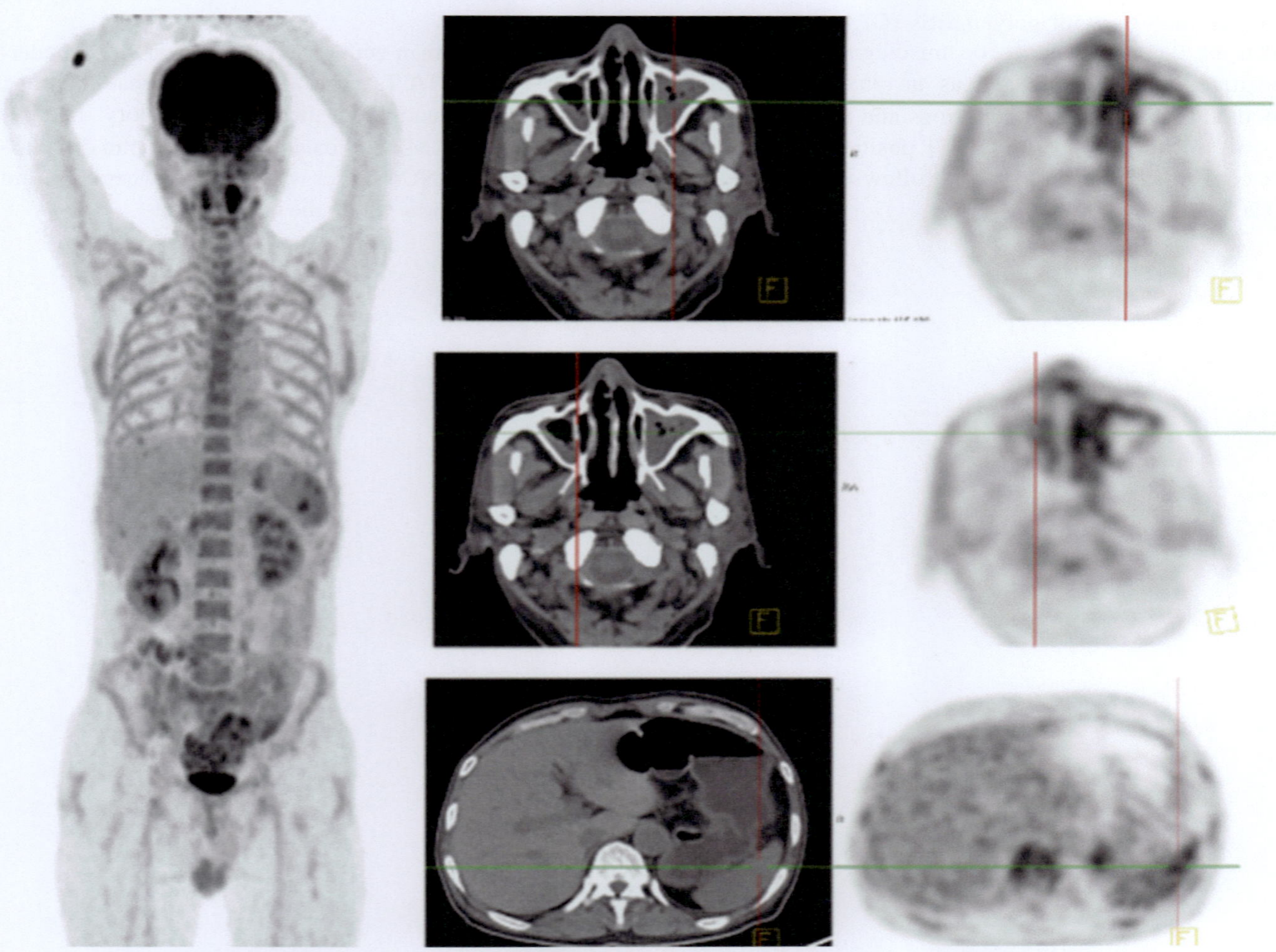

Fig. 6.15 ^{18}F-FDG PET/CT image

6.11.2 Technique

- Patient preparation: patient should not take anything by mouth for 6 h before administration of radiopharmaceutical.
- 185 MBq of 18F-FDG administered intravenously.
- Imaging device: whole body PET/CT camera (Siemens biograph) with resolution of 5.0 mm FWHM,

6.11.3 Differential Diagnosis

- Primary muscle tumor.
- Sarcoidosis.

6.11.4 Diagnosis and Clinical Follow-Ups

Bone marrow puncture showed reactive hyperplasia. After hormone therapy, the symptoms relieved significantly.

6.11.5 Discussion

Granulomatosis with polyangiitis (GPA) involves nasopharynx, so it is easy to be misdiagnosed. PET/CT is positive in GPA and used as an auxiliary diagnostic method to assess extent of lesions and range of systemic involvement [118, 119]. PET/CT positive lesions need to be confirmed by pathology and follow-up after treatment [120, 121].

6.12 Granulomatosis with Polyangiitis 2

Kimiteru Ito

Abstract Granulomatosis with polyangiitis (GPA), also known as Wegener's granulomatosis, is a rare disease characterized by granulomatous necrotizing vasculitis, which primarily involves small- and medium-sized blood vessels. GPA is a rare type of systemic vasculitis that involves the upper and lower respiratory tracts and the kidneys. Severe inflammation and renal failure rapidly develops in untreated patients and can be life-threatening. Therefore, early diagnosis is essential to improve prognosis. A considerably high ^{18}F-FDG uptake is exhibited in GPA before treatment; however, the uptake promptly decreases after treatment. In this study, ^{18}F-FDG PET/CT was used in the diagnosis and follow-up of patients with GPA.

Keywords: Granulomatosis with polyangiitis, Wegener's granuloma, Vasculitis, ANCA, PET/CT

6.12.1 Clinical Presentation

A 79-year-old woman with fever of unknown origin underwent ^{18}F-FDG PET/CT. Chest X-ray showed that both lung lesions resisted antibiotic therapy. Laboratory findings showed that serum MPO-circulating antineutrophil cytoplasmic antibodies (ANCAs) titer was elevated, whereas serum PR3–ANCA titer was within the normal limits.

6.12.2 Key Images (Fig. 6.16–6.19)

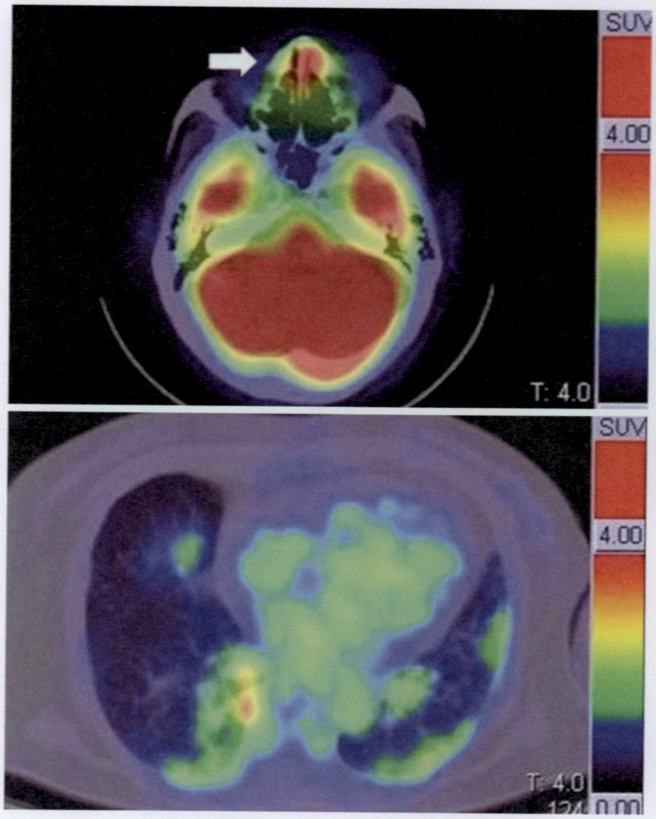

Fig. 6.16 Axial ^{18}F-FDG PET/CT showed abnormal ^{18}F-FDG uptake in the nasal wall (white arrow; SUV_{max}, 5.1). Axial ^{18}F-FDG PET/CT showed increased ^{18}F-FDG uptake in the opacities in both lungs (SUV_{max}, 4.0) in this figure.

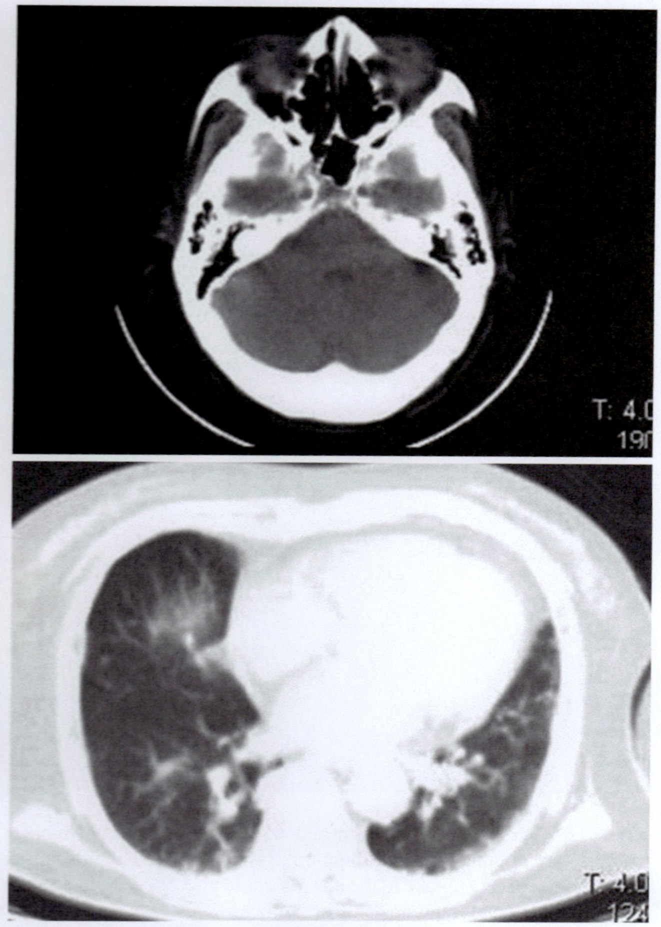

Fig. 6.17 Nonenhanced CT alone did not show the nasal lesion in this figure

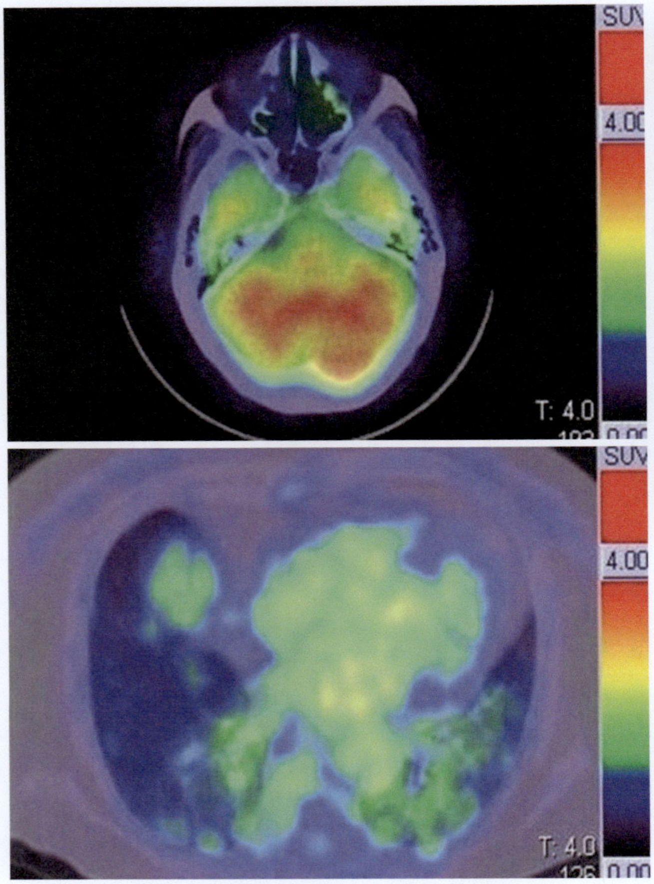

Fig. 6.18 The patient was diagnosed with GPA using nasal biopsy from ^{18}F-FDG uptake area. A follow-up ^{18}F-FDG PET/CT in this figure showed no ^{18}F-FDG uptake in the nasal mucosa after the administration of prednisolone and immunosuppressant therapy

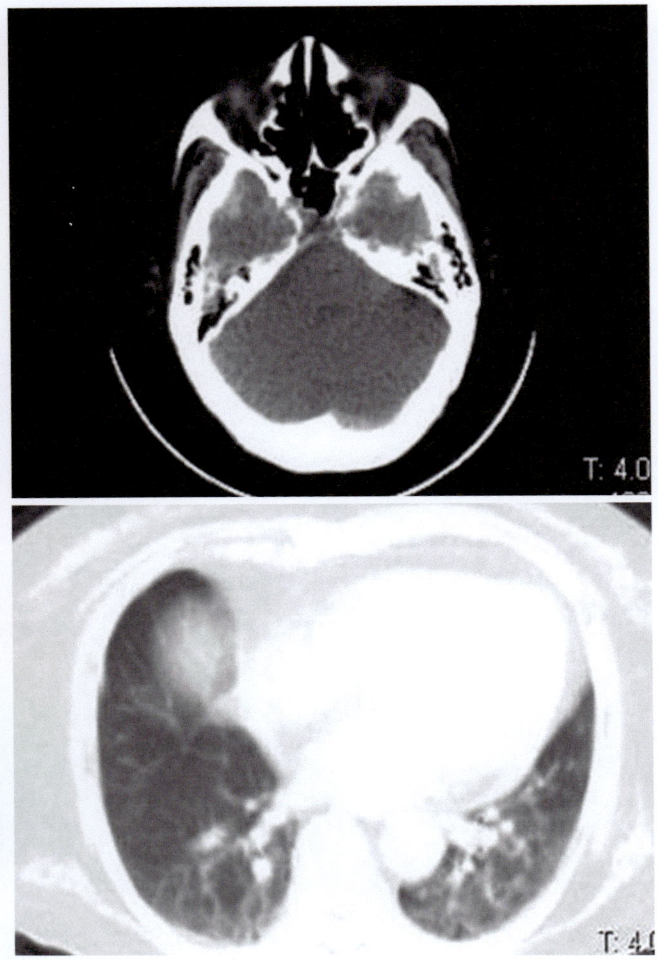

Fig. 6.19 ^{18}F-FDG uptake in the opacities in both lungs decreased

6.12.3 Technique

- Patient preparation: The patient should not take anything orally up to 4 h before the administration of ^{18}FDG.
- 4–6 MBq/kg of ^{18}F-FDG was intravenously administered.
- Imaging device: Whole body PET/CT camera (Siemens biograph 16) with a resolution of 3.75 mm FWHM was used.

6.12.4 Differential Diagnosis

- Various malignancies (for example, lymphoma and lung cancer)
- Sarcoidosis
- Mycobacterium
- Other collagen diseases

6.12.5 Discussion

Active GPA lesions were detected using ^{18}F-FDG PET/CT in our case. GPA lesions in the upper respiratory tract were easier to detect using ^{18}F-FDG PET/CT than using nonenhanced CT alone [122–125]. Notably, all radiologists must be familiar with the clinical features and ^{18}F-FDG PET of GPA.

6.13 Systemic Lupus Erythematosus

Xuena Li

Abstract Systemic lupus erythematosus (SLE) is an autoimmune connective tissue disease involving organs and systems. A 35-year-old female appeared with lumbago without incentives. Main clinical symptoms were bilateral renal pain, bilateral elbows, shoulders and knees pain, stiffness, and fever. Laboratory tests showed positive antinuclear antibody, anti-Smith, anti-U1RNP, and increased immunoglobulin IgG, CK, and LDH. PET/CT showed increased FDG uptake in lymph nodes in bilateral cervical, supraclavicular, inguinal, mediastinal, retroperitoneal, and left axillary regions, some of which were enlarged, diffusely elevated uptake in spleen and patchy increased-density shadow in both lungs with uneven rising metabolism. Symptoms improved by hormone, cyclophosphamide, and immunomodulatory therapy.

Keywords: Systemic lupus erythematosus, FDG, PET

6.13.1 Clinical Presentation

A 35-year-old female appeared with lumbago without obvious incentives. The main clinical symptoms were bilateral renal pain, bilateral elbows, shoulders and knees pain, stiffness, and fever. Laboratory tests showed positive antinuclear antibody (ANA), anti-Smith, anti-U1RNP, and increased immunoglobulin IgG, CK, and LDH.

6.13.2 Key Images

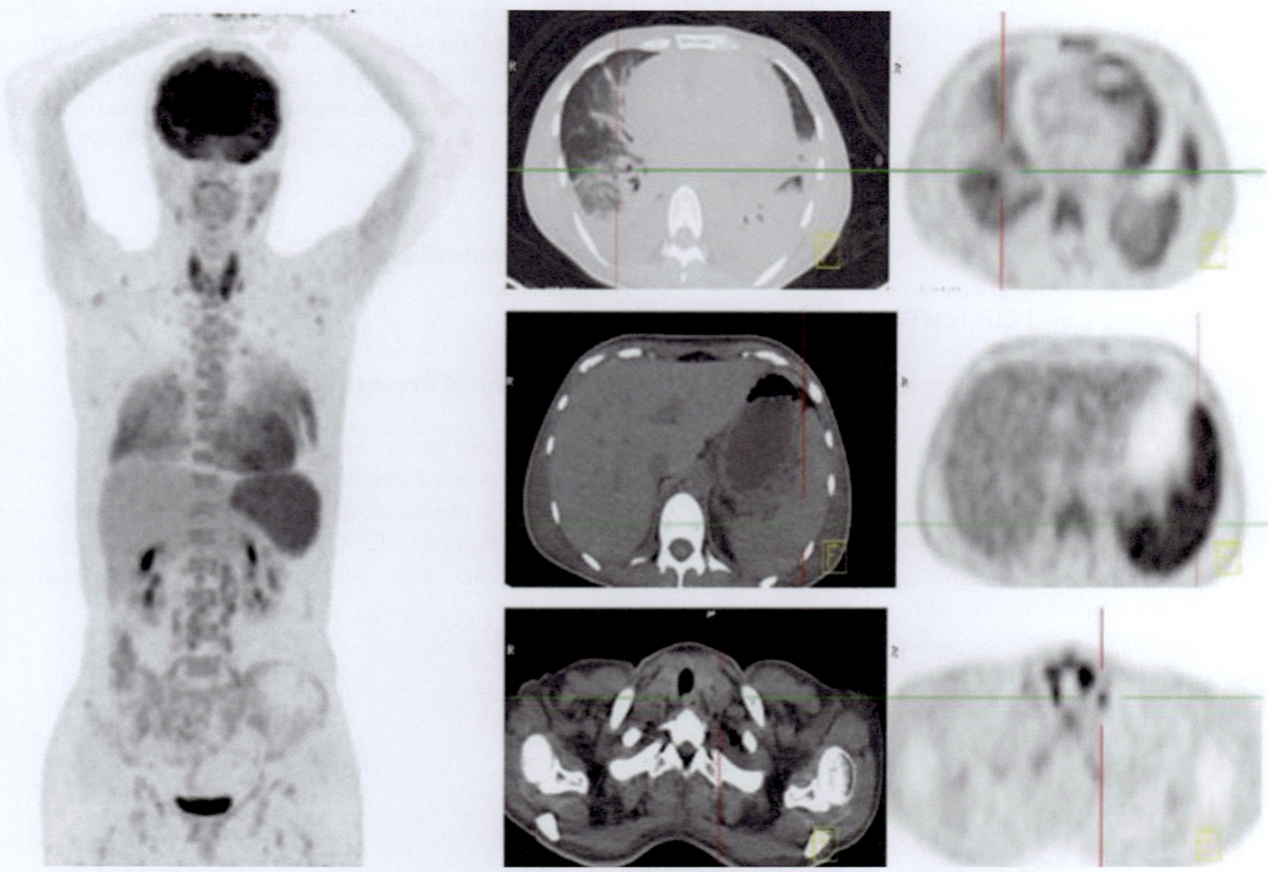

Fig. 6.20 ^{18}F-FDG PET/CT image

PET/CT shows increased FDG uptake in lymph nodes in bilateral cervical, supraclavicular, inguinal, mediastinal, retroperitoneal, and left axillary regions, some of which are enlarged, diffusely elevated uptake in spleen and patchy increased-density shadow in both lungs with uneven rising metabolism

6.13.3 Technique

- Patient preparation: patient should not take anything by mouth for 6 h before administration of radiopharmaceutical.
- 185 MBq of 18F-FDG administered intravenously.
- Imaging device: whole body PET/CT camera (Siemens biograph) with resolution of 5.0 mm FWHM,

6.13.4 Differential Diagnosis

- Primary muscle tumor
- Sarcoidosis

6.13.5 Diagnosis and Clinical Follow-Ups

The symptoms improved after hormone, cyclophosphamide, and immunomodulatory therapy.

6.13.6 Discussion

SLE is an autoimmune connective tissue disease involving multiple organs. Chest is often involved because it is rich in connective tissue. The early diagnosis of SLE is vital for its clinically acute onset, rapid progress, and high mortality. PET/CT of pulmonary lesions can present positive changes that reflect disease activity [126–128].

6.14 IgG4-Related Diseases; Autoimmune Pancreatitis and Lymphadenitis

Kazuhiro Oguchi

Case 1. Abstract An 80-year-old man received FDG-PET/CT for preoperative staging of gastric cancer. PET/CT images showed diffuse pancreatic FDG uptake as well as abnormal uptake into the bilateral supraclavicular, mediastinal, hilar, and abdominal lymph nodes and retroperitoneal soft tissue. His serum IgG4 was elevated. Pathological examination of a gastro-duodenal specimen revealed infiltration of numerous IgG4-positive plasma cells to confirm a diagnosis of IgG4-related disease. Diffuse or multifocal pancreatic FDG uptake is a characteristic finding of IgG4-related autoimmune pancreatitis. Extra-pancreatic uptake in specific organs is also helpful to identify IgG4-related disease.

Keywords: Autoimmune pancreatitis, IgG4-related disease, lymphadenopathy

6.14.1 Clinical Presentation

An 80-year-old man complained of abdominal pain. CT images revealed swelling of the pancreas. Blood testing showed slight elevation of serum IgG4. Ten months later, he underwent FDG-PET/CT for preoperative staging of gastric cancer. His serum IgG4 was elevated at 873 mg/dL.

6.14.2 Key Images (Fig. 6.21)

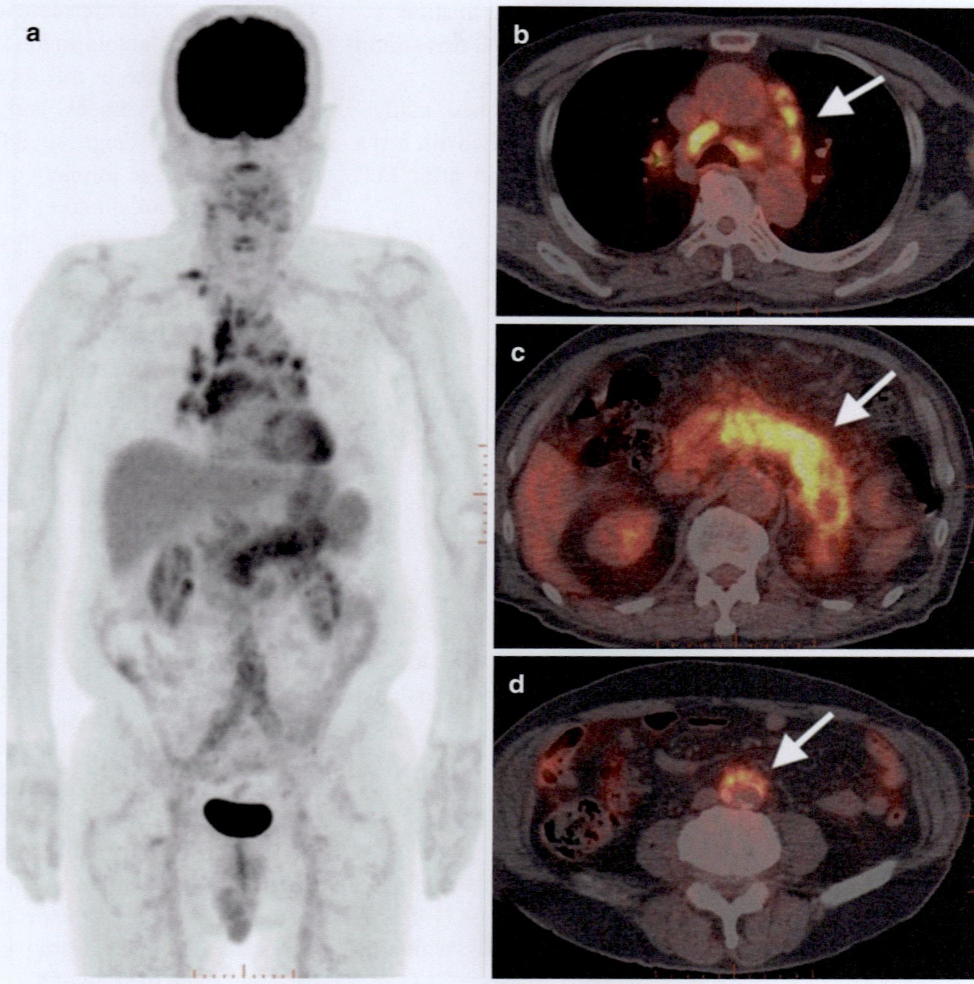

Fig. 6.21 Case 1 ^{18}F-FDG PET/CT

6.14.3 Technique

The patient fasted for over 5 h before PET examination.

A total of 264 MBq (4 MBq/kg) of F-18 FDG was administrated intravenously.

Whole-body PET/CT images were obtained using a PET/CT scanner (Discovery PET/CT 600, GE) with a spatial resolution of 5.1 mm FWHM at 60 min after FDG injection.

6.14.4 Image Interpretation

A swollen pancreas and diffuse FDG uptake were seen (c). Bilateral supraclavicular, mediastinal (b), and hilar lymph nodes displayed swelling and increased FDG uptake. Abnormal FDG uptake in the abdominal lymph nodes and retroperitoneal soft tissue (d) were also evident.

6.14.5 Differential Diagnosis

IgG4-related disease, malignant lymphoma, pancreatic cancer with metastases, sarcoidosis, multicentric Castleman disease.

6.14.6 Diagnosis and Clinical Follow-Up

The patient received surgery for gastric cancer. Pathological examination confirmed the infiltration of IgG4-positive plasma cells in the duodenum and pyloric walls, which met the diagnostic criteria for IgG4-related disease.

6.14.7 Discussion

Diffuse or multifocal pancreatic FDG uptake is a hallmark of IgG4-related autoimmune pancreatitis [129]. Extra-pancreatic uptake in the submandibular gland, mediastinal and hilar lymph nodes, and retroperitoneal soft tissue are also helpful to diagnose IgG4-related disease [129–131]. Abnormal uptake in many other organs, including the pituitary gland, cranial nerve, biliary tract, kidney, and prostate gland, has been reported in patients with IgG4-related disease [131, 132].

Case 2. Abstract A 78-year-old man was referred to an institution for anemia and renal dysfunction. FDG-PET/CT showed abnormal FDG uptake in the pancreas, salivary glands, systemic lymph nodes, para-aortic soft tissue, prostate gland, and kidneys. IgG4-related disease was diagnosed after pathological examination of a renal biopsy revealed IgG4-related tubulointerstitial nephritis. Special attention should be paid for abnormal uptake of FDG in the cortical region of the kidney or prostate gland.

Keywords: Autoimmune pancreatitis, IgG4-related disease, lymphadenopathy, Renal FDG uptake

6.14.8 Clinical Presentation

A 78-year-old man under treatment for diabetes mellitus was referred to a hospital for examination of anemia. CT images revealed swelling of the pancreas, liver, spleen, and bilateral kidneys. Serological testing showed IgG4 elevation (420 mg/dL) and renal dysfunction.

6.14.9 Key Images (Fig. 6.22)

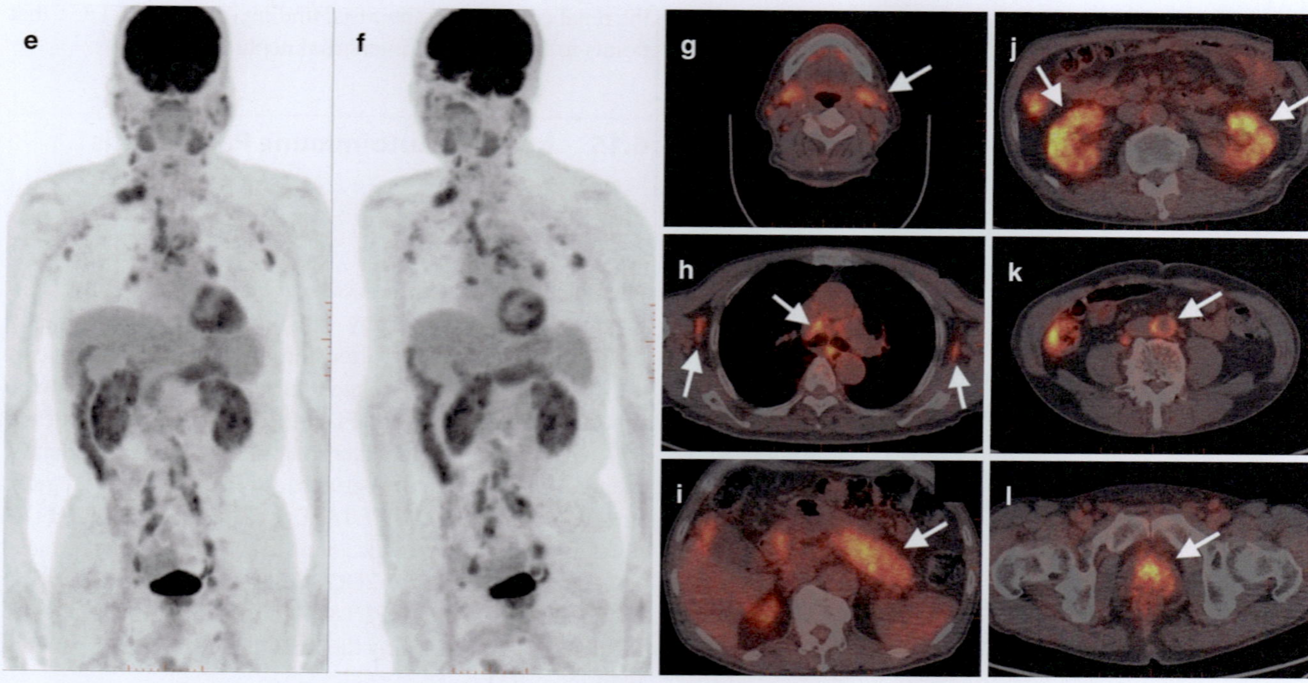

Fig. 6.22 Case 2 ^{18}F-FDG PET/CT

6.14.10 Technique

The patient fasted for over 5 h prior to PET examination.

A total of 249 MBq (4 MBq/kg) of F-18 FDG was administrated intravenously.

Whole-body PET/CT images were obtained using a PET/CT camera (Discovery PET/CT 600, GE) with a spatial resolution of 5.1 mm FWHM at 60 min after FDG injection.

6.14.11 Image Interpretation

A swollen pancreatic tail and diffuse FDG uptake were seen (i). The salivary glands, especially the submandibular glands (g), systemic lymph nodes (h), para-aortic soft tissue (k), and prostate gland (l), all displayed abnormal FDG uptake. Bilateral swelling of the kidneys and abnormal accumulation in the cortical region were apparent (j). Physiological uptake in the ascending colon was seen.

6.14.12 Differential Diagnosis

IgG4-related disease, malignant lymphoma, pancreatic cancer with metastases, sarcoidosis, multicentric Castleman disease, vasculitis.

6.14.13 Diagnosis and Clinical Follow-Up

Kidney biopsy due to renal dysfunction revealed pathological findings of IgG4-related tubulointerstitial nephritis. Accordingly, he was diagnosed as having IgG4-related disease. Subsequent corticosteroid therapy improved his anemia and renal dysfunction.

6.14.14 Discussion

IgG4-related disease can manifest as autoimmune pancreatitis, sclerosing cholangitis, sialoadenitis, retroperitoneal fibrosis, interstitial nephritis, and other forms [133–135]. Excreted urinary FDG usually indicates high uptake in the kidney and urinary system. Moreover, high accumulation in the renal cortex is an abnormal finding on FDG-PET/CT that points to IgG4-related interstitial nephritis [136].

6.15 IgG4RD: Autoimmune Pancreatitis

Masatoyo Nakajo

Abstract The F-18-fluorodeoxyglucose (^{18}F-FDG) positron emission tomography (PET)/computed tomography (CT) findings before and after steroid treatment in a 69-year-old man with IgG4-related disease (IgG4-RD) were reported. Pretreatment ^{18}F-FDG PET/CT revealed abnormal ^{18}F-FDG uptake in the lacrimal glands, salivary glands, pleura, pancreas, and periaortic retroperitoneal region. Posttreatment ^{18}F-FDG PET/CT revealed reduced ^{18}F-FDG uptake in the lesions with abnormal ^{18}F-FDG uptake mentioned above. These ^{18}F-FDG PET/CT findings suggest the usefulness of ^{18}F-FDG PET/CT for assessing the extent of the disease and evaluating the treatment response of patients with IgG4-RD.

Keywords: IgG4-related disease, ^{18}F-FDG PET/CT, Diagnosis, Monitoring

6.15.1 Clinical Presentation

A 69-year-old man presented with a right upper eyelid mass. Excisional biopsy revealed the infiltration of IgG4-positive plasma cells with an IgG4/IgG ratio > 40%. Serum IgG4 was elevated at 1020 mg/dL (reference range: 4.8–105 mg/dL). Therefore, the patient was diagnosed with IgG4-RD, and a systematic work-up with ^{18}F-FDG PET/CT was performed.

6.15.2 Key Images (Fig. 6.23)

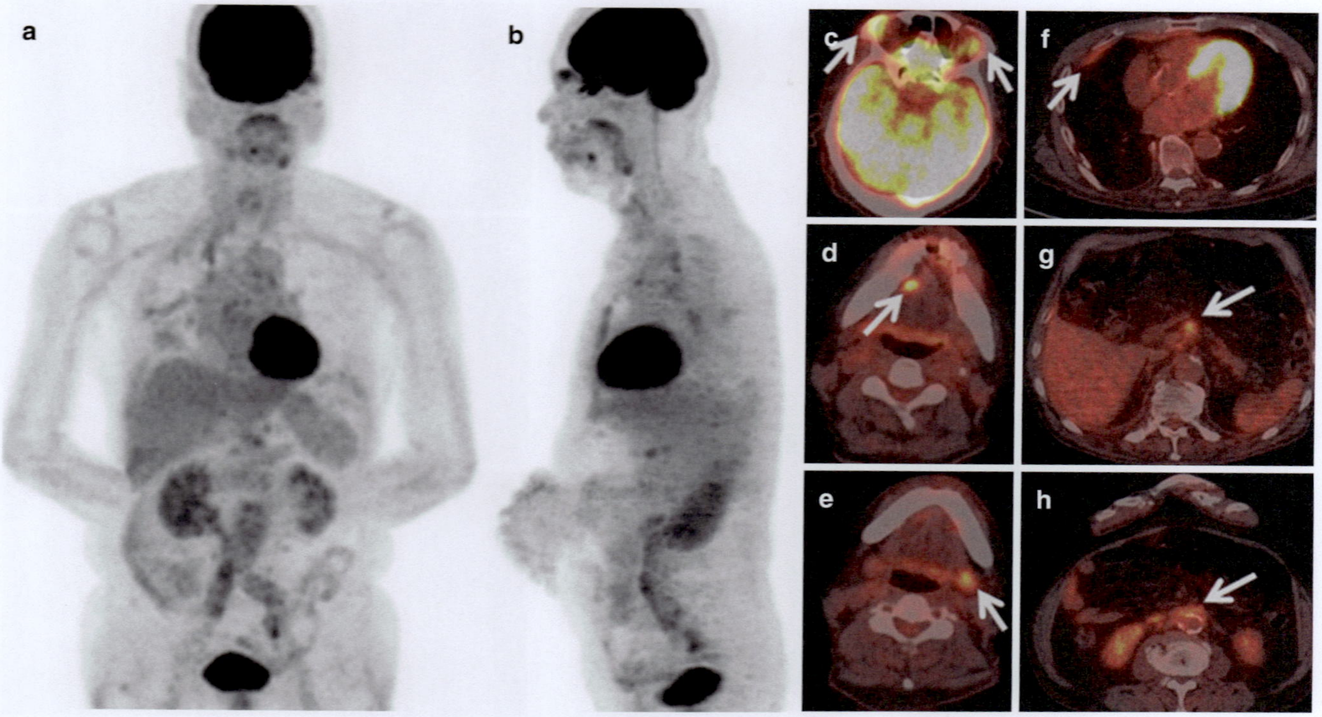

Fig. 6.23 18F-FDG PET/CT image

6.15.3 Technique

- Patient preparation: The patient was instructed to fast for ≥5 h before the administration of ^{18}F-FDG.
- Administrated dose of ^{18}F-FDG: 250 MBq.
- Imaging device: Whole-body PET/CT camera (Discovery 600 M PET/CT, GE Medical Systems) with a resolution of 5.1 mm of full-width at half-maximum.
- Image acquisition: Acquisition began 1 h after the intravenous injection of ^{18}F-FDG, and the images were obtained from brain to feet (acquisition time was 2.5 min per bed position with 14 bed positions) after CT using a 16-slice CT scanner (slice thickness, 3.75 mm; pitch, 1.75 mm; 120 keV; auto mA [35–100 mA depending on the patient body mass]).
- Reconstruction: Three-dimensional ordered-subset expectation maximization algorithm (image matrix size, 192 × 192; 16 subsets, 2 iterations: VUE Point Plus).

6.15.4 Image Interpretation

Pretreatment ^{18}F-FDG PET/CT maximum intensity projection (MIP) (Fig. 6.23a,b) and fused images showed increased abnormal ^{18}F-FDG uptake in the bilateral lacrimal glands (Fig. 6.23c, arrows), right sublingual gland (Fig. 6.23d, arrow), left submandibular gland (Fig. 6.23e, arrow), right pleura (Fig. 6.23f, arrow), proximal part of the pancreatic body (Fig. 6.23g, arrow), and periaortic retroperitoneal region (Fig. 6.23h, arrow).

6.15.5 Differential Diagnosis [137]

- Lymphoproliferative disorders
  - Malignant lymphoma
  - Multicentric Castleman disease
- Examples of other autoimmune diseases
  - Retroperitoneal fibrosis
  - Autoimmune pancreatitis

6.15.6 Diagnosis and Clinical Follow-Up (Fig. 6.24)

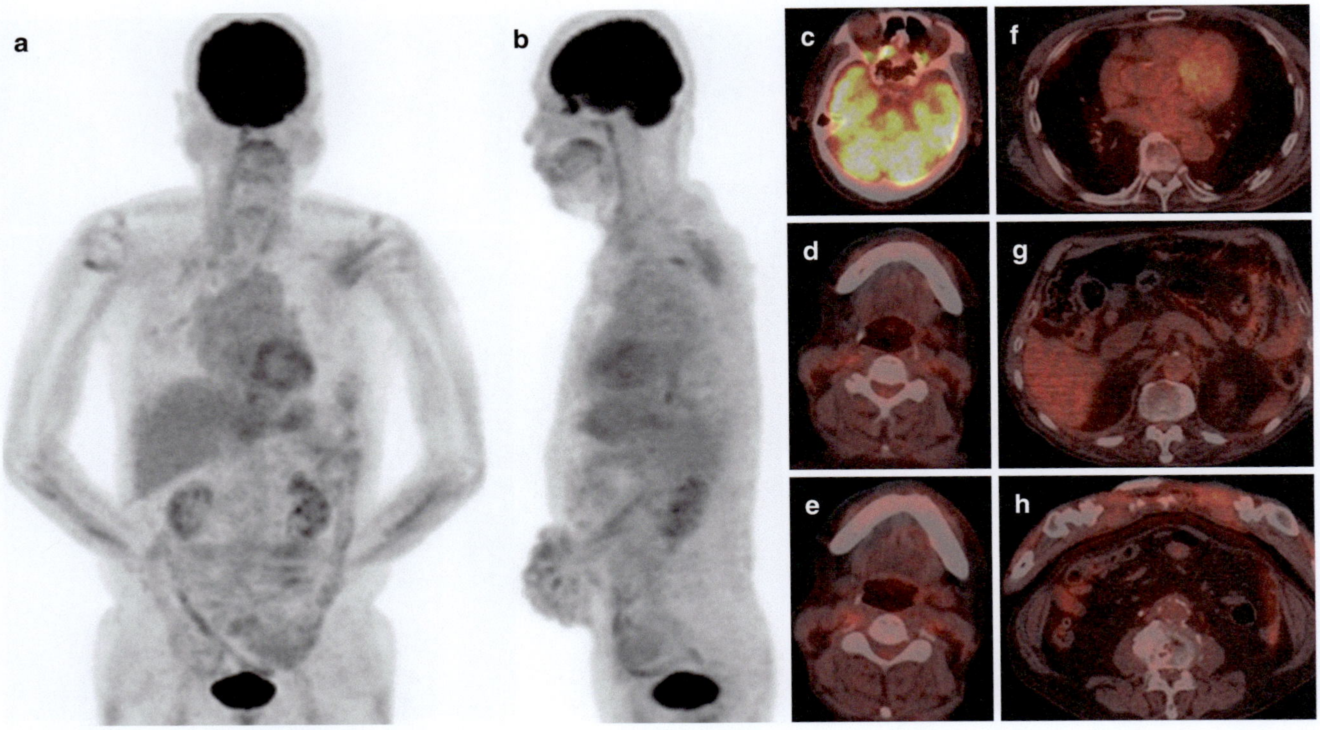

Fig. 6.24 Biopsy of the lacrimal glands confirmed the diagnosis of IgG4-RD, and oral glucocorticoid therapy was initiated. ^{18}F-FDG PET/CT MIP (**a**, **b**) with fused images after 6 months of treatment revealed that the abnormal uptake in the lacrimal glands (**c**), salivary glands (**d**, **e**), pleura (**f**), pancreas (**g**), and periaortic retroperitoneal region (**h**) almost completely disappeared, indicating a good treatment response. The serum IgG4 levels were normalized

6.15.7 Discussion

IgG4-RD is a systemic inflammatory disorder characterized by swollen lesions with lymphoplasmacytic infiltration of IgG4-positive plasma cells [138]. ^{18}F-FDG PET/CT is a whole-body examination that provides metabolic information about disease activity [139] The present case demonstrated the usefulness of ^{18}F-FDG PET/CT for assessing the extension disease and evaluating the treatment response of patients with IgG4-RD.

6.16 IgG4-Related Cardiovascular Disease (IgG4-CVD)

Noriko Oyama-Manabe

Abstract Immunoglobulin G4 (IgG4)–related disease can affect the cardiovascular system, including the coronary arteries and pericardium and especially the walls of large- and medium-sized vessels. The features of IgG4-related cardiovascular disease (IgG4-CVD) on CT include arterial wall thickening and homogeneous wall enhancement. Inflammatory abdominal aortic aneurysms are also attributed to a manifestation of IgG4-CVD. The entire aorta and major branches can be involved with more than twofold the FDG uptake of the venous background pool. Combining the metabolic information from FDG-PET/CT with the thickened vessel wall data from co-registered CECT could be a powerful method for evaluating inflammatory IgG4-CVD.

Keywords: IgG4-related disease, CT, FDG PET, Aortitis, Inflammatory aortic aneurysm

6.16.1 Clinical Presentation

83-year-old woman presenting with diabetes mellitus. Screening CT showed infra-renal abdominal aorta aneurysm (AAA).

6.16.2 Key Images

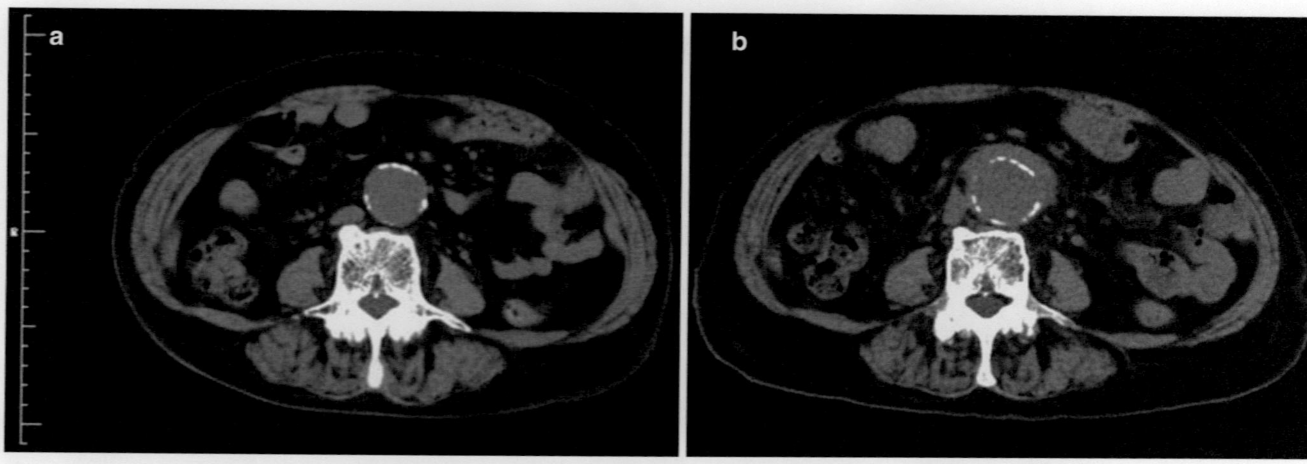

Fig. 6.25 Noncontrast CT

6.16.3 Technique

- Patient preparation: patient should not take anything by mouth for 6 h before administration of radiopharmaceutical.
- PET images were acquired 60 min after an intravenous injection of FDG (4–5 MBq/kg).
- Imaging device: whole body PET/CT camera (Biograph 64 with TrueV and high-definition PET, Siemens Japan, Tokyo).
- Emission scanning for 3 min per bed position was carried out following the CT image acquisition for attenuation corrections.

6.16.4 Image Interpretation

Initial noncontrast CT (Fig. 6.25a) demonstrates infra-renal AAA (31 × 30 mm). Four years later, follow-up CT (Fig. 6.25b) showed diffuse aortic wall thickness (maximal thickness 8 mm) and rapid progression in size (inner diameter 34 × 35 mm, outer diameter 46 × 42 mm).

6.16.5 Differential Diagnosis

- Atherosclerotic aortic aneurysm
- Infectious aortic aneurysm
- Inflammatory aortic aneusysm
- Impending rupture of the aortic aneurysm

6.16.6 Diagnosis and Clinical Follow-Ups (Fig. 6.26)

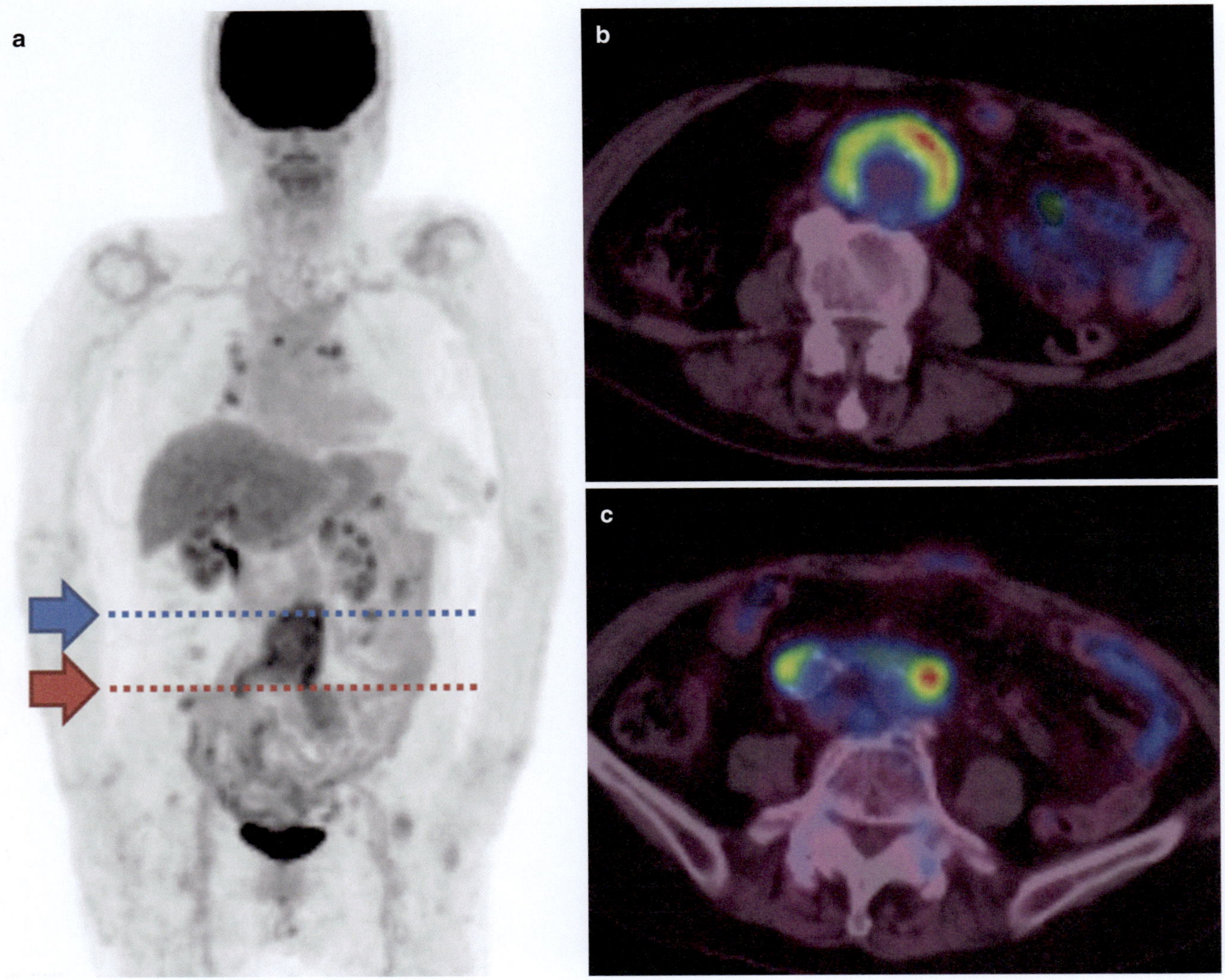

Fig. 6.26 Maximum intensity projection image (**a**) and axial fused images at AAA (**b**, blue arrow level) and common iliac arteries (**c**, red arrow level) are displayed. Strong focal uptakes on AAA ($SUV_{max} = 4.9$) and common iliac arteries ($SUV_{s} = 5.9$) which represented the active inflammation. Aortic replacement was held. There were lymphoplasmacytic infiltration and extensive dense infiltration of IgG4-positive plasma cells within the aortic wall, mainly in the adventitia, which was concordant with IgG4-related inflammatory aneurysm

6.16.7 Discussion

The metabolic information from FDG-PET/CT could be a powerful method for evaluating inflammatory IgG4-aortitis [140, 141]. The infra-renal abdominal aorta and iliac arteries were the most commonly involved sites with more than twice the FDG uptake as compared to the venous blood pool, which could form aneurysmal change [141].

References

1. Boers M, Verhoeven AC, Markusse HM, van de Laar MA, Westhovens R, van Denderen JC, et al. Randomised comparison of combined step-down prednisolone, methotrexate and sulphasalazine with sulphasalazine alone in early rheumatoid arthritis. Lancet. 1997;350:309–18.
2. Landewé RB, Boers M, Verhoeven AC, Westhovens R, van de Laar MA, Markusse HM, , et al. COBRA combination therapy in patients with early rheumatoid arthritis: long-term structural benefits of a brief intervention. Arthritis Rheum 2002;46: 347–356.
3. McQueen FM, Stewart N, Crabbe J, Robinson E, Yeoman S, Tan PL, et al. Magnetic resonance imaging of the wrist in early rheumatoid arthritis reveals a high prevalence of erosions at four months after symptom-onset. Ann Rheum Dis. 1998;57: 350–6.
4. Ostergaard M, Hansen M, Stoltenberg M, Gideon P, Klarlund M, Jensen KE, et al. Magnetic resonance imaging-determined synovial membrane volume as a marker of disease activity and a predictor of progressive joint destruction in the wrists of patients with rheumatoid arthritis. Arthritis Rheum. 1999;42:918–29.
5. Kane D, Balint PV, Sturrock RD. Ultrasonography is superior to clinical examination in the detection and localization of knee joint effusion in rheumatoid arthritis. J Rheumatol. 2003;30:966–71.
6. Koenigkam-Santos M, Sharma P, Kalb B, Oshinski JN, Weyand CM, Goronzy JJ, et al. Magnetic resonance angiography in extracranial giant cell arteritis. J Clin Rheumatol. 2011;17:306–10.
7. Kubota R, Yamada S, Kubota K, Ishiwata K, Tamahashi N, Ido T. Intratumoral distribution of flurine-18-fluorodeoxyglucose in vivo: high accumulation in macrophages and granulation tissues studied by microautoradiography. J Nucl Med. 1992;33:1972–80.
8. Yamada S, Kubota K, Kubota R, Ido T, Tamahashi N. High accumulation of fluorine-18-fluorodeoxyglucose in turpentine-induced inflammatory tissue. J Nucl Med. 1995;36:1301–6.
9. Matsui T, Nakata N, Nagai S, Nakatani A, Takahashi M, Momose T, et al. Inflammatory cytokines and hypoxia contribute to 18F-FDG uptake by cells involved in pannus formation in rheumatoid arthritis. J Nucl Med. 2009;50:920–6.
10. Palmer WE, Rosenthal DI, Schoenberg OI, Fischman AJ, Simon LS, Rubin RH, et al. Quantification of inflammation in the wrist with gadolinium-enhanced MR imaging and PET with 2-[F-18]-fluoro-2-deoxy-D-glucose. Radiology. 1995;196:647–55.
11. Beckers C, Ribbens C, André B, Marcelis S, Kaye O, Mathy L, et al. Assessment of disease activity in rheumatoid arthritis with (18)F-FDG PET. J Nucl Med. 2004;45:956–64.
12. Kubota K, Ito K, Morooka M, Mitsumoto T, Kurihara K, Yamashita H, et al. Whole-body FDG-PET/CT on rheumatoid arthritis of large joints. Ann Nucl Med. 2009;23:783–91.
13. Goerres GW, Forster A, Uebelhart D, Seifert B, Treyer V, Michel B, , et al. F-18 FDG whole-body PET for the assessment of disease activity in patients with rheumatoid arthritis. Clin Nucl Med 2006;31:386–390.
14. Elzinga EH, van der Laken CJ, Comans EF, Lammertsma AA, Dijkmans BA, Voskuyl AE. 2-Deoxy-2-[F-18]fluoro-D-glucose joint uptake on positron emission tomography images: rheumatoid arthritis versus osteoarthritis. Mol Imaging Biol. 2007;9:357–60.
15. Ostendorf B, Mattes-György K, Reichelt DC, Blondin D, Wirrwar A, Lanzman R, et al. Early detection of bony alterations in rheumatoid and erosive arthritis of finger joints with high-resolution single photon emission computed tomography, and differentiation between them. Skelet Radiol. 2010;39:55–61.
16. Okabe T, Shibata H, Shizukuishi K, Yoneyama T, Inoue T, Tateishi U. F-18 FDG uptake patterns and disease activity of collagen vascular diseases-associated arthritis. Clin Nucl Med. 2011;36:350–4.
17. Beckers C, Jeukens X, Ribbens C, André B, Marcelis S, Leclercq P, et al. (18)F-FDG PET imaging of rheumatoid knee synovitis correlates with dynamic magnetic resonance and sonographic assessments as well as with the serum level of metalloproteinase-3. Eur J Nucl Med Mol Imaging. 2006;33:275–80.
18. Sato M, Inubushi M, Shiga T, Hirata K, Okamoto S, Kamibayashi T, et al. Therapeutic effects of acupuncture in patients with rheumatoid arthritis: a prospective study using (18)F-FDG-PET. Ann Nucl Med. 2009;23:311–6.
19. Brown AK, Conaghan PG, Karim Z, Quinn MA, Ikeda K, Peterfy CG, et al. An explanation for the apparent dissociation between clinical remission and continued structural deterioration in rheumatoid arthritis. Arthritis Rheum. 2008;58:2958–67.
20. Elzinga EH, van der Laken CJ, Comans EF, Boellaard R, Hoekstra OS, Dijkmans BA, et al. 18F-FDG PET as a tool to predict the clinical outcome of infliximab treatment of rheumatoid arthritis: an explorative study. J Nucl Med. 2011;52:77–80.
21. Polisson RP, Schoenberg OI, Fischman A, Rubin R, Simon LS, Rosenthal D, et al. Use of magnetic resonance imaging and positron emission tomography in the assessment of synovial volume and glucose metabolism in patients with rheumatoid arthritis. Arthritis Rheum. 1995;38:819–25.
22. Adams MC, Turkington TG, Wilson JM, Wong TZ. A systematic review of the factors affecting accuracy of SUV measurements. AJR Am J Roentgenol. 2010;195:310–20.
23. Szkudlarek M, Court-Payen M, Jacobsen S, Klarlund M, Thomsen HS, Østergaard M. Interobserver agreement in ultrasonography of the finger and toe joints in rheumatoid arthritis. Arthritis Rheum. 2003;48:955–62.
24. Kubota K, Ito K, Morooka M, Minamimoto R, Miyata Y, Yamashita H, et al. FDG PET for rheumatoid arthritis: basic considerations and whole-body PET/CT. Ann N Y Acad Sci. 2011;1228:29–38.
25. Miese F, Scherer A, Ostendorf B, Heinzel A, Lanzman RS, Kröpil P, et al. Hybrid 18F-FDG PET-MRI of the hand in rheumatoid arthritis: initial results. Clin Rheumatol. 2011;30:1247–50.
26. Suto T, Okamura K, Yonemoto Y, Okura C, Tsushima Y, Takagishi K. Prediction of large joint destruction in patients with rheumatoid arthritis using 18F-FDG PET/CT and disease activity score. Medicine (Baltimore). 2016;95:e2841.
27. Suto T, Yonemoto Y, Okamura K, Okura C, Kaneko T, Kobayashi T, et al. Predictive factors associated with the progression of large-joint destruction in patients with rheumatoid arthritis after biologic therapy: a post-hoc analysis using FDG-PET/CT and the ARASHI (assessment of rheumatoid arthritis by scoring of large-joint destruction and healing in radiographic imaging) scoring method. Mod Rheumatol. 2017;27:820–7.
28. Chuang TY, Hunder GG, Ilstrup DM, Kurland LT. Polymyalgia rheumatica: a 10-year epidemiologic and clinical study. Ann Intern Med. 1982;97:672–80.
29. Healey LA. Long-term follow-up of polymyalgia rheumatica: evidence for synovitis. Semin Arthritis Rheum. 1984;13:322–8.
30. Salvarani C, Cantini F, Olivieri I, Hunder GS. Polymyalgia rheumatica: a disorder of extraarticular synovial structures? J Rheumatol. 1999;26:517.

31. Salvarani C, Cantini F, Olivieri I, Barozzi L, Macchioni L, Niccoli L, et al. Proximal bursitis in active polymyalgia rheumatica. Ann Intern Med. 1997;127:27–31.
32. Cantini F, Salvarani C, Olivieri I, Niccoli L, Padula A, Macchioni L, et al. Shoulder ultrasonography in the diagnosis of polymyalgia rheumatica: a case–control study. J Rheumatol. 2001;28:1049–55.
33. Moosig F, Czech N, Mehl C, Henze E, Zeuner RA, Kneba M, et al. Correlation between 18-fluorodeoxyglucose accumulation in large vessels and serological markers of inflammation in polymyalgia rheumatica: a quantitative PET study. Ann Rheum Dis. 2004;63:870–3.
34. Blockmans D, De Ceuninck L, Vanderschueren S, Knockaert D, Mortelmans L, Bobbaers H. Repetitive 18-fluorodeoxyglucose positron emission tomography in isolated polymyalgia rheumatica: a prospective study in 35 patients. Rheumatology (Oxford). 2007;46:672–7.
35. Yamashita H, Kubota K, Takahashi Y, Minamimoto R, Morooka M, Ito K, et al. Whole-body fluorodeoxyglucose positron emission tomography/computed tomography in patients with active polymyalgia rheumatica: evidence for distinctive bursitis and large-vessel vasculitis. Mod Rheumatol. 2012;22:705–11.
36. Takahashi H, Yamashita H, Kubota K, Miyata Y, Okasaki M, Morooka M, et al. Differences in fluorodeoxyglucose positron emission tomography/computed tomography findings between elderly onset rheumatoid arthritis and polymyalgia rheumatica. Mod Rheumatol. 2015;25:546–51.
37. Cimmino MA, Camellino D, Paparo F, Morbelli S, Massollo M, Cutolo M, et al. High frequency of capsular knee involvement in polymyalgia rheumatica/giant cell arteritis patients studied by positron emission tomography. Rheumatology (Oxford). 2013;52:1865–72.
38. Wakura D, Kotani T, Takeuchi T, Komori T, Yoshida S, Makino S, et al. Differentiation between polymyalgia rheumatica (PMR) and elderly-onset rheumatoid arthritis using 18F-Fluorodeoxyglucose positron emission tomography/computed tomography: is enthesitis a new pathological lesion in PMR? PLoS One. 2016;11:e0158509.
39. Owen CE, Poon AMT, Lee ST, Yap LP, Zwar RB, McMenamin CM, et al. Fusion of positron emission tomography/computed tomography with magnetic resonance imaging reveals hamstring peritendonitis in polymyalgia rheumatica. Rheumatology (Oxford). 2018;57:345–53.
40. Rehak Z, Vasina J, Nemec P, Fojtik Z, Koukalova R, Bortlicek Z, et al. Various forms of (18)F-FDG PET and PET/CT findings in patients with polymyalgia rheumatica. Biomed Pap Med Fac Univ Palacky Olomouc Czech Repub. 2015;159:629–36.
41. Rehak Z, Sprlakova-Pukova A, Bortlicek Z, Fojtik Z, Kazda T, Joukal M, et al. PET/CT imaging in polymyalgia rheumatica: praepubic 18F-FDG uptake correlates with pectineus and adductor longus muscles enthesitis and with tenosynovitis. Radiol Oncol. 2017;51:8–14.
42. Camellino D, Paparo F, Morbelli S, Cutolo M, Sambuceti G, Cimmino MA. Interspinous bursitis is common in polymyalgia rheumatica, but is not associated with spinal pain. Arthritis Res Ther. 2014;16:492.
43. Palard-Novello X, Querellou S, Gouillou M, Saraux A, Marhadour T, Garrigues F, et al. Value of (18)F-FDG PET/CT for therapeutic assessment of patients with polymyalgia rheumatica receiving tocilizumab as first-line treatment. Eur J Nucl Med Mol Imaging. 2016;43:773–9.
44. Nash P, Mease PJ, Braun J, van der Heijde D. Seronegative spondyloarthropathies: to lump or split? Ann Rheum Dis. 2005;64(Suppl. II):9–13.
45. Godfrin B, Zabraniecki L, Lamboley V, Bertrand-Latour F, Sans N, Fournié B. Spondyloarthropathy with entheseal pain. A prospective study in 33 patients. Joint Bone Spine. 2004;71:557–62.
46. Taniguchi Y, Arii K, Kumon Y, Fukumoto M, Ohnishi T, Horino T, et al. Positron emission tomography/computed tomography: a clinical tool for evaluation of enthesitis in patients with spondyloarthritides. Rheumatology (Oxford). 2010;49:348–54.
47. Strobel K, Fischer DR, Tamborrini G, Kyburz D, Stumpe KD, Hesselmann RG, et al. 18F-fluoride PET/CT for detection of sacroiliitis in ankylosing spondylitis. Eur J Nucl Med Mol Imaging. 2010;37:1760–5.
48. Yamashita H, Kubota K, Takahashi Y, Minamimoto R, Morooka M, Kaneko H, et al. Similarities and differences in fluorodeoxyglucose positron emission tomography/computed tomography findings in spondyloarthropathy, polymyalgia rheumatica and rheumatoid arthritis. Joint Bone Spine. 2013;80:171–7.
49. Vijayant V, Sarma M, Aurangabadkar H, Bichile L, Basu S. Potential of (18)F-FDG-PET as a valuable adjunct to clinical and response assessment in rheumatoid arthritis and seronegative spondyloarthropathies. World J Radiol. 2012;4:462–8.
50. Bruijnen ST, van der Weijden MA, Klein JP, Hoekstra OS, Boellaard R, van Denderen JC, et al. Bone formation rather than inflammation reflects ankylosing spondylitis activity on PET-CT: a pilot study. Arthritis Res Ther. 2012;14:R71.
51. Lee SG, Kim IJ, Kim KY, Kim HY, Park KJ, Kim SJ, et al. Assessment of bone synthetic activity in inflammatory lesions and syndesmophytes in patients with ankylosing spondylitis: the potential role of 18F-fluoride positron emission tomography-magnetic resonance imaging. Clin Exp Rheumatol. 2015;33:90–7.
52. Buchbender C, Ostendorf B, Ruhlmann V, Heusch P, Miese F, Beiderwellen K, et al. Hybrid 18F-labeled fluoride positron emission tomography/magnetic resonance (MR) imaging of the sacroiliac joints and the spine in patients with axial Spondyloarthritis: a pilot study exploring the link of MR bone pathologies and increased Osteoblastic activity. J Rheumatol. 2015;42:1631–7.
53. Takata T, Takahashi A, Taniguchi Y, Terada Y, Sano S. Detection of asymptomatic enthesitis in psoriasis patients: an onset of psoriatic arthritis? J Dermatol. 2016;43:650–4.
54. Chaudhari AJ, Ferrero A, Godinez F, Yang K, Shelton DK, Hunter JC, et al. High-resolution (18)F-FDG PET/CT for assessing disease activity in rheumatoid and psoriatic arthritis: findings of a prospective pilot study. Br J Radiol. 2016;89:20160138.
55. Idolazzi L, Salgarello M, Gatti D, Viapiana O, Vantaggiato E, Fassio A, et al. 18F-fluoride PET/CT for detection of axial involvement in ankylosing spondylitis: correlation with disease activity. Ann Nucl Med. 2016;30:430–4.
56. Park EK, Pak K, Park JH, Kim K, Kim SJ, Kim IJ, et al. Baseline increased 18F-fluoride uptake lesions at vertebral corners on positron emission tomography predict new syndesmophyte development in ankylosing spondylitis: a 2-year longitudinal study. Rheumatol Int. 2017;37:765–73.
57. Sawicki LM, Lütje S, Baraliakos X, Braun J, Kirchner J, Boos J, et al. Dual-phase hybrid 18 F-fluoride positron emission tomography/MRI in ankylosing spondylitis: investigating the link between MRI bone changes, regional hyperaemia and increased osteoblastic activity. J Med Imaging Radiat Oncol. 2018;62:313–9.
58. Yamashita H, Takahashi Y, Kubota K, et al. Utility of fluorodeoxyglucose positron emission tomography/computed tomography for early diagnosis and evaluation of disease activity of relapsing polychondritis: a case series and literature review. Rheumatology (Oxford). 2014;53:1482–90.
59. Lei W, Zeng H, Zeng DX, Zhang B, Zhu YH, Jiang JH, et al. (18) F-FDG PET-CT: a powerful tool for the diagnosis and treatment of relapsing polychondritis. Br J Radiol. 2016;89(1057):20150695. https://doi.org/10.1259/bjr.20150695. Epub 2015 Nov 3.5
60. Yamashita H, Kubota K, Takahashi Y, et al. Clinical value of 18F-fluoro-dexoxyglucose positron emission tomography/computed tomography in patients with adult-onset Still's disease: a

seven-case series and review of the literature. Mod Rheumatol. 2013;24:645–50.
61. Dong MJ, Wang CQ, Zhao K, Wang GL, Sun ML, Liu ZF, et al. 18F-FDG PET/CT in patients with adult-onset Still's disease. Clin Rheumatol. 2015;34:2047–56.
62. Treglia G, Mattoli MV, Leccisotti L, Ferraccioli G, Giordano A. Usefulness of whole-body fluorine-18-fluorodeoxyglucose positron emission tomography in patients with large-vessel vasculitis: a systematic review. Clin Rheumatol. 2011;30:1265–75.
63. Muto G, Yamashita H, Takahashi Y, Miyata Y, Morooka M, Minamimoto R, Kubota K, Kaneko H, Kano T, Mimori A. Large vessel vasculitis in elderly patients: early diagnosis and steroid-response evaluation with FDG-PET/CT and contrast-enhanced CT. Rheumatol Int. 2014;34:1545–54.
64. Umehara H, Okazaki K, Masaki Y, Kawano M, Yamamoto M, Saeki T, et al. A novel clinical entity, IgG4-related disease (IgG4RD): general concept and details. Mod Rheumatol. 2012;22:1–14.
65. Shigekawa M, Yamao K, Sawaki A, Hara K, Takagi T, Bhatia V, et al. Is 18F-fluorodeoxyglucose positron emission tomography meaningful for estimating the efficacy of corticosteroid therapy in patients with autoimmune pancreatitis? J Hepatobiliary Pancreat Sci. 2010;17:269–74.
66. Ozaki Y, Oguchi K, Hamano H, Arakura N, Muraki T, Kiyosawa K, et al. Differentiation of autoimmune pancreatitis from suspected pancreatic cancer by fluorine-18 fluorodeoxyglucose positron emission tomography. J Gastroenterol. 2008;43:144–51.
67. Ebbo M, Grados A, Guedj E, Gobert D, Colavolpe C, Zaidan M, et al. 18F-FDG PET/CT for staging and evaluation of treatment response in IgG4-related disease: a retrospective multicenter study. Arthritis Care Res (Hoboken). 2014;66:86–96.
68. Takahashi H, Yamashita H, Morooka M, Kubota K, Takahashi Y, Kaneko H, Kano T, Mimori A. The utility of FDG-PET/CT and other imaging techniques in the evaluation of IgG4-related disease. Joint Bone Spine. 2014. pii: S1297-319X(14)00031-1. [Epub ahead of print]; https://doi.org/10.1016/j.jbspin.2014.01.010.
69. Tokue A, Higuchi T, Arisaka Y, Nakajima T, Tokue H, Tsushima Y. Role of F-18 FDG PET/CT in assessing IgG4-related disease with inflammation of head and neck glands. Ann Nucl Med. 2015;29:499–505.
70. Lauwyck J, Piette Y, Van Walleghem L, De Geeter F. IgG4-related disease: the utility of (18)F-FDG PET/CT in diagnosis and treatment. Hell J Nucl Med. 2015;18(Suppl 1):155–9.
71. Zhao Z, Wang Y, Guan Z, Jin J, Huang F, Zhu J. Utility of FDG-PET/CT in the diagnosis of IgG4-related diseases. Clin Exp Rheumatol. 2016;34:119–25.
72. Lee J, Hyun SH, Kim S, Kim DK, Lee JK, Moon SH, et al. Utility of FDG PET/CT for differential diagnosis of patients clinically suspected of IgG4-related disease. Clin Nucl Med. 2016;41:e237–43.
73. Martinez-Pimienta G, Noriega-Álvarez E, Simó-Perdigó M. Study of systemic disease IgG4. Usefulness of 2-[18F]-fluoro-2-deoxy-D-glucose -positron emission tomography/computed tomography for staging, selection of biopsy site, evaluation of treatment response and follow-up. Eur J Rheumatol. 2017;4:222–5.
74. Berti A, Della-Torre E, Gallivanone F, Canevari C, Milani R, Lanzillotta M, et al. Quantitative measurement of 18F-FDG PET/CT uptake reflects the expansion of circulating plasmablasts in IgG4-related disease. Rheumatology (Oxford). 2017;56:2084–92.
75. Takano K, Yajima R, Kamekura R, Yamamoto M, Takahashi H, Yama N, et al. Clinical utility of 18 F-fluorodeoxyglucose/positron emission tomography in diagnosis of immunoglobulin G4-related sclerosing sialadenitis. Laryngoscope. 2018;128:1120–5.
76. Owada T, Maezawa R, Kurasawa K, Okada H, Arai S, Fukuda T. Detection of inflammatory lesions by f-18 fluorodeoxyglucose positron emission tomography in patients with polymyositis and dermatomyositis. J Rheumatol. 2012;39:1659–65.
77. Tanaka S, Ikeda K, Uchiyama K, et al. [18F]FDG uptake in proximal muscles assessed by PET/CT reflects both global and local muscular inflammation and provides useful information in the management of patients with polymyositis/dermatomyositis. Rheumatology (Oxford). 2013;52:1271–8.
78. Matuszak J, Blondet C, Hubelé F, Gottenberg JE, Sibilia J, Bund C, et al. Muscle fluorodeoxyglucose uptake assessed by positron emission tomography-computed tomography as a biomarker of inflammatory myopathies disease activity. Reumatology (Oxford). 2019. pii: kez040. [Epub ahead of print]; https://doi.org/10.1093/rheumatology/kez040.
79. Motegi SI, Fujiwara C, Sekiguchi A, Hara K, Yamaguchi K, Maeno T. Clinical value of 18 F-fluorodeoxyglucose positron emission tomography/computed tomography for interstitial lung disease and myositis in patients with dermatomyositis. J Dermatol. 2019;46:213–8.
80. Sun L, Dong Y, Zhang N, Lv X, Chen Q, Wei W. [18F] Fluorodeoxyglucose positron emission tomography/computed tomography for diagnosing polymyositis/dermatomyositis. Exp Ther Med. 2018;15:5023–8.
81. Tateyama M, Fujihara K, Misu T, Arai A, Kaneta T, Aoki M. Clinical values of FDG PET in polymyositis and dermatomyositis syndromes: imaging of skeletal muscle inflammation. BMJ Open. 2015;5:e006763.
82. Soussan M, Abisror N, Abad S, Nunes H, Terrier B, Pop G, et al. FDG-PET/CT in patients with ANCA-associated vasculitis: case-series and literature review. Autoimmun Rev. 2014;13:125–31.
83. Nelson DR, Johnson GB, Cartin-Ceba R, Specks U. Characterization of F-18 fluorodeoxyglucose PET/CT in granulomatosis with polyangiitis. Sarcoidosis Vasc Diffuse Lung Dis. 2016;32:342–52.
84. Kemna MJ, Bucerius J, Drent M, Vöö S, Veenman M, van Paassen P, et al. Aortic ^{18}F-FDG uptake in patients suffering from granulomatosis with polyangiitis. Eur J Nucl Med Mol Imaging. 2015;42:1423–9.
85. Lei J, Yan X, Taoying G, et al. Imaging characteristics of adult onset Still's disease demonstrated with ^{18}F-FDG PET/CT. Mol Med Rep. 2017;16(3):3680–6.
86. Yaguchi D, Inoue N, Koike W, et al. FDG-PET/CT findings in adult-onset Still's disease. QJM. 2019;112:705–6. pii: hcz057
87. Owada T, Maezawa R, Kurasawa K, et al. Detection of inflammatory lesions by F-18 Fluorodeoxyglucose positron emission tomography in patients with polymyositis and dermatomyositis. J Rheumatol. 2012;39(8):1659–65.
88. Sun L, Dong Y, Zhang N, et al. [^{18}F]Fluorodeoxyglucose positron emission tomography/computed tomography for diagnosing polymyositis/dermatomyositis. Exp Ther Med. 2018;15(6):5023–8.
89. Maliha PG, Hudson M, Abikhzer G, et al. ^{18}F-FDG PET/CT versus conventional investigations for cancer screening in autoimmune inflammatory myopathy in the era of novel myopathy classifications. Nucl Med Commun. 2019;40(4):377–82.
90. Tateyama M, Fujihara K, Misu T, et al. Clinical values of FDG PET in polymyositis and dermatomyositis syndromes: imaging of skeletal muscle inflammation. BMJ Open. 2015;5(1):e006763.
91. Bai X, Tie N, Wang X, et al. Intense muscle activity due to polymyositis incidentally detected in a patient evaluated for possible malignancy by FDG PET/CT imaging. Clin Nucl Med. 2017;42(8):647–8.
92. Khan S, Christopher-Stine L. Polymyositis, dermatomyositis, and autoimmune necrotizing myopathy; clinical features. Rheum Dis Clin N Am. 2011;37(2):143–58.
93. Horino T, Matsumoto T, Ichii O, et al. Long-term imaging findings on serial FDG PET/CT scans in a patient with polymyositis. J Clin Rheumatol. 2019;. [Epub ahead of print]

94. Tanaka S, Ikeda K, Uchiyama K, et al. [18 F] FDG uptake in proximal muscles assessed by PET/CT reflects both global and local muscular inftammation and provides useful information in the management of patients with polymyositis/dermatomyositis. Rheumatology. 2013;52(7):1271–8.
95. Matuszak J, Blondet C, Hubelé F, et al. Muscle fluorodeoxyglucose uptake assessed by positron emission tomography-computed tomography as a biomarker of inflammatory myopathies disease activity. Rheumatology (Oxford). 2019 Mar 8. pii: kez040.
96. Mahmood S, Rodríguez Martínez de Llano S. ^{18}F-FDG PET detection of unknown primary malignancy in dermatomyositis. Clin Nucl Med. 2012;37(8):e204–5.
97. Pei L, Guan ZW, Ji XJ, et al. The application of ^{18}F fluorodeoxyglucose-positron emission tomography/computed tomography in the diagnosis and treatment of dermatomyositis. Zhonghua Nei Ke Za Zhi. 2016;55(7):525–30.
98. Motegi SI, Fujiwara C, Sekiguchi A, et al. Clinical value of ^{18}F-fluorodeoxyglucose positron emission tomography/computed tomography for interstitial lung disease and myositis in patients with dermatomyositis. J Dermatol. 2019;46(3):213–8.
99. Tanaka S, Ikeda K, Uchiyama K, et al. ^{18}FDG uptake in proximal muscles assessed by PET/CT reflects both global and local muscular inflammation and provides useful information in the management of patients with polymyositis/dermatomyositis. Rheumatology. 2013;52(7):1271–8.
100. Kundrick A, Kirby J, Ba D, et al. Positron emission tomography costs less to patients than conventional screening for malignancy in dermatomyositis. Semin Arthritis Rheum. 2018;49:140–4. S0049-0172(18)30107-0
101. Lazarou IN, et al. Classification, diagnosis, and management of idiopathic inflammatory myopathies. J Rheumatol. 2013;40:550–64.
102. Hill C, et al. Frequency of specific cancer types in dermatomyositis and polymyositis: a population based study. Lancet. 2001;357:96–100.
103. Tateyama M, et al. Clinical values of FDG PET in polymyositis and dermatomyositis syndromes: imaging of skeletal muscle inflammation. BMJ Open. 2015;12:5.
104. Li Y, et al. Multiple values of (18)F-FDG PET/CT in idiopathic inflammatory myopathy. Clin Rheumatol. 2017;36:2297–305.
105. Motegi S, et al. Clinical value of (18)F-fluorodeoxyglucose positron emission tomography/computed tomography for interstitial lung disease and myositis in patients with dermatomyositis. J Dermatol. 2019;46:213–8.
106. Kubota K, et al. Whole-body FDG-PET/CT on rheumatoid arthritis of large joints. Ann Nucl Med. 2009;23:783–91.
107. Kubota K, et al. FDG PET for rheumatoid arthritis: basic considerations and whole-body PET/CT. Ann N Y Acad Sci. 2011;1228:29–38.
108. Goerres GW, et al. F-18 FDG whole-body PET for the assessment of disease activity in patients with rheumatoid arthritis. Clin Nucl Med. 2006;31:386–90.
109. Yamashita H, et al. Clinical value of whole-body PET/CT in patients with active rheumatic diseases. Arthritis Res Ther. 2014;16:423.
110. Beckers C, Ribbens C, André B, et al. Assessment of disease activity in rheumatoid arthritis with ^{18}F-FDG PET. J Nucl Med. 2004;45(6):956–64.
111. Goerres GW, Forster A, Uebelhart D, et al. F-18 FDG whole-body PET for the assessment of disease activity in patients with rheumatoid arthritis. Clin Nucl Med. 2006;31(7):386–90.
112. Matsui T, Nakata N, Nagai S, et al. Inflammatory cytokines and hypoxia contribute to ^{18}F-FDG uptake by cells involved in pannus formation in rheumatoid arthritis. J Nucl Med. 2009;50(6):920–6.
113. Lee SJ, Jeong JH, Lee CH, et al. Development and validation of an ^{18}F-FDG PET/CT-based tool for the evaluation of joint counts and disease activity in patients with rheumatoid arthritis. Arthritis Rheumatol. 2019;71:1232–40. [Epub ahead of print]
114. Yamashita H, et al. Whole-body fluorodeoxyglucose positron emission tomography/computed tomography in patients with active polymyalgia rheumatica: evidence for distinctive bursitis and large-vessel vasculitis. Mod Rheumatol. 2012;22: 705–11.
115. Takahashi H, et al. Differences in fluorodeoxyglucose positron emission tomography/computed tomography findings between elderly onset rheumatoid arthritis and polymyalgia rheumatica. Mod Rheumatol. 2015;25(54):6–51.
116. Yamashita H, et al. Utility of fluorodeoxyglucose positron emission tomography/computed tomography for early diagnosis and evaluation of disease activity of relapsing polychondritis: a case series and literature review. Rheumatology (Oxford). 2014;53:1482.
117. Deng H, et al. Relapsing polychondritis on PET/CT. Clin Nucl Med. 2012;37:712.
118. De Geeter F, Gykiere P. 18F-FDG PET/CT imaging in granulomatosis with polyangiitis. Hell J Nucl Med. 2016;19(1):5–6.
119. De Geeter F, Gykiere P. 18F-FDG PET imaging of granulomatosis with polyangiitis –Wegener's syndrome. Hell J Nucl Med. 2016;19(1):53–6.
120. Bonnet P, Abisror N, Fain O, et al. 18FDG PET for detecting renal granulomatous localization: illustration of granulomatosis with polyangiitis and sarcoidosis. J Clin Rheumatol. 2019;. [Epub ahead of print]
121. Fu Z, Liu M, Li Z, et al. Occult renal granulomatous inflammatory lesions in granulomatosis with polyangiitis detected by 18F-FDG PET/CT. Clin Nucl Med. 2017;42(9):707–8.
122. Ito K, et al. Evaluation of Wegener's granulomatosis using 18F-fluorodeoxyglucose positron emission tomography/computed tomography. Ann Nucl Med. 2013;27(3):209–16.
123. Ozmen O, et al. Integration of 2-deoxy-2-[18F] fluoro-D-glucose PET/CT into clinical management of patients with Wegener's granulomatosis. Ann Nucl Med. 2013;27(10):907–15.
124. Kemna MJ, et al. Aortic ^{18}F-FDG uptake in patients suffering from granulomatosis with polyangiitis. Eur J Nucl Med Mol Imaging. 2015;42(9):1423–9.
125. Nelson DR, et al. Characterization of F-18 fluorodeoxyglucose PET/CT in granulomatosis with polyangiitis. Sarcoidosis Vasc Diffuse Lung Dis. 2016;32(4):342–52.
126. Perel-Winkler A, Bokhari S, Perez-Recio T, et al. Myocarditis in systemic lupus erythematosus diagnosed by ^{18}F-fluorodeoxyglucose positron emission tomography. Lupus Sci Med. 2018;5(1):e000265.
127. Makis W, Ciarallo A, Gonzalez-Verdecia M, et al. Systemic lupus Erythematosus associated pitfalls on ^{18}F-FDG PET/CT: reactive follicular hyperplasia, Kikuchi-Fujimoto disease, inflammation and lymphoid hyperplasia of the spleen mimicking lymphoma. Nucl Med Mol Imaging. 2018;52(1):74–9.
128. Girard A, Ohnona J, Bernaudin JF, et al. Generalized lymph node FDG uptake as the first manifestation of systemic lupus erythematosus. Clin Nucl Med. 2017;42(10):787–9.
129. Ozaki Y, et al. Differentiation of autoimmune pancreatitis from suspected pancreatic cancer by floutrine-18 fluorodeoxylucose positron emission tomogramphy. J Gastroenterol. 2008;43(2):144–51.
130. Sato M, et al. Extrapancreatic F-18 FDG accumulateon in autoimmune pancreastitis. Ann Nucl Med. 2008;22(3):215–9.
131. Umehara H, et al. Comprehensive diagnostic criteria for IgG4-related disease (IgG4-RD), 2011. Mod Rheumatol. 2012;22(1):21–30.

132. Hamano H, et al. IgG4-related disease – a systemic disease that deserves attension regardess of one's subspecialty. Intern Med. 2018;57(9):1201–7.
133. Ozaki Y, et al. Differentiation of autoimmune pancreatitis from suspected pancreatic cancer by floutrine-18 fluorodeoxylucose positron emission tomography. J Gastroenterol. 2008;43(2):144–51.
134. Zhang J, et al. Characterizing IgG4-related disease with ^{18}F-FDG PET/CT: a prospective cohort study. Eur J Nucl Med Mol Imaging. 2014;41(8):1624–34.
135. Tokue A, et al. Role of F-18 FDG PET/CT in assessing IgG4-related disease with inflammation of head and neck glands. Ann Nucl Med. 2015;29(6):499–505.
136. Krebs S, et al. IgG4-related kidney disease in a patient with history of breast cancer: findings on ^{18}F-FDG PET/CT. Clin Nucl Med. 2016;41(8):e388–9.
137. Nakatani K, et al. Utility of FDG PET/CT in IgG4-relayed systemic disease. Clin Radiol. 2012;67(4):297–305.
138. Kamisawa T, et al. IgG4-related disease. Lancet. 2015;385(9976):1460–71.
139. Nakajo M, et al. The efficacy of whole-body FDG PET or PET/CT for autoimmune pancreatitis and associated extrapancreatic autoimmune lesions. Eur J Nucl Med Mol Imaging. 2007;34(12):2088–95.
140. Oyama-Manabe N, et al. IgG4-related cardiovascular disease from the aorta to coronary artery: utility of multidetector CT and PET/CT in diagnosis and follow-up. Radiographics. 2018; https://doi.org/10.1148/rg.2018180049. 180049. [Epub ahead of print]
141. Yabusaki S, et al. Characteristics of immunoglobulin G4-related aortitis/periaortitis and periarteritis on flu orodeoxyglucose positron emission tomography/computed tomography co-registered with contrast-enhanced computed tomography. EJNMMI Res. 2017;7(1):20.

FDG PET/CT for Sarcoidosis

7

Masao Miyagawa, Emiri Watanabe, Naoto Kawaguchi, Rami Tashiro, Masayoshi Sarai, Osamu Manabe, Noriko Oyama-Manabe, Ayumi Watanabe, and Hiroshi Toyama

7.1 Role of FDG PET/CT in Diagnosis of Cardiac Sarcoidosis

Masao Miyagawa

Abstract Recently, remarkable progress in cardiac imaging with FDG PET and MRI has been made. FDG PET detects active inflammatory lesions in cardiac sarcoidosis (CS) as hot spots with a better sensitivity than ^{67}Ga scintigraphy. The new guidelines for diagnosis and treatment of CS were published by the Heart Rhythm Society in 2014, and more recently revised by the Japanese Circulation Society in 2017. In the past few years, many studies have demonstrated the diagnostic utility of FDG PET in patients with CS; therefore, abnormally high FDG accumulation in the heart was adopted as the major criteria for cardiac involvement of sarcoidosis. At present, FDG PET/CT is considered mandatory in the clinical diagnosis group of the updated guidelines.

Keywords: Cardiac sarcoidosis, FDG PET, Guidelines, Myocardial FDG uptake, Glucose transporter, Image interpretation

7.1.1 Introduction

Sarcoidosis is a systemic inflammatory disorder of unknown etiology whose clinical presentation is characterized by heterogeneous distribution of epithelioid granulomatous inflammation without caseous necrosis and concomitant fibrosis. Multiple organs, including the lungs, lymph nodes, eyes, bones, liver, spleen, skin, muscles, nervous system, and heart, are involved. Although about 20% of patients are chronically progressive, spontaneous remission is generally observed. However, cardiac involvement is a signal of poor prognosis, accounting for 25% of deaths from sarcoidosis. The most common causes of death are fatal ventricular arrhythmias and heart failure. Therefore, early detection and treatment are crucial. The diagnosis of CS is still challenging because histological detection rate by endomyocardial biopsy is as low as 20%.

Guidelines for the diagnosis of CS were initially published in 1992 and revised in 2006 in Japan [1]. Cardiac involvement had been considered an infrequent manifestation; however, an autopsy investigation reported a higher occurrence up to 50% in Japan. Myocardial perfusion SPECT using ^{201}Tl or ^{99m}Tc-agents can detect scarring as perfusion defect, but both sensitivity and specificity are low to detect CS. It is important to detect inflammatory activity and severity in order to decide treatment strategy. For this purpose, ^{67}Ga citrate scintigraphy has traditionally been used. However, since it has inherent low spatial resolution,

M. Miyagawa (✉)
Department of Radiology, Ehime University Hospital, Toon, Ehime, Japan

Department of Radiology, Ehime University Graduate School of Medicine, Toon, Ehime, Japan
e-mail: miyagawa@m.ehime-u.ac.jp

E. Watanabe · N. Kawaguchi · R. Tashiro
Department of Radiology, Ehime University Graduate School of Medicine, Toon, Ehime, Japan
e-mail: emirim.0911@gmail.com; kawaguchi.naoto.vv@ehime-u.ac.jp; rami0528@m.ehime-u.ac.jp

M. Sarai
Department of Cardiology, Fujita Health University Hospital, Toyoake, Aichi, Japan
e-mail: msarai@fujita-hu.ac.jp

O. Manabe
Department of Nuclear Medicine, Hokkaido University Graduate School of Medicine, Sapporo, Japan
e-mail: osamumanabe817@med.hokudai.ac.jp

N. Oyama-Manabe
Department of Diagnostic and Interventional Radiology, Hokkaido University Hospital, Sapporo, Hokkaido, Japan
e-mail: norikooyama@med.hokudai.ac.jp

A. Watanabe · H. Toyama
Department of Radiology, Fujita Health University, Toyoake, Aichi, Japan
e-mail: awat@fujita-hu.ac.jp; htoyama@fujita-hu.ac.jp

H. Toyama et al. (eds.), *PET/CT for Inflammatory Diseases*, https://doi.org/10.1007/978-981-15-0810-3_7

it is less sensitive to detect mild-to-moderate active CS. Recently, remarkable progress in FDG PET imaging and MRI has been made. FDG PET detects active inflammatory lesions in CS as hot spots with a better sensitivity than ^{67}Ga scintigraphy.

7.1.2 Latest Diagnostic Guidelines for Cardiac Sarcoidosis

The new guidelines for diagnosis and treatment of CS were published by the Heart Rhythm Society in 2014 [2], and more recently revised by the Japanese Circulation Society (JCS) in 2017 [3]. New guidelines described how to diagnose CS for the histological diagnosis group (those with positive myocardial biopsy findings) and for the clinical diagnosis group. Isolated CS was introduced as a new entity because it was more common than previously reported, occupying 20–50% of all sarcoidosis cases [4]. Thus, diagnostic guidelines for isolated CS were also created.

In the JCS guidelines, major criteria for cardiac involvement were defined as follows: (1) high-grade atrioventricular block or fatal ventricular arrhythmia as sustained ventricular tachycardia; (2) basal thinning of the ventricular septum or abnormal ventricular wall anatomy; (3) left ventricular ejection fraction (LVEF) less than 50%; (4) ^{67}Ga scintigraphy or FDG PET reveals abnormally high tracer accumulation in the heart; (5) MRI reveals late gadolinium enhancement (LGE) of the myocardium.

As there are currently no specific biomarkers available to diagnose CS, clinicians place expectations on imaging modalities such as cardiac MRI and FDG PET. Cardiac MRI has good spatial resolution enough to discern the location of LGE not only horizontal distribution but also vertical involvement of myocardial layer. In the past few years, many studies have shown the diagnostic utility of FDG PET in CS; therefore, FDG PET is included in the major criteria. While FDG PET is considered mandatory in the clinical diagnosis group, it has been pointed out that physiological FDG uptake in the myocardium would be an obstacle to making a correct diagnosis.

7.1.3 Optimal Preparation for Detection of Cardiac Sarcoidosis by FDG-PET

In 2012, the Japanese Ministry of Health, Labor and Welfare (JMHLW) had approved reimbursement coverage for FDG PET usage to detect inflammation sites in CS firstly in the world. However, there was not enough consensus on the preparation method and image interpretation for FDG-PET/CT. Thus, the guidelines for FDG-PET imaging for CS were published by the Japanese Society of Nuclear Cardiology in 2014 [1] and revised in 2019 [5]. In the guidelines, the high sensitivity but great variability in specificity in the diagnosis of CS probably due to various preparation methods of FDG-PET was reported.

FDG accumulates in the cells where glucose metabolism is enhanced, such as cancer cells and inflammatory cells. "Pathological" glucose uptake is mainly regulated by glucose transporter (GLUT) 1 and 3. These are increased on the cell membrane in patients with cancers and inflammatory diseases such as sarcoidosis. On the other hand, physiological glucose uptake by myocardial cells is regulated mainly by GLUT4. As the blood glucose level and/or insulin level increases, the physiological glucose uptake increases by GLUT4. Therefore, long fasting preparation suppresses blood glucose level and makes it possible to distinguish "pathological" from "physiological" FDG uptake. The suppression of physiological FDG uptake is the key to assess inflammatory activity of CS [6].

There are three main methods to minimize physiological FDG uptake in the normal myocardium [7]. In the first place is to prolong intervals of fasting, which leads to a decrease in blood glucose and insulin levels and, eventually, an increase in blood FFA levels. Although most of papers discussed fasting conditions in more than 12 h, several studies confirmed that more than 18 h of fasting made an improvement in specificity for detecting CS [8, 9]. In the second place is dietary modification prior to FDG-PET. A low-carbohydrate diet (LCD) <5 g the night before FDG PET is highly recommended to minimize blood glucose and insulin levels [10]. Additionally, a LCD together with a high-fat diet 3–6 h before PET was also recommended to suppress physiological FDG uptake in the myocardium [11]. However, the efficacy of high-fat diet by itself in increasing serum FFA levels has yet to be established. In the last place, intravenous injection of unfractionated heparin activates the serum lipoprotein lipase to increase FFA, resulting in suppression of myocardial glucose utilization. The protocol of heparin injection at a dose of 50 IU/kg 15 min prior to FDG administration has been adopted, which increases serum FFA levels rapidly thereafter [12]. However, it is contraindicated in patients with a bleeding tendency. Care must be taken to prevent the occurrence of heparin-induced thrombocytopenia (HIT). The incidence of HIT has been reported to vary from 0.5% to 5% [13]. Since we do not have enough data regarding an appropriate dose and regimen of heparin injection at this moment, future studies comparing different doses and regimen are needed.

7.1.4 FDG PET/CT Image Interpretation

Image assessment is conducted comprehensively, using whole-body maximum intensity projection (MIP) images, axial transverse tomography, LV short-axis, LV vertical long-axis, and LV horizontal long-axis images, in addition to bull's eye map display. Axial transverse images are helpful for observing the presence of abnormal FDG uptake in the right ventricular wall or atrial walls. Since CS is considered to be a systemic disease, abnormal FDG uptake in the lungs, lymph nodes, spleen, liver, muscles, eyes, and skin should be observed using whole-body MIP images. However, the presence of isolated CS, in which such abnormal FDG uptake is not observed, has been reported.

Myocardial FDG distribution observed in CS has been visually analyzed on the basis of some classifications. Ishimaru et al. proposed a classification into four types of patterns [12]: none, focal, focal on diffuse, and diffuse. A focal pattern is considered to be a characteristic finding of FDG uptake in the active inflammatory lesion in CS. A focal on diffuse pattern is considered to be a finding of focal FDG uptake on a background of mild diffuse uptake, either due to physiological uptake or heart failure as the heart metabolism shifts from fatty acid to glucose metabolism. Thus, the focal on diffuse pattern could be included as part of the focal one, which was determined as being positive for CS. On the other hand, diffuse FDG distribution pattern generally does not indicate an abnormality, since it is pathologically known that the CS lesion is not diffuse but localized. Applying this classification, the sensitivity and specificity of FDG PET/CT imaging for detection of CS were reported to be 100% and 81%, respectively [12].

7.1.5 Quantitative Analysis and Assessment of Treatment Response by FDG PET/CT

Yokoyama et al. reported that the myocardial SUVmax with a cutoff value of 4.0 provided a sensitivity of 97.3% with a specificity of 83.6% for diagnosing CS under the strictest preparation method for FDG PET [14]. However, there are problems with the use of SUV in the diagnosis of CS which have yet to be solved. SUVmax captures a voxel with the highest intensity of FDG uptake but does not delineate whether the FDG uptake is focal or involves a large volume of myocardium. The extent of FDG-positive lesions can be measured by identifying voxels with an SUV intensity above a predefined threshold value. Ahmadian et al. proposed a new method to quantify the FDG volume intensity, that is, cardiac metabolic volume (CMV; cm^3) and cardiac metabolic activity (CMA; g glucose) [15].

FDG PET is reported to be useful for assessing the effects of immunosuppressive therapies. Serial FDG PET studies should be performed with precisely the same preparation and data acquisition protocols. Osborne et al. examined 23 patients who had undergone a total of 90 serial PET examinations during treatment for CS [16]. In a longitudinal cohort, a reduction in the intensity and extent of myocardial inflammation area on FDG PET was associated with improvement in LVEF. Ahmadian et al. also performed serial FDG PET/CT studies before and after immunosuppression therapy [17]. FDG uptake was analyzed visually and quantitatively using SUVmax, CMV, and CMA with volume above SUV thresholds of 2.7 and 4.1 g/mL. Complete resolution of FDG uptake was common using CMA and CMV, but a 2.7 g/mL SUV threshold and SUVmax were more likely to reveal partial responses. In this way, quantitative interpretation of PET/CT can detect changes in myocardial FDG uptake in response to immunosuppression. However, it should be acknowledged that a reduction in it has not been proven to change the disease progression or natural history of CS [18]. Larger, multicenter imaging studies in CS are needed to see if quantitative changes in FDG uptake are associated with its outcomes.

7.2 Cardiac Sarcoidosis Case 1

Masao Miyagawa, Emiri Watanabe, and Naoto Kawaguchi

Abstract New guidelines describe how to diagnose cardiac sarcoidosis (CS) of the histological diagnosis group with positive biopsy findings and of the clinical diagnosis group. Many studies have demonstrated the diagnostic utility of ^{18}F-FDG (FDG) PET in CS; therefore, abnormal FDG accumulation in the heart is adopted as one of the major criteria [3]. The suppression of physiological FDG uptake in the myocardium is the key to assess inflammatory lesions of CS. Properly prepared FDG PET can be an aid in the determination of biopsy sites as it is a biomarker of active myocardial inflammation.

Keywords: Cardiac sarcoidosis, ^{18}F-FDG PET/CT, Endomyocardial biopsy, Active inflammation

7.2.1 Clinical Presentation

A 56-year-old woman with complete atrioventricular block (AVB) on electrocardiogram. Echocardiographic findings showed a basal thinning of interventricular septum and abnormal wall motion with left ventricular ejection fraction of 34%. The result of endomyocardial biopsy revealed granulomatous lymphadenitis without caseation necrosis, which was compatible with sarcoidosis (Fig. 7.1e).

7.2.2 Key Images

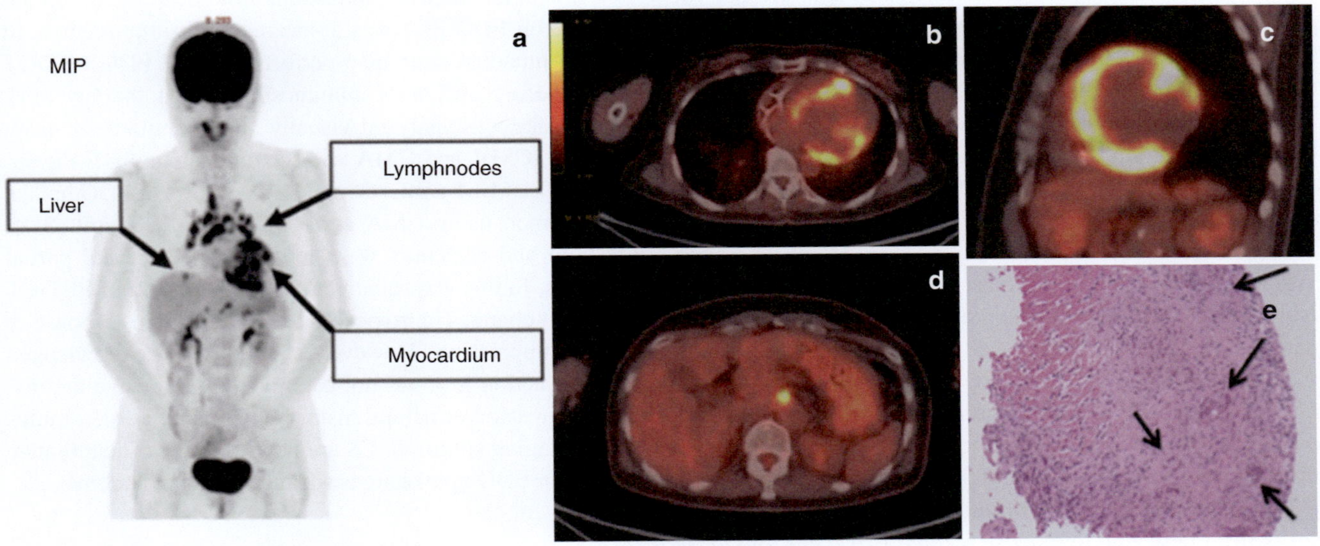

Fig. 7.1 Maximum intensity projection (MIP) view of the FDG PET (**a**). There are abnormal uptake in lymph nodes of mediastinum, hilar, and para-aortic regions. Trans-axial views at cardiac level (**b**) and abdomen (**d**), and short-axis view at basal myocardium (**c**). PET shows significant accumulation including interventricular septal wall. (**e**) Myocardial tissue from endomyocardial biopsy reveals granuloma without caseation necrosis, which is compatible with sarcoidosis (arrows: Langerhans giant cells)

7.2.3 Protocol of FDG PET/CT for CS

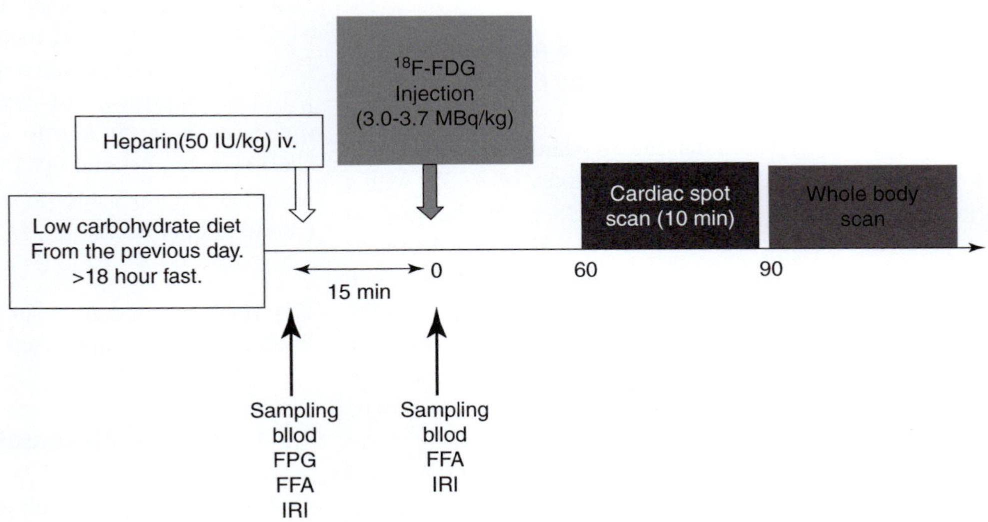

Fig. 7.2 Patient preparation: a low-carbohydrate diet (<5 g) followed by an overnight fasting ≥18 h. 50 IU/kg of unfractionated heparin injected intravenously and 15 min later, 3.0–3.7 MBq of FDG administered. Blood sampling for plasma free fatty acid (FFA), immune-reactive insulin (IRI), and fasting plasma glucose (FPG) levels before and 15 min after heparin injection. Cardiac spot scan and whole-body PET/CT using Discovery PET/CT 600 (GE Healthcare).

7.2.4 Image Interpretation

Maximum intensity projection (MIP) view of the FDG PET (Fig. 7.1a). There are abnormal uptake in lymph nodes of mediastinum, hilar, and para-aortic regions. Trans-axial views at cardiac level (b) and abdomen (d), and short-axis view at basal myocardium (c). PET shows significant accumulation including interventricular septal wall.

7.2.5 Indications of Cardiac PET/CT for CS

There are three clinical Indications of cardiac PET/CT for CS [2, 18]: (1) Patients with an unexplained, new onset of advanced AVB or ventricular tachycardia under 60 years old. (2) In patients with biopsy-proven extra-CS with one or more abnormalities detected on initial screening by symptoms/ECG/echocardiography. (3) Follow-up examinations for patients with proven CS. The patient of Fig. 7.1 matches the first indication.

7.2.6 The Histological Diagnosis Group (Those with Positive Myocardial Biopsy Findings)

The diagnosis of CS is challenging because histological detection rate by endomyocardial biopsy is as low as 20%. In this patient, active inflammatory lesions with relatively high FDG accumulation in the interventricular septum are found on PET/CT, which may have led to positive histological findings, since the septum is a suitable site for biopsy.

7.2.7 Discussion

FDG PET detects active inflammatory lesions in CS as hot spots with a better sensitivity than ^{67}Ga scintigraphy. Although histological detection rate by myocardial biopsy is very low, properly prepared FDG PET can be an aid in determination of endomyocardial biopsy sites as it is a biomarker of active inflammation.

7.3 Cardiac Sarcoidosis Case 2

Masao Miyagawa, Rami Tashiro, and Naoto Kawaguchi

Abstract New guidelines describe how to diagnose cardiac sarcoidosis (CS) of the clinical diagnosis group. In combined usage of PET and MRI, we can detect myocardial tissue characterization in CS. FDG PET detects active inflammation and a focal uptake pattern is considered as a characteristic finding of CS, while late gadolinium enhancement (LGE) on cardiac MRI can detect fibrosis, which is usually located in the mid and/or epicardial layer rather than endocardial layer in CS. In addition, perfusion defect on resting SPECT myocardial perfusion imaging (MPI) reflects irreversible scarring due to local inflammation.

Keywords: Cardiac sarcoidosis, ^{18}F-FDG PET/CT, Cardiac MRI, Myocardial perfusion imaging

7.3.1 Clinical Presentation

A 61-year-old man had been noted bilateral hilar lymphadenopathy and diagnosed with sarcoidosis by mediastinoscopy. Three years later, there was cardiac dysfunction due to ECG abnormalities of Q wave with T-wave inversion at II, III, aVF, and V4~V6 leads, which were suspected of old inferior myocardial infarction.

7.3.2 Technique

Protocol of FDG PET/CT for CS was performed in the same way as the CS Case 7.2.1.

7.3.3 Image Interpretation

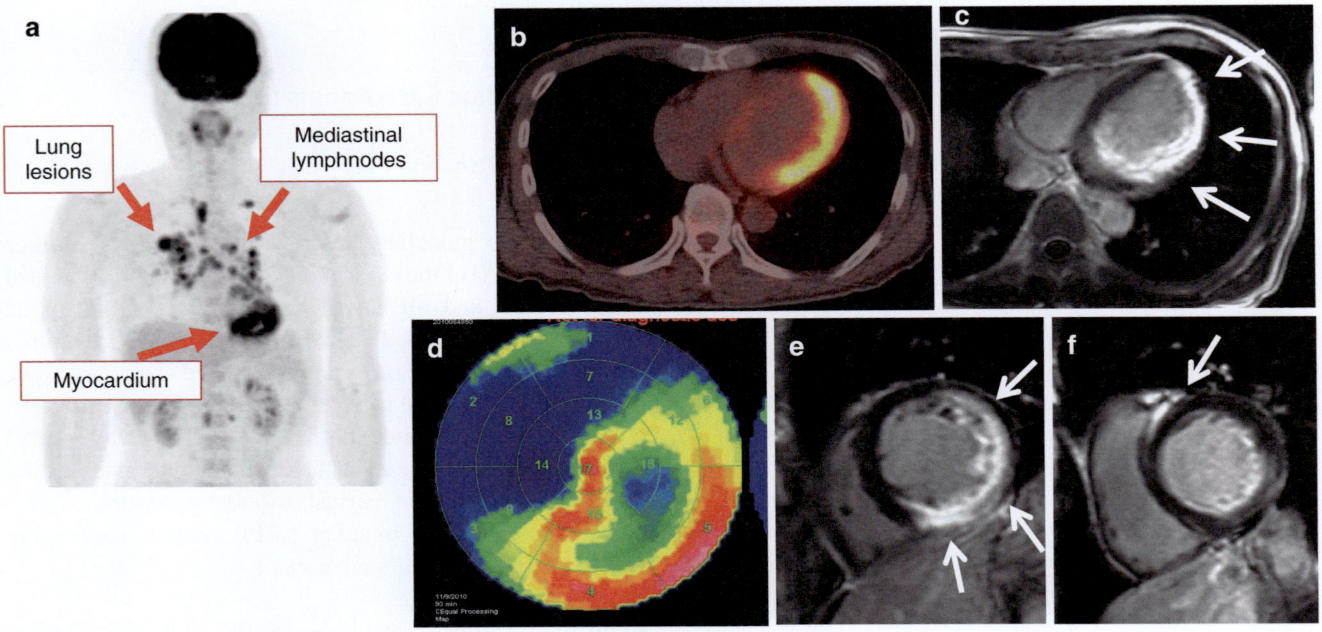

Fig. 7.3 Maximum intensity projection (MIP) view of the FDG PET (**a**). There are abnormal uptake in right upper lung lesions, mediastinal lymph nodes, and left myocardium. PET/CT shows significant FDG accumulation in the apico-lateral myocardial wall on trans-axial view (**b**). On the same view, MRI shows LGE in the similar regions including posterior wall (**c**). Bull's-eye polar map display of the left ventricle (LV) is useful for detailed assessment of FDG distribution (**d**). On short-axis views, MRI shows LGE in the posterolateral wall (**e**) and the right ventricular side of septum including epicardium (**f**)

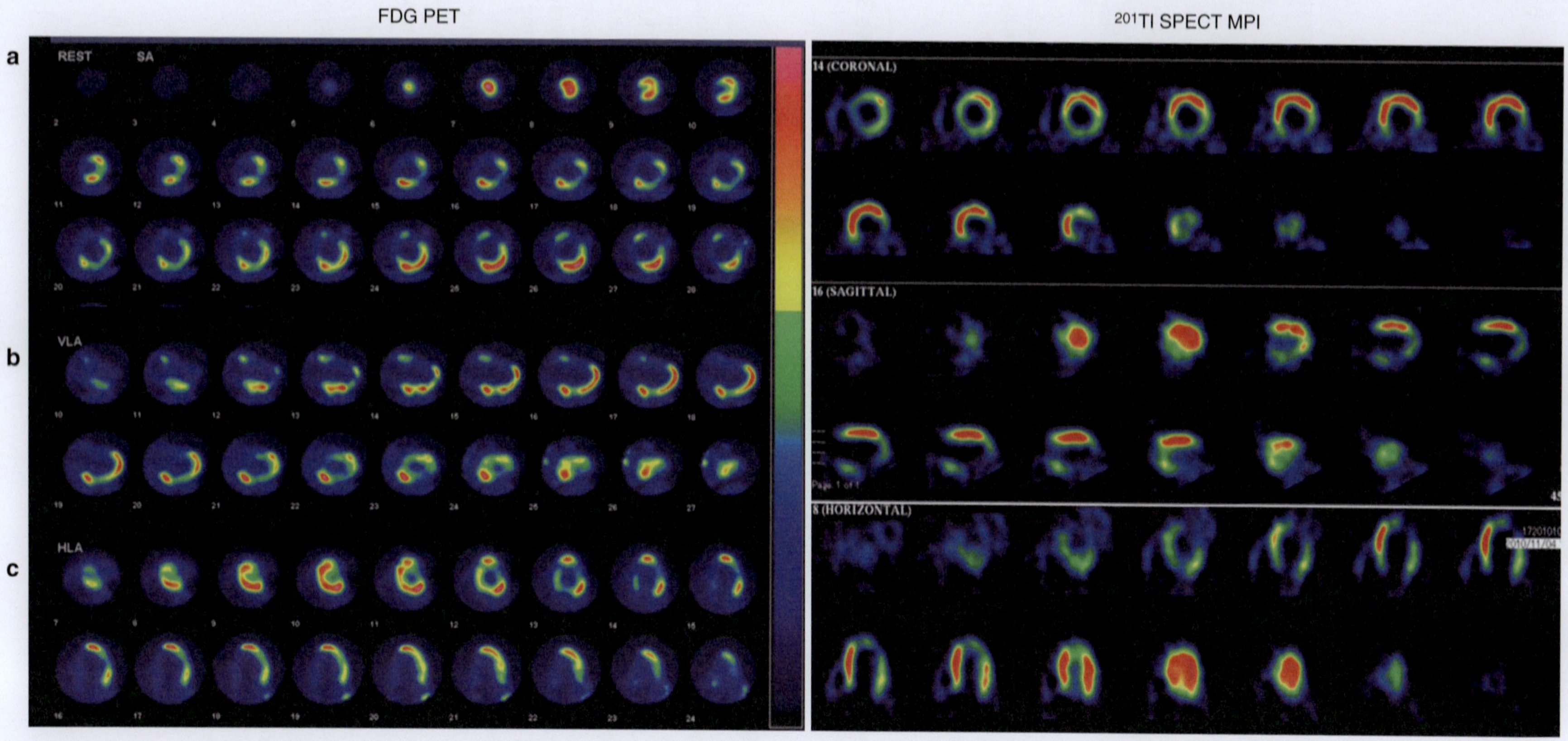

Fig. 7.4 The left is myocardial FDG PET and the right is resting thallium-201 (^{201}Tl) SPECT MPI. **a**: LV short-axis, **b**: vertical long-axis, and **c**: horizontal long-axis images. The myocardial FDG PET has a focal on diffuse pattern. In addition, a mismatch pattern between perfusion defect on ^{201}Tl SPECT MPI and FDG uptake on PET is also observed. Resting perfusion defects can either be due to compression of the microvasculature by inflammation or be due to scarring [19]

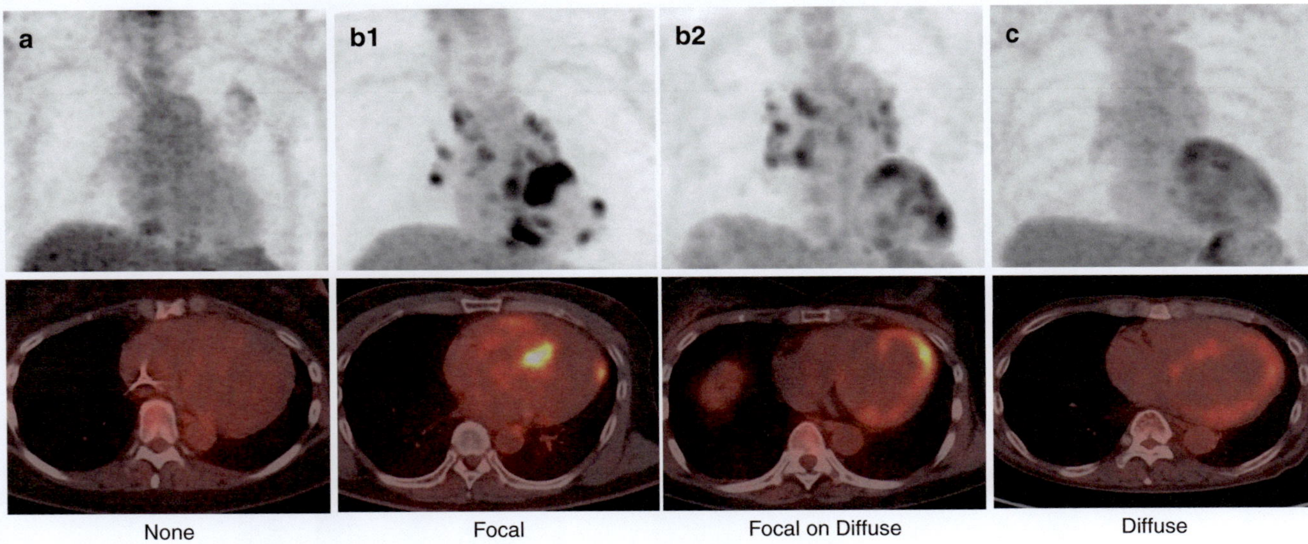

Fig. 7.5 The upper row is MIP images and the lower row is PET/CT fusion images. FDG uptake in the LV myocardium is classified into three patterns (**a**, **b**, **c**) and a focal pattern is considered as a characteristic finding of CS [5, 20]. A focal on diffuse pattern is considered as a finding of localized abnormal uptake on a background of mild physiological uptake of FDG; therefore, it would be rather included in a part of the focal pattern. A diffuse pattern generally does not indicate an abnormality, as it is known that the CS lesion is not pathologically diffuse but localized

7.3.4 Diagnostic Criteria of FDG PET/CT Imaging in CS

7.3.5 The Clinical Diagnosis Group

New guidelines describe how to diagnose CS of the clinical diagnosis group [3]. Biopsy-proven extra-CS patients with one or more abnormalities detected on screening by symptoms/ECG/echocardiography such as this patient are clinical indication of FDG PET/CT. Then, the patient met the two of five major criteria, which are positive for clinical diagnosis of CS: (1) FDG PET reveals abnormally high tracer accumulation in the heart; and (2) the LGE on cardiac MRI.

7.3.6 Discussion

In combined usage of PET and SPECT MPI, we can determine the stage of CS, because those provide data on the state of myocardial tissue disorder. (1) Early stage: normal perfusion and positive FDG uptake. (2) Advanced stage: perfusion defect and positive FDG uptake including a mismatch pattern. (3) End stage: perfusion defect and negative FDG uptake [19].

7.4 Cardiac Sarcoidosis Case 3

Masayoshi Sarai

Abstract Guidelines for the diagnosis and treatment of cardiac sarcoidosis were recently updated by the Japanese Circulation Society and published in 2017 [3]. Among them, late-gadolinium enhancement (LGE) of the myocardium in gadolinium-enhanced magnetic resonance imaging (MRI) and ^{18}F-fluorodeoxyglucose (FDG) positron emission tomography (PET) were upgraded to major criteria as new features. ^{18}F-FDG reflects the activity of inflammation in cardiac sarcoidosis (CS). LGE in MRI is considered an important index of tissue damage and fibrosis in CS. It is critically important to diagnose the disease at an early stage to ensure effective treatment and a positive outcome.

Keywords: Cardiac sarcoidosis, ^{18}F-FDG-PET, LGE-MRI, Corticosteroid therapy

7.4.1 Clinical Presentation

A 63-year-old man presenting with right mediastinal lymph node swelling by X-ray examination. Mediastinal lymph node biopsy was not diagnostic, but sarcoidosis was diagnosed from nodular erythema in the lower right thigh. After that, a complete right bundle block appeared on the electrocardiogram.

7.4.2 Key Images

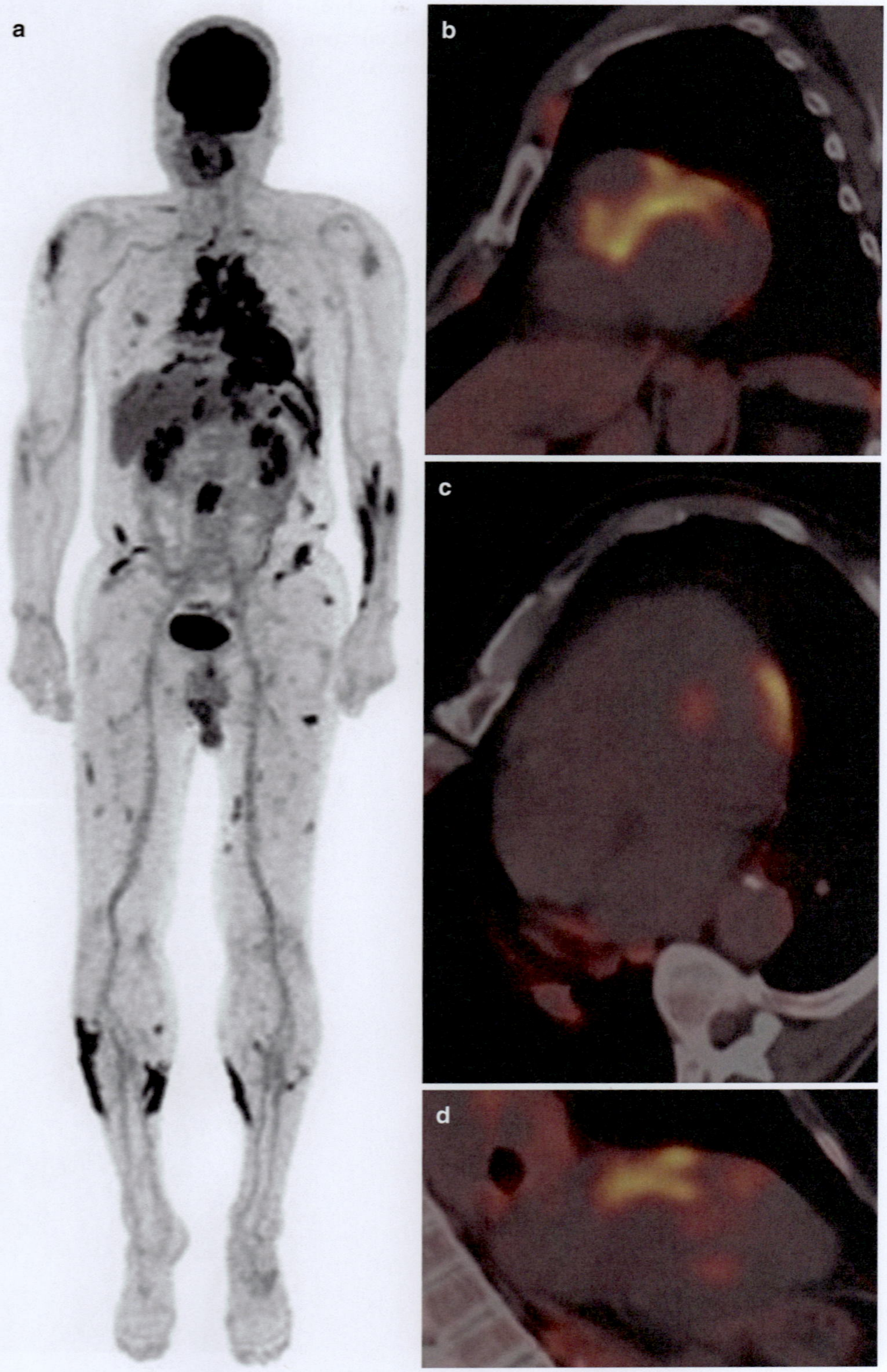

Fig. 7.6 ^{18}F-FDG-PET images before treatment. (**a**) Whole body, (**b**) cardiac short axis, (**c**) cardiac horizontal long axis, (**d**) cardiac vertical long axis

7.4.3 Technique

- Patient preparation: patient fasted for 18 h after a 6-h high-fat, high-protein, and low-carbohydrate diet and received intravenous unfractionated heparin (50 IU/kg) 15 min prior to ^{18}F-FDG injection [21].
- FDG PET/CT scanning: cardiac spot scan and whole-body scan were performed 60 min after ^{18}F-FDG injection using a PET/CT scanner (Biograph mCT, Siemens).

7.4.4 Image Interpretation

Whole-body FDG/PET scanning showed multiple high accumulations of tracer in the lymph nodes in the right supraclavicular, mediastinum, and bilateral hila. Multiple nodular accumulations in the lung, muscle, skin, and bone were also detected (Fig. 7.6a). There was high uptake in the left ventricle (LV), mainly the basal level of anteroseptal and lateral wall (Fig. 7.6b–d). The SUVmax value of LV was 24.8.

7.4.5 Diagnosis and Clinical Follow-ups

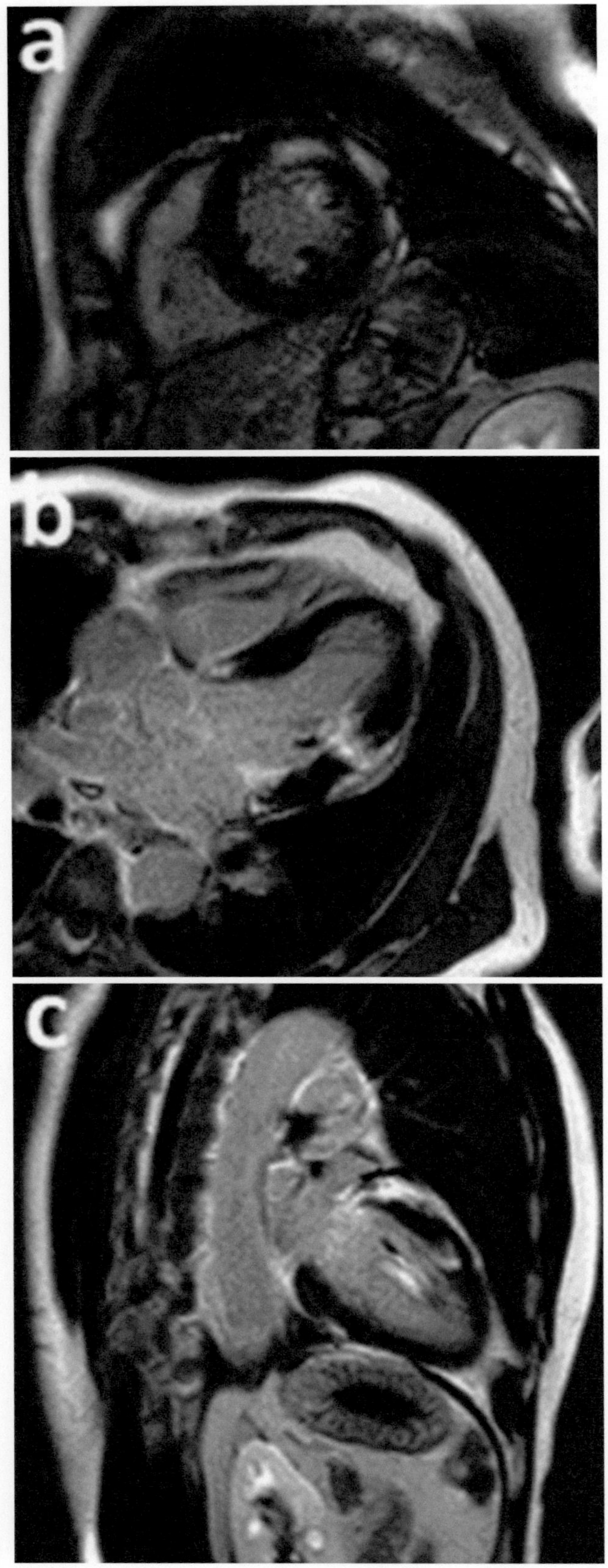

Fig. 7.7 Late gadolinium enhancement in the cardiac MRI images before treatment. (**a**) Cardiac short axis, (**b**) cardiac horizontal long axis, (**c**) cardiac vertical long axis

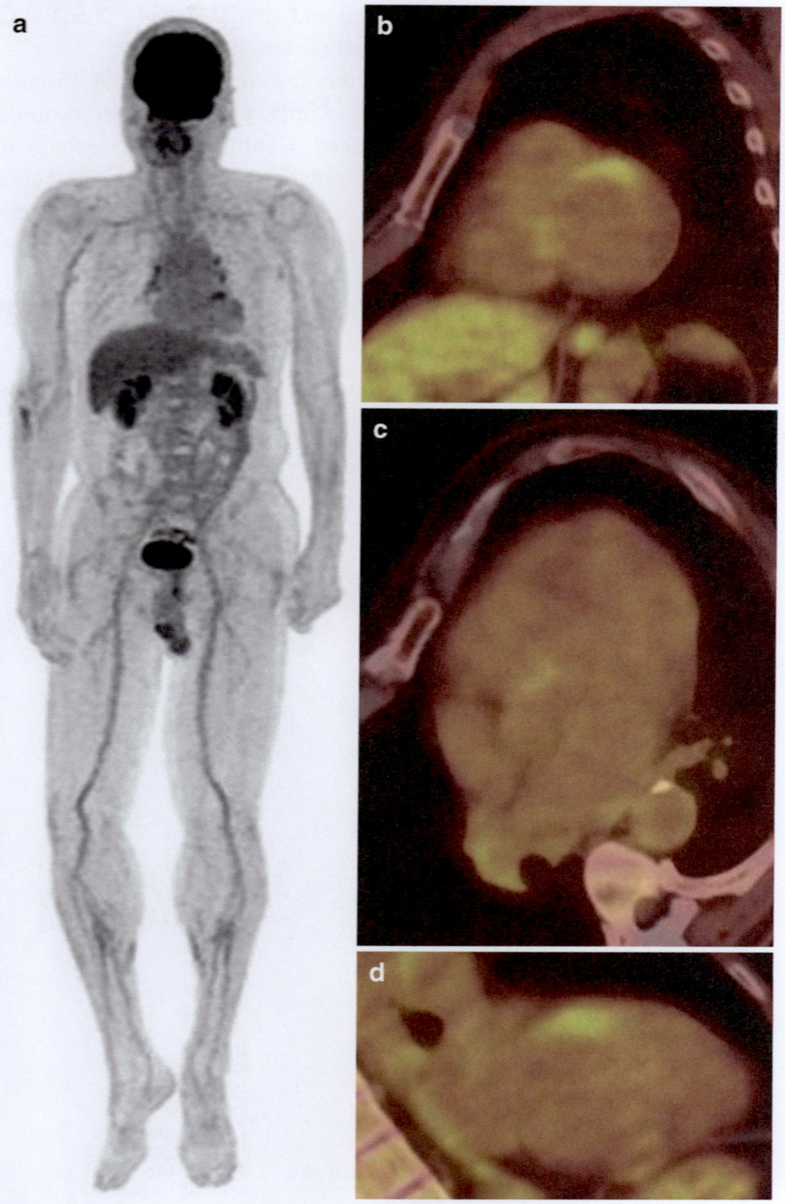

Fig. 7.8 ^{18}F-FDG-PET images after treatment. (**a**) Whole body, (**b**) cardiac short axis, (**c**) cardiac horizontal long axis, (**d**) cardiac vertical long axis

LGE was seen in the MRI imaging. Several patchy abnormal intensity areas matched the accumulation site of FDG (Fig. 7.7a–c). From the above results, the patient was diagnosed with CS with active inflammation and was therefore treated with 30 mg/day of corticosteroid. Follow-up FDG PET/CT performed 3 months after the initiation of the corticosteroid therapy showed clearly reduced FDG uptake in the myocardium (Fig. 7.8b–d). The SUVmax value of LV after corticosteroid therapy decreased from 24.8 to 4.1. The FDG uptake of other sites was reduced (Fig. 7.8a).

7.4.6 Discussion

In this case, the corticosteroid therapy significantly improved not only the extracardiac accumulation of FDG but also cardiac accumulation. Serial quantitative FDG-PET/CT can help guide monitoring and be a surrogate biomarker of corticosteroid therapy to prevent cardiac involvement of sarcoidosis [22].

7.5 Cardiac Sarcoidosis Case 4

Masayoshi Sarai

Abstract Sarcoidosis is a rare multi-organ system granulomatous disease of uncertain etiology. The disease may affect nearly any organ system, but most frequently the lymph nodes and lungs. The diagnosis of sarcoidosis is often delayed due to absent or nonspecific symptom(s).

Sarcoidosis is characterized by temporal and spatial variations in the onset pattern. The clinical course and prognosis are highly variable and dependent on the disease severity and organ involvement. Early detection is important, especially because cardiac involvement is fatal. Cardiac manifestations range widely from asymptomatic to sudden cardiac death [23].

Keywords: Cardiac sarcoidosis, ^{18}F-FDG-PET, Corticosteroid therapy

7.5.1 Clinical Presentation

A 46-year-old man was diagnosed with lung sarcoidosis by transbronchial lung biopsy 6 years earlier. Recently, he presented with complete right bundle block and left ventricular contraction failure. He was diagnosed with cardiac sarcoidosis by endomyocardial biopsy.

7.5.2 Key Images

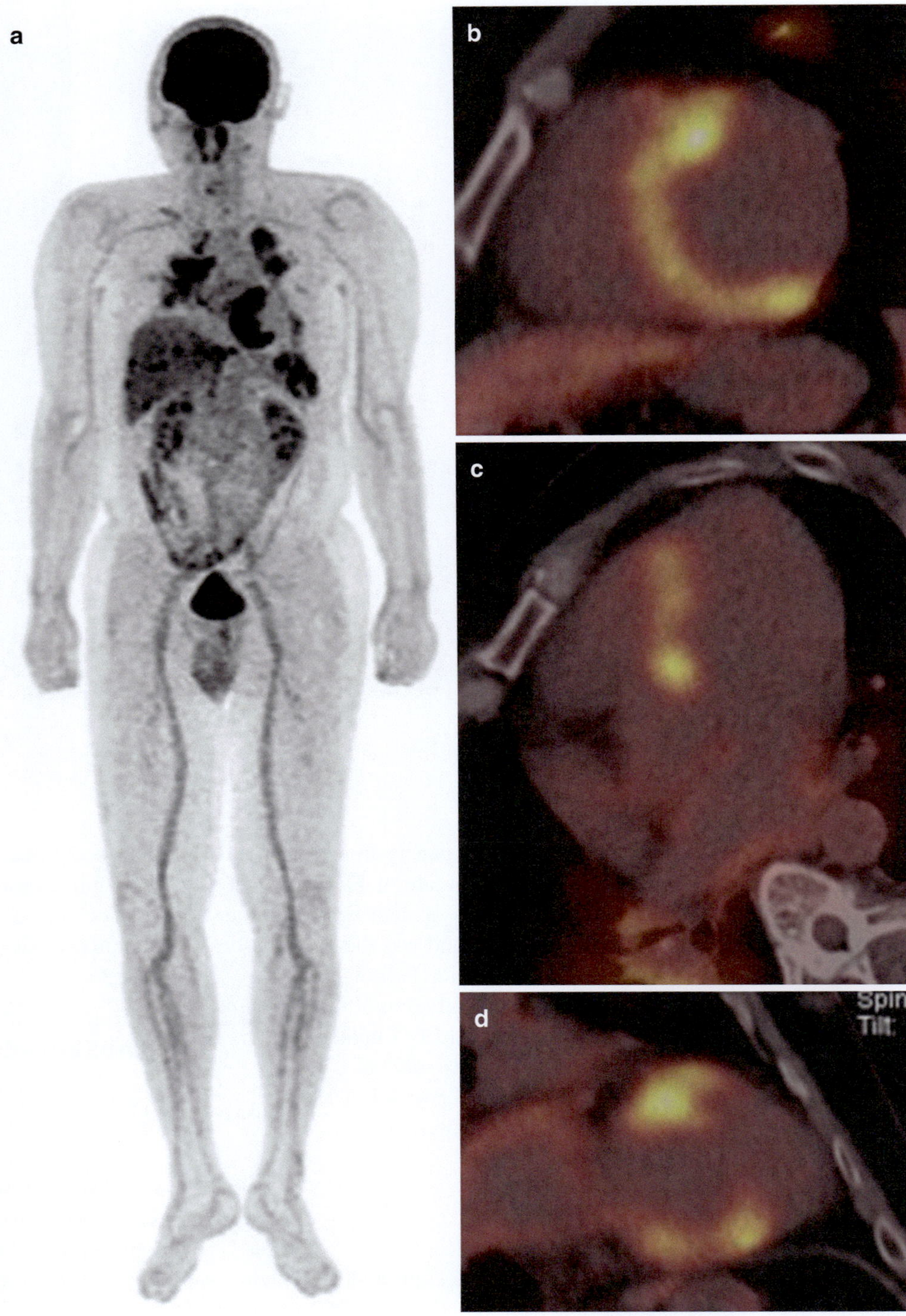

Fig. 7.9 ^{18}F-FDG-PET images before treatment. (**a**) Whole body, (**b**) cardiac short axis, (**c**) cardiac horizontal long axis, (**d**) cardiac vertical long axis

7.5.3 Technique

- Patient preparation: patient fasted for 18 h after a 6-h high-fat, high-protein, and low-carbohydrate diet and received intravenous unfractionated heparin (50 IU/kg) 15 min prior to ^{18}F-FDG injection.
- FDG PET/CT scanning: cardiac spot scan and whole-body scan were performed 60 min after ^{18}F-FDG injection using a PET/CT scanner (Biograph mCT, Siemens).

7.5.4 Image Interpretation

Whole-body FDG/PET scanning showed multiple high accumulations of tracer in the lymph nodes in the right supraclavicular, mediastinum, and bilateral hilum (Fig. 7.9a). Multiple nodular accumulations in the lung, muscle, skin, and bone were also detected. There was high uptake in the left ventricle (LV), mainly the basal level of anteroseptal and lateral wall (Fig. 7.9b–d). The SUVmax value of LV was 24.8.

7.5.5 Diagnosis and Clinical Follow-ups

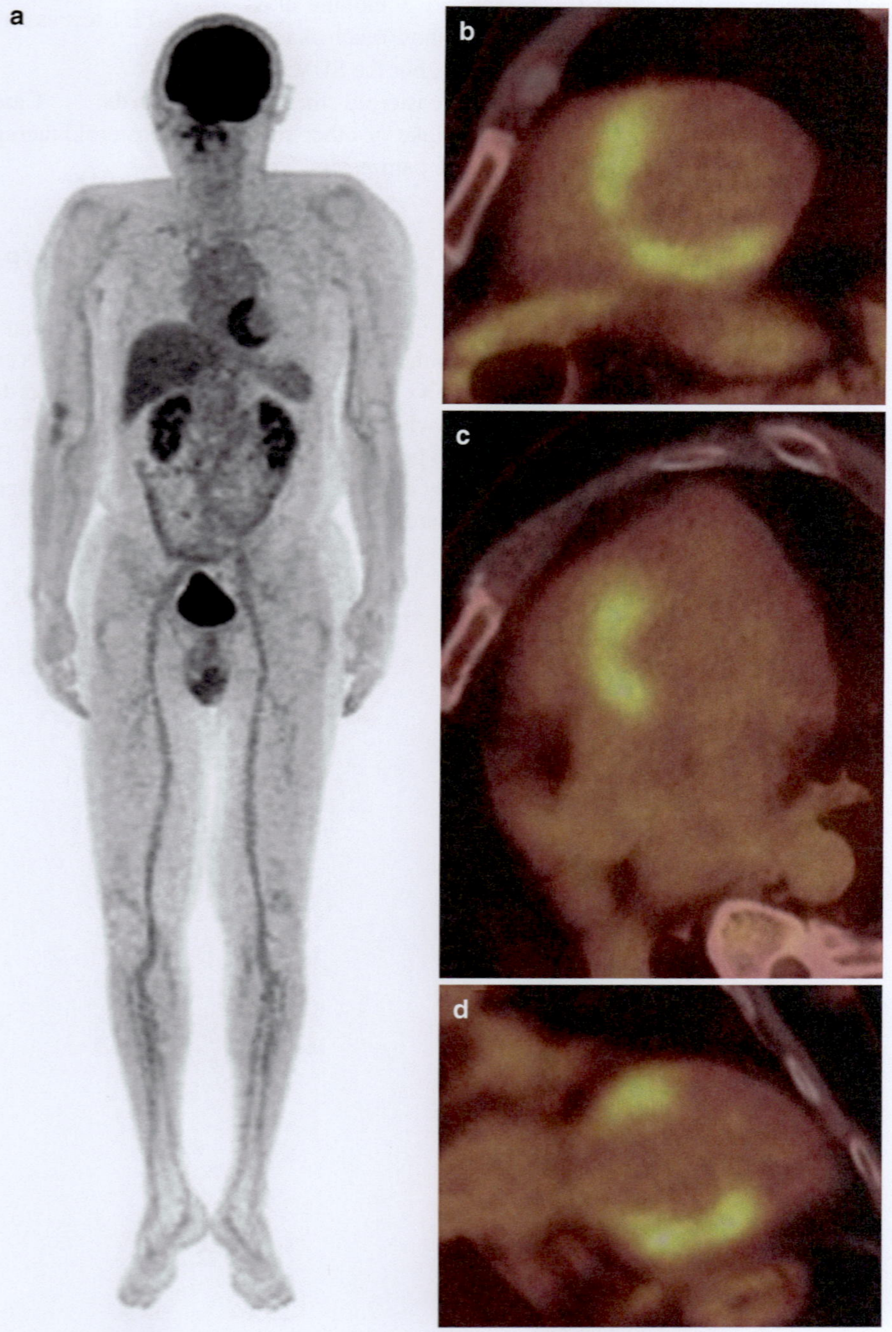

Fig. 7.10 ^{18}F-FDG-PET images after treatment. (**a**) Whole body, (**b**) cardiac short axis, (**c**) cardiac horizontal long axis, (**d**) cardiac vertical long axis

Table 7.1 Clinical parameters before and after treatment

	Pretreatment	Posttreatment
EF (%)	40	45
CTR (%)	53	47
ACE (U/L)	22.6	10.3
Troponin I (ng/mL)	0.041	< 0.006
NT-proBNP (pg/mL)	649	169
SUVmax	15.0	5.5

EF ejection fraction of left ventricle, *CTR* cardiothoracic ratio, *ACE* angiotensin converting enzyme

The patient was diagnosed with CS with active inflammation and was therefore treated with 30 mg/day of corticosteroid. Follow-up FDG PET/CT performed 3 months after initiation of corticosteroid therapy did not show much change visually in the left ventricle (Fig. 7.10b–d), but the SUVmax value of the left ventricle after corticosteroid therapy decreased from 15.0 to 5.5. The FDG uptake of other sites was reduced (Fig. 7.10a). Other clinical parameters were also improved (Table 7.1).

7.5.6 Discussion

In this case, the corticosteroid therapy significantly improved the extracardiac accumulation of FDG. FDG uptake did not show much change visually in the left ventricle. Serial quantitative FDG-PET/CT like SUVmax can help guide monitoring and be a surrogate biomarker of the efficacy of corticosteroid therapy to prevent cardiac involvement of sarcoidosis [24].

7.6 Cardiac Sarcoidosis Case 5

Masayoshi Sarai

Abstract In some cardiac sarcoidosis (CS) cases a re-increase in cardiac FDG accumulation has been documented after treatment initiation [24]. It is unclear whether the decline in cardiac FDG accumulation reflects long-term CS progression and natural history. In CS, it has not yet been examined whether the spread of cardiac lesions with FDG accumulation and SUVmax are associated with prognosis. It is necessary to study in future whether corticosteroid therapy should be performed using the inflammation findings in the FDG-PET test as an index.

Keywords: Cardiac sarcoidosis, ^{18}F-FDG-PET, Corticosteroid therapy, Prognosis

7.6.1 Clinical Presentation

A 67-year-old man with a complete atrioventricular block appeared 20 years earlier, followed by pacemaker implantation. Soon, he was diagnosed with CS and started corticosteroid therapy. This time, the patient's pacemaker was upgraded to CRT-D due to the appearance of ventricular tachycardia. Corticosteroid therapy has been continued at maintenance dose.

7.6.2 Key Images

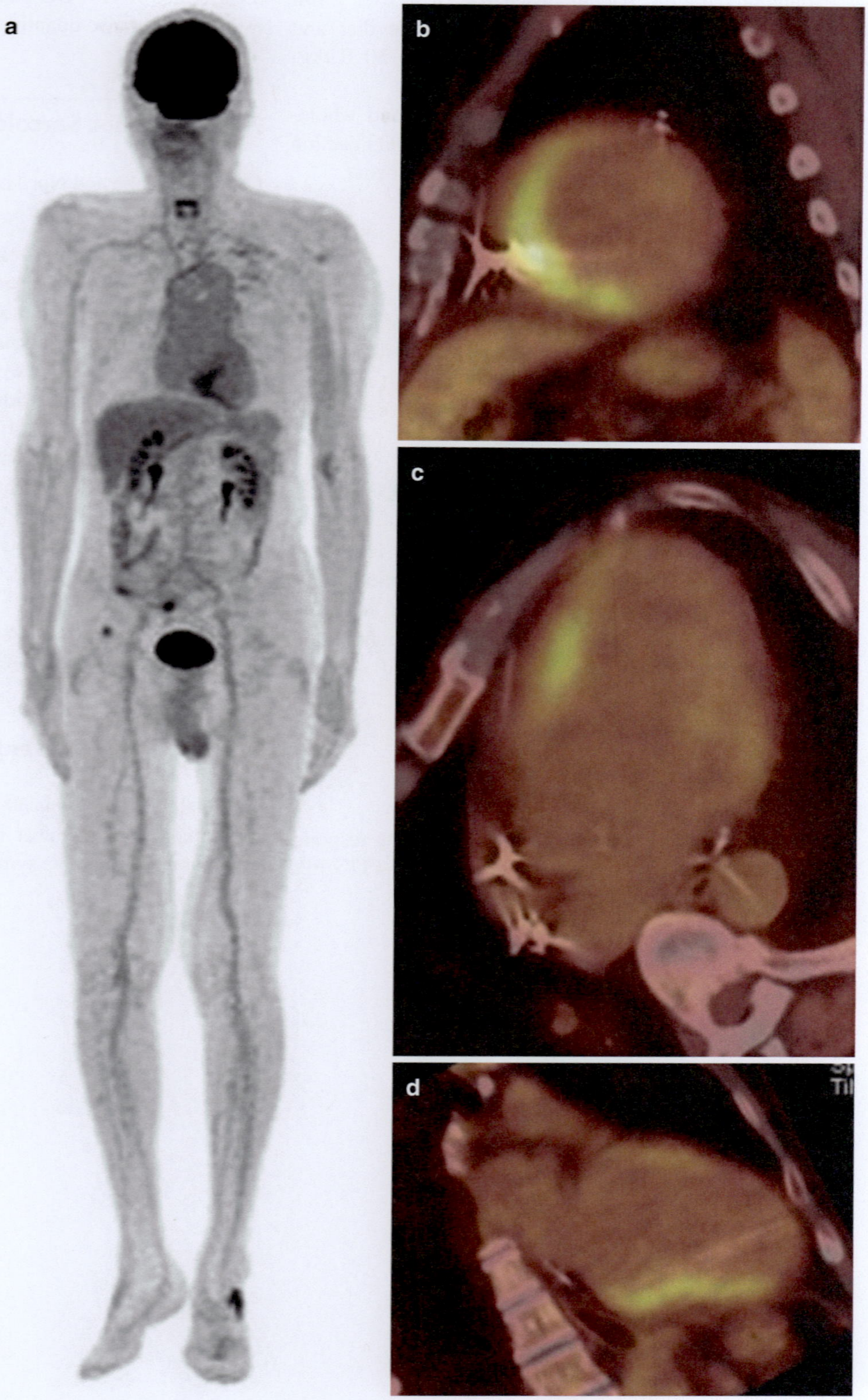

Fig. 7.11 ^{18}F-FDG-PET images 12 years after initiation of treatment. (**a**) Whole body, (**b**) cardiac short axis, (**c**) cardiac horizontal long axis, (**d**): cardiac vertical long axis

7.6.3 Technique

- Patient preparation: patient fasted for 18 h after a 6-h high-fat, high-protein, and low-carbohydrate diet and received intravenous unfractionated heparin (50 IU/kg) 15 min prior to ^{18}F-FDG injection.
- FDG PET/CT scanning: cardiac spot scan and whole-body scan were performed 60 min after ^{18}F-FDG injection using a PET/CT scanner (Biograph mCT, Siemens).

7.6.4 Image Interpretation

Whole-body FDG/PET scanning showed little accumulation other than in the heart (Fig. 7.11a). Focal accumulation was found in the septal and inferior wall in the left ventricle (Fig. 7.11b–d). The SUVmax value of LV was 7.0.

7.6.5 Diagnosis and Clinical Follow-ups

Recently, the clinical findings for several years have been stable. Corticosteroid therapy has also been continued at a maintenance dose. The only parameter indicating activation of cardiac sarcoidosis was cardiac FDG accumulation. However, corticosteroid is not being increased, and the patient is under observation.

7.6.6 Discussion

^{18}F-FDG PET is reported to be useful in assessing response to immunosuppressive treatment [25]. When ^{18}F-FDG PET is repeatedly applied, inspection conditions should be standardized as much as possible. For the judgment of the treatment effect of ^{18}F-FDG PET in CS patients, not only visual evaluation but also quantitative evaluation is desirable.

7.7 Cardiac Sarcoidosis Case 6

Osamu Manabe and Noriko Oyama-Manabe

Abstract Cardiac involvement is the most serious manifestation of sarcoidosis. The etiology of sarcoidosis and its disease progression is unknown, but ^{18}F-fluorodeoxyglucose (FDG) positron emission tomography (PET)/computed tomography (CT) and cardiac magnetic resonance (CMR) can provide sufficient evidence for the diagnosis of cardiac sarcoidosis (CS). An insufficient suppression of the physiological myocardial uptake is one of the causes of misdiagnosis by FDG PET/CT. We present herein a patient's case that highlights the scenario of isolated CS presentation, along with a discussion of FDG PET/CT and CMR imaging in such cases.

Keywords: Cardiac sarcoidosis, ^{18}F-FDG PET, Cardiac magnetic resonance, Isolated cardiac sarcoidosis

7.7.1 Clinical Presentation

The male patient, in his 30s, was identified as having lymphadenopathy of the lower neck by a physical examination, without any subjective symptoms.

7.7.2 Key Images and Image Interpretations

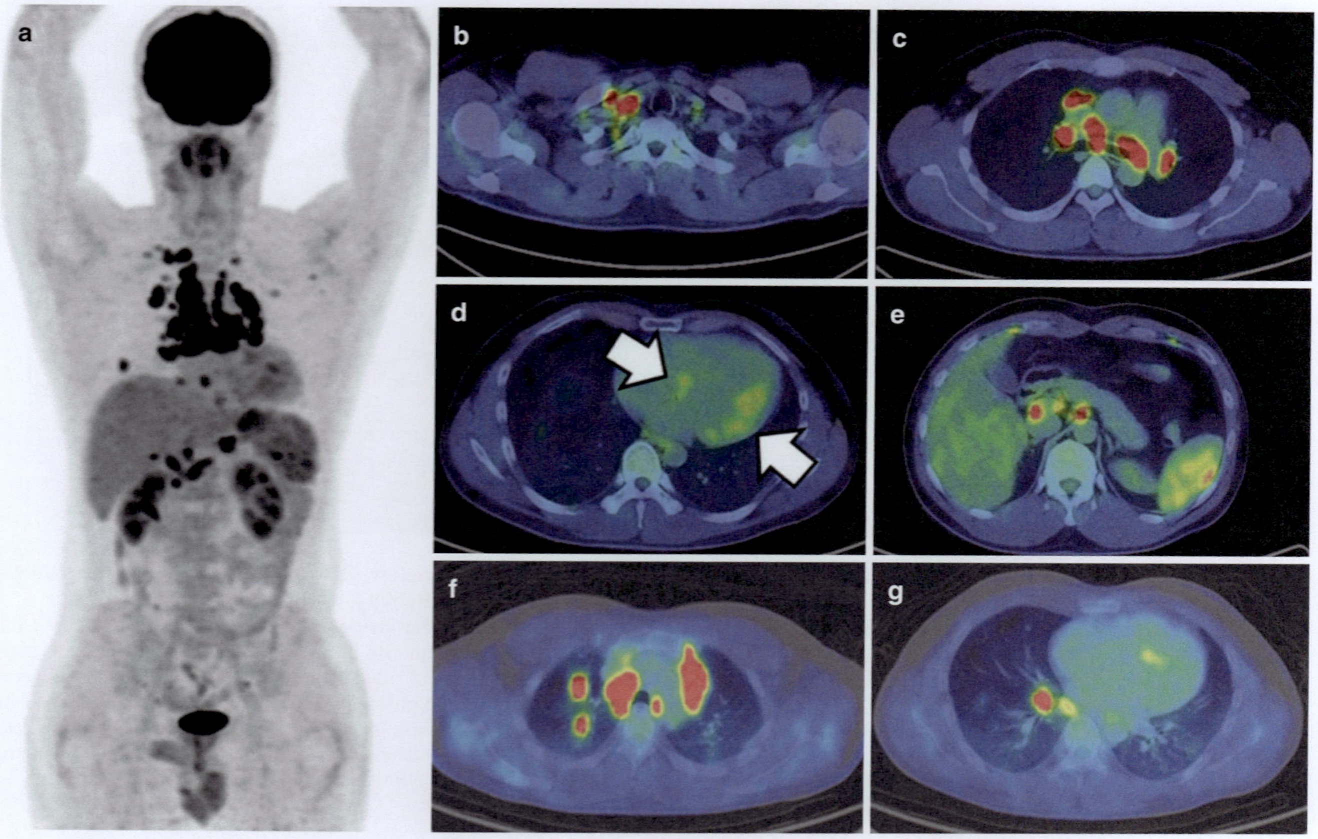

Fig. 7.12 FDG PET/CT at the patient's initial visit
Whole-body FDG PET/CT scanning revealed multiple high accumulations of tracer in the lymph nodes in the bilateral but right-dominant supraclavicular (**b**), mediastinum (**c**), bilateral hilum (**c**), left axilla (**a**), abdominal para-aorta (**e**), and surrounding inferior vena cava (**e**). Multiple nodular accumulations in the lung (**f, g**) and heterogeneous uptake in the spleen (**e**) were also detected. There was slight uptake in the left ventricle (LV), mainly the basal level and lateral wall (**d**; white arrows), which was sometimes seen for the physiological uptake. The fasting period was 18 h before the PET/CT scan, but no special preparation such as a low-carbohydrate diet or injection of unfractionated heparin was conducted. Sarcoidosis was suspected due to the distribution of the FDG uptakes, and then confirmed by bronchoalveolar lavage (BAL) and transbronchial needle aspiration (TBNA).

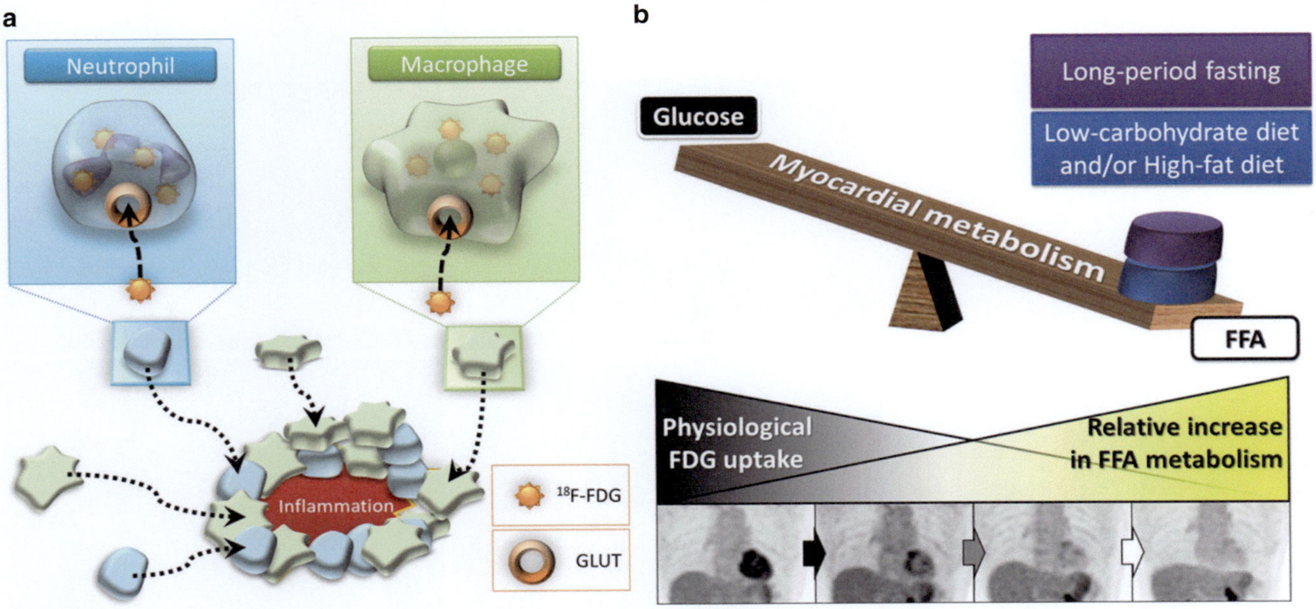

Fig. 7.13 Schema of the FDG accumulation and pre-imaging preparation
FDG uptake in the inflammatory foci is due to the activation of inflammatory cells (e.g., lymphocytes and macrophages) that accumulate sequentially following inflammation including active cardiac sarcoidosis (CS). Cellular activation increases the expression of glucose transporter (GLUT) in these cells. Once taken up into the cells via the GLUT, FDG is phosphorylated to FDG-6-phosphate by hexokinase as well as glucose. After entry into cells, FDG becomes phosphorylated to FDG-6-phosphate by hexokinase without being metabolized further along the glycolytic pathway. Therefore, FDG-6-phosphate accumulates intracellularly, in a condition referred to as "metabolic trapping"(**a**)
The pitfall of FDG is that living myocardial cells use the glucose for their energy source, requiring patient pre-imaging preparation to suppress the physiological myocardial glucose metabolism. Several approaches to reducing physiological myocardial glucose metabolism have been reported, such as long-period fasting and a low-carbohydrate diet and/or high-fat diet. These approaches lead to myocardial free fatty acid (FFA) metabolism dominance (**b**) [21]

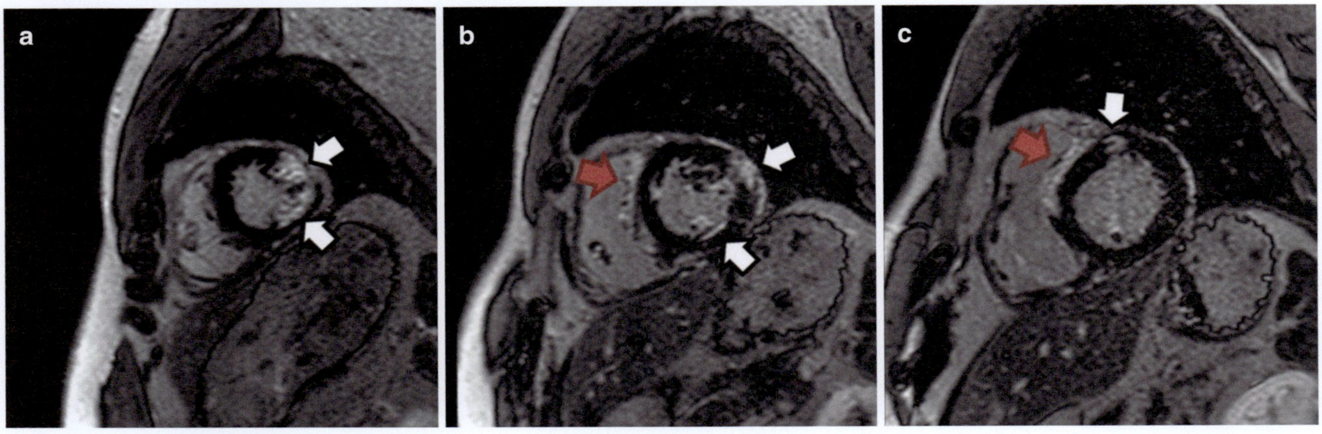

Fig. 7.14 Late gadolinium-enhanced cardiac MRI
Five years after the first FDG PET/CT scan, complete left bundle branch block (CLBBB) was detected by a scheduled electrocardiography. There was no clinical symptom, but echocardiography showed the hypokinesis of the septal wall compared to the patient's previous examinations. Late gadolinium enhancement was seen in the CMR imaging. Short-axis images at the apical (**a**), mid- (**b**), and basal (**c**) level are displayed. A band-like intensity area in the outer layer of the septal wall (red arrows) and several patchy abnormal intensity areas (white arrows) were compatible with CS

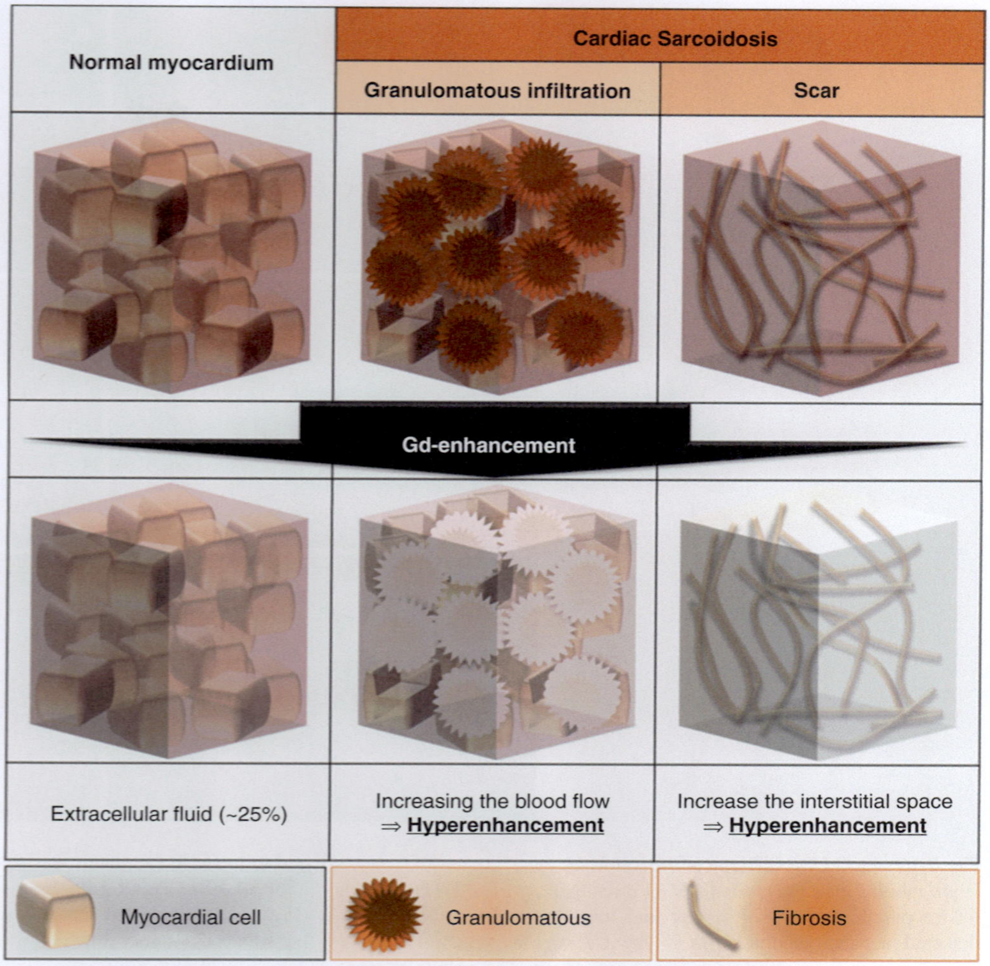

Fig. 7.15 Schema of the late gadolinium enhancement
In normal myocardium, myocardial cells (*left panel*) are highly dense, and the interstitial space with extracellular fluid that can be enhanced is limited. The infiltrated granulomas in the active phase of CS (*center panel*) are well enhanced after gadolinium injection. The scar formation with fibrosis in the chronic phase is well enhanced due to the spread of the interstitial space [26].

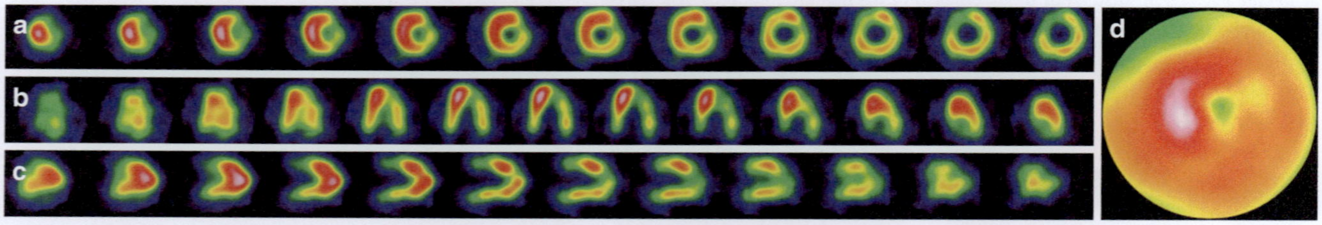

Fig. 7.16 ^{99m}Tc-MIBI scintigraphy
Short axis (**a**), horizontal long axis (**b**), vertical long axis (**c**), and polar map (**d**) are displayed. Perfusion decreases at the apex, lateral wall at the distal-to-basal level, and anterior to septal wall at the basal level are revealed (**a**–**d**). The left ventricular ejection fraction estimated from quantitative gated SPECT was 47%. Injected ^{99m}Tc-MIBI distributes in the myocardium according to the regional myocardial perfusion, and its uptake to the myocardium is related to the presence of intact mitochondria. Therefore, the infiltrated granulomas in CS are delineated by the perfusion decrease region.

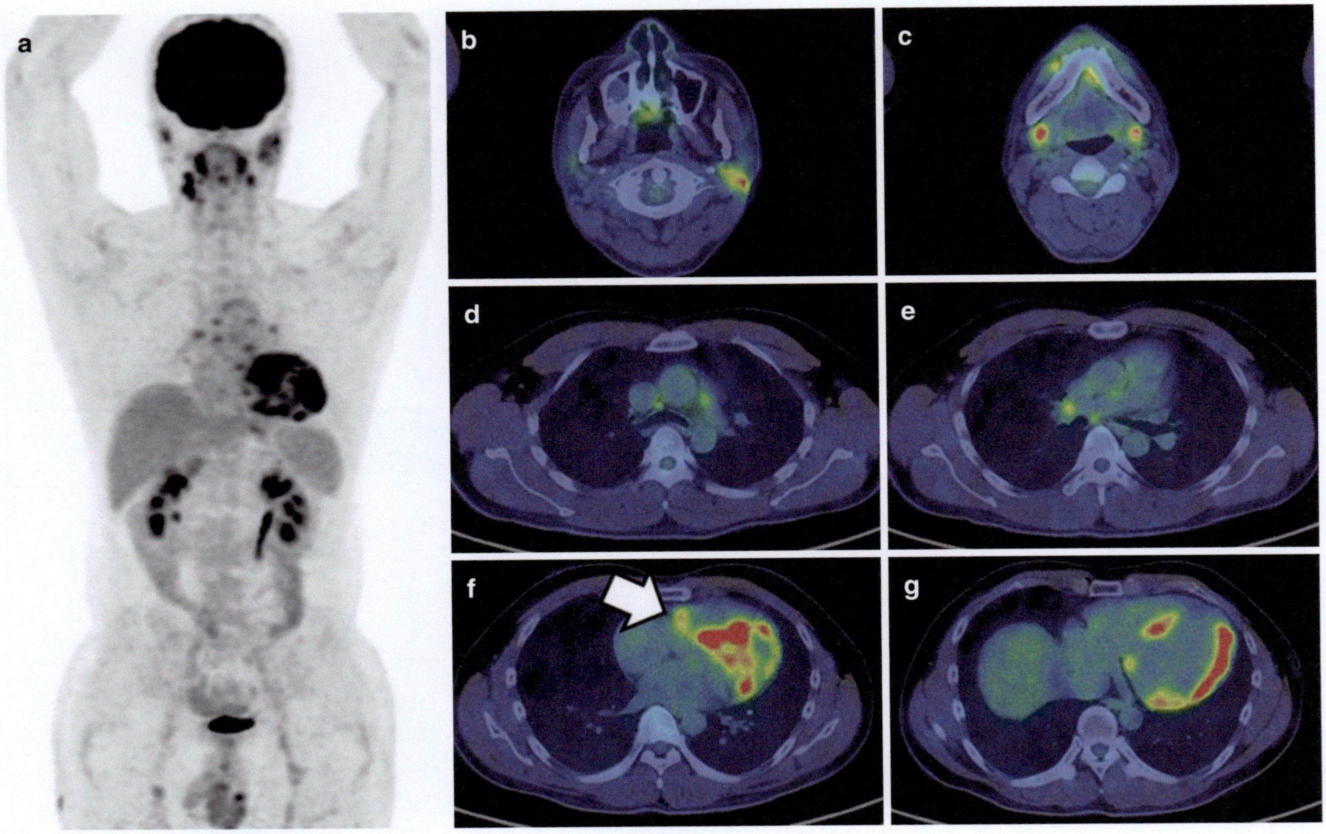

Fig. 7.17 FDG PET/CT scan at the follow-up
Eight months later the patient's MRI investigation, FDG PET/CT with the preparation of >18-h fasting and low-carbohydrate food intake detected a clear accumulation in the LV regions which was well accorded with the perfusion decrease area (**f**, **g**). The uptake of right ventricle also indicates the active CS (**f**; *white arrow*). Interestingly, the accumulations of the other sites were quite different from the previous scan (*see* Fig. 7.12). Instead of the decreased or disappeared uptakes of the lymph nodes, lung, and spleen (**a**, **d**, **e**), accumulation at the parotid and submandibular glands was observed (**b**, **c**). The retrospective evaluation of FDG PET/CT findings in this case at the first examination (Fig. 7.12) suggested that the slight uptake of myocardium might be silent CS rather than physiological. The patient did not show any clinical symptoms even with CLBBB and abnormal CMR findings. If the patient had not undergone the physical checkup and there had been only the second FDG PET/CT scan, this case might have been misdiagnosed as isolated CS because there were few findings in the other extracardiac sites.

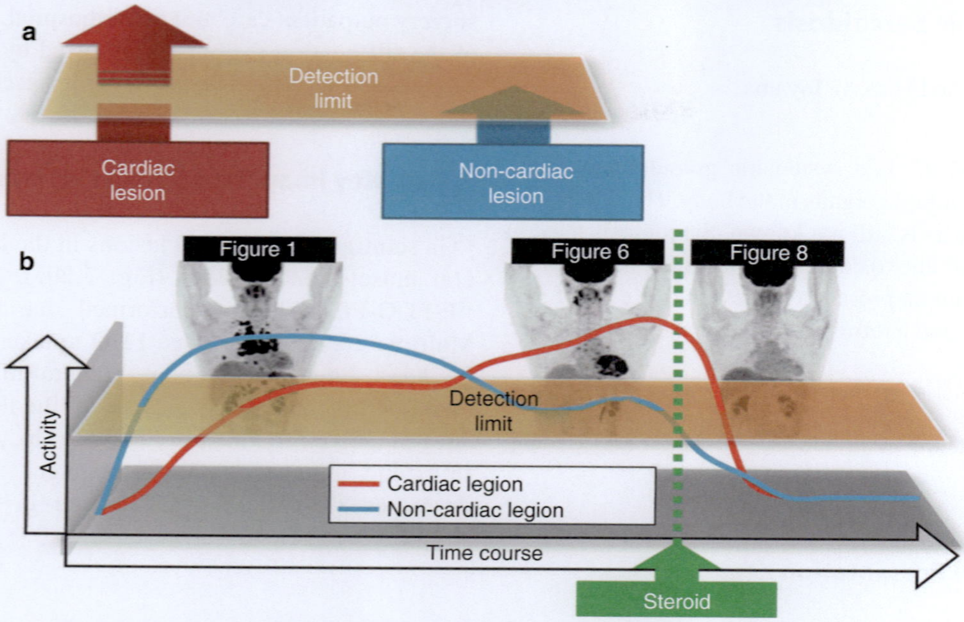

Fig. 7.18 Natural course of the sarcoidosis and isolated CS [27, 28] Sarcoidosis is a granulomatous inflammatory disorder of unknown etiology which is known to affect any organ systems including the heart. Nearly two-thirds of patients with sarcoidosis achieve spontaneous remission within a decade after their initial diagnosis. However, a certain few patients experience a chronic or progressive course. Cardiac involvement is the most serious manifestation of sarcoidosis. Possible mechanisms of isolated CS might be explained by the following clinical situations: (**a**) sarcoidosis first occurs in the myocardium, and it does not spread to other lesions, or (**b**) sarcoidosis spreads to cardiac and other lesions, but only the cardiac lesion is detected clinically (this may include the patients with inactivated sarcoidosis of the other organs but activity remaining in only a cardiac lesion). In the present patient's case, he might have been misdiagnosed as having isolated CS if he had not undergone the physical examination, because he had no clinical symptoms and the follow-up FDG PET/CT demonstrated that the uptake of lymph nodes and the other organs such as lung and spleen had disappeared without treatment.

Fig. 7.19 FDG PET/CT imaging after the corticosteroid therapy The patient was diagnosed with CS with active inflammation and was therefore treated with 30 mg/day of corticosteroid. Follow-up FDG PET/CT with >18-h fasting combined with a low-carbohydrate diet preparation performed 1 month after the initiation of the corticosteroid therapy showed obviously reduced FDG uptake in the myocardium (slight remaining uptake in the lateral wall) (**b**, **c**). The FDG uptake of the other sites had disappeared (**a**). FDG PET is useful to not only diagnose but also monitor treatment effects in patients with CS [29].

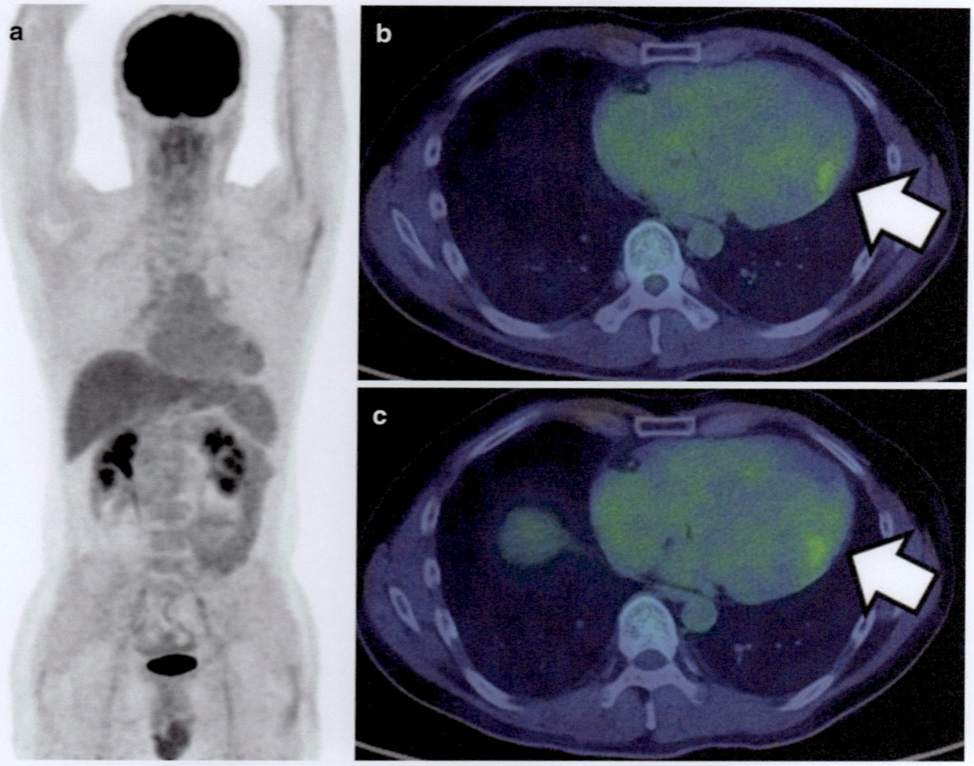

7.8 Systemic Sarcoidosis

Ayumi Watanabe and Hiroshi Toyama

Abstract Sarcoidosis is a systematic granulomatous disease that affects multiple organs in the body. The etiology of systemic sarcoidosis is still not known. Sarcoidosis may, in rare cases, be fatal due to complications in the heart, lungs, and brain. The authors present a representative case of systemic sarcoidosis and a retrospective review of our systemic sarcoidosis cases.

Keywords: Systemic sarcoidosis, ^{18}F-FDG PET, Lung, Muscle

7.8.1 Clinical Presentation

A 62-year-old woman experiencing stiffness in the right vastus intermedius muscle presented to the orthopedic surgery outpatient care unit at our hospital. After a biopsy of the stiffness on the muscle followed by a diagnosis of sarcoidosis, she was referred to cardiovascular medicine.

7.8.2 Key Images and Image Interpretation

^{67}Ga scintigraphy detected lesions in the heart and bilateral muscles of the legs (Fig. 7.20a). After 2 years, ^{18}F-FDG-PET/CT was performed due to palpitation. Multiple areas of increased FDG uptake were found in the heart, lung, mediastinum, bilateral hilum, retroperitoneal lymph nodes, and muscles of the limbs indicating sites of active inflammatory activity (b). After 3 months following prednisolone treatment, significantly decreased ^{18}F-FDG-PET/CT uptake in multiple areas was observed (c).

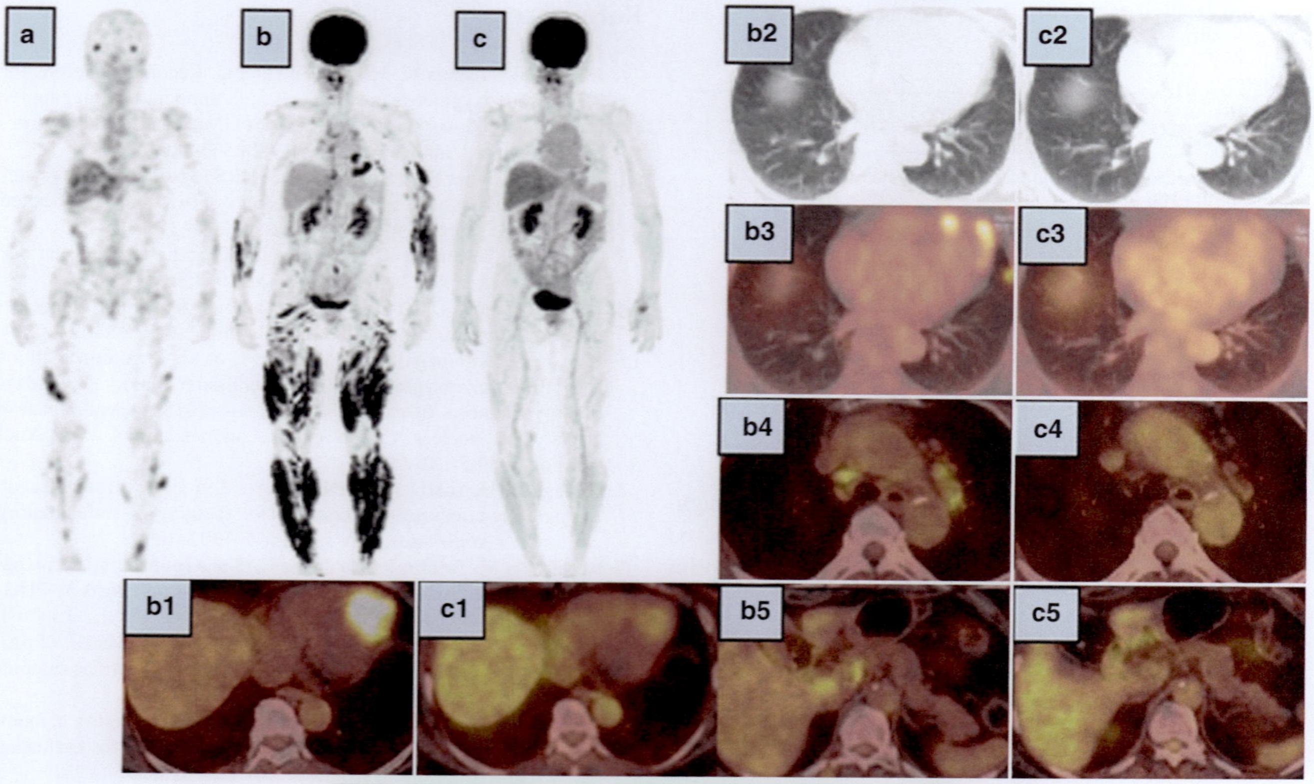

regions	%
heart	67.4
salivary glands	14.0
lungs	39.5
mediastinum and hilum lymph nodes	76.7
retroperitoneal lymph nodes	27.9
liver	14.0
spleen	23.3
muscles of limbs	20.9

Fig. 7.20 ^{67}Ga SPECT (**a**), pre- (**b**) and post- (**c**) steroid treatment ^{18}F- FDG-PET

Table 7.2 Percentage (%) of patients with increased uptake in each region

Regions	%
Heart	67.4
Salivary glands	14.0
Lungs	39.5
Mediastinum and hilum lymph nodes	76.7
Retroperitoneal lymph nodes	27.9
Liver	14.0
Spleen	23.3
Muscles of limbs	20.9

7.8.3 Technique

Patient preparation: patient fasted for 18 h after a 6-h high-fat, high-protein, and low-carbohydrate diet and received intravenous unfractionated heparin (50 IU/kg) 15 min prior to ^{18}F-FDG injection.

FDG PET/CT scanning: Whole-body imaging was performed from head to toe 60 min after ^{18}F-FDG injection using a PET/CT scanner (Biograph mCT, Siemens).

7.8.4 Regional Incidence of Increased Uptakes on ^{18}F-FDG PET/CT in Systemic Sarcoidosis

We analyzed 70 ^{18}F-FDG PET/CT studies in patients with cardiac sarcoidosis and evaluated incidence of increased uptakes in each patient (Table 7.2). However, the real incidence of accumulation in the salivary glands and mediastinal/hilar lymph nodes may be lower due to including physiological accumulation.

7.8.5 Discussion

Sarcoidosis has complications, such as lung or eye lesions, that may not cause morbidity but may significantly impair the patient's quality of life. Therefore, it is important to evaluate not only cardiac lesions but also active lesions that may occur in other organs. ^{18}F-FDG-PET/CT can evaluate the whole-body active lesion distribution via whole-body scanning in addition to cardiac scanning and has high accuracy compared to ^{67}Ga scintigraphy. It has been reported that the FDG accumulation is consistent with the high infiltration of inflammatory cells. Detecting the lesion uptake may be useful as additional confirmation of the biopsy result. ^{18}F-FDG-PET/CT may also be useful for assessing the efficacy of sarcoidosis treatment.

References

1. Ishida Y, Yoshinaga K, Miyagawa M, et al. Recommendations for ^{18}F-fluorodeoxyglucose positron emission tomography imaging for cardiac sarcoidosis: Japanese Society of Nuclear Cardiology recommendations. Ann Nucl Med. 2014;28:393–403.
2. Birnie DH, Sauer WH, Bogun F, et al. HRS expert consensus statement on the diagnosis and management of arrhythmias associated with cardiac sarcoidosis. Heart Rhythm. 2014;11:1305–23.
3. Terasaki F, Yoshinaga K. New guidelines for diagnosis of cardiac sarcoidosis in Japan. Ann Nucl Cardiol. 2017;3:42–5.
4. Isobe M, Tezuka D. Isolated cardiac sarcoidosis: clinical characteristics, diagnosis and treatment. Int J Cardiol. 2015;182:132–40.
5. Kumita S, Yoshinaga K, Miyagawa M, et al. Recommendations for ^{18}F-fluorodeoxyglucose positron emission tomography imaging for diagnosis of cardiac sarcoidosis—2018 update: Japanese Society of Nuclear Cardiology Recommendations. Ann Nucl Cardiol. 2019;5:141–59.
6. Miyagawa M, Yokoyama R, Nishiyama Y, et al. Positron emission tomography-computed tomography for imaging of inflammatory cardiovascular diseases. Circ J. 2014;78:1302–10.
7. Miyagawa M, Tashiro R, Watanabe E, et al. Optimal patient preparation for detection and assessment of cardiac sarcoidosis by FDG-PET. Ann Nucl Cardiol. 2017;3:113–6.
8. Langah R, Spicer K, Gebregziabher M, et al. Effectiveness of prolonged fasting ^{18}F-FDG PET-CT in the detection of cardiac sarcoidosis. J Nucl Cardiol. 2009;16:801–10.
9. Morooka M, Moroi M, Uno K, et al. Long fasting is effective in inhibiting physiological myocardial -^{18}F-FDG uptake and for evaluating active lesions of cardiac sarcoidosis. EJNMMI Res. 2014;4:1–11.
10. Coulden R, Chung P, Sonnex E, et al. Suppression of myocardial ^{18}F-FDG uptake with a preparatory "Atkins-style" low-carbohydrate diet. Eur Radiol. 2012;22:2221–8.
11. Williams G, Kolodny GM. Suppression of myocardial ^{18}F-FDG uptake by preparing patients with a high-fat, low carbohydrate diet. AJR Am J Roentgenol. 2008;190:W151–6.
12. Ishimaru S, Tsujino I, Takei T, et al. Focal uptake on ^{18}F-fluoro-2-deoxyglucose positron emission tomography images indicates cardiac involvement of sarcoidosis. Eur Heart J. 2005;26:1538–43.
13. Jang IK, Hursting MJ. When heparins promote thrombosis: review of heparin-induce thrombocytopenia. Circulation. 2005;111:2671–83.
14. Yokoyama R, Miyagawa M, Okayama H, et al. Quantitative analysis of myocardial ^{18}F-fluorodeoxyglucose uptake by PET/CT for detection of cardiac sarcoidosis. Int J Cardiol. 2015;195:180–7.
15. Ahmadian A, Brogan A, Berman J, et al. Quantitative interpretation of FDG PET/CT with myocardial perfusion imaging increases diagnostic information in the evaluation of cardiac sarcoidosis. J Nucl Cardiol. 2014;21:925–39.
16. Osborne MT, Hulten EA, Singh A, et al. Reduction in ^{18}F-fluorodeoxyglucose uptake on serial cardiac positron emission tomography is associated with improved left ventricular ejection fraction in patients with cardiac sarcoidosis. J Nucl Cardiol. 2014;21:166–74.
17. Ahmadian A, Pawar S, Govender P, Berman J, Ruberg FL, Miller EJ. The response of FDG uptake to immunosuppressive treatment on FDG PET/CT imaging for cardiac sarcoidosis. J Nucl Cardiol. 2017;24:413–24.
18. Chareonthaitawee P, Beanlands RS, Chen W, et al. Joint SNMMI–ASNC expert consensus document on the role of ^{18}F-FDG PET/CT in cardiac sarcoid detection and therapy monitoring. J Nucl Med. 2017;58:1341–53.
19. Blankstein R, Waller AH. Evaluation of known or suspected cardiac sarcoidosis. Circ Cardiovasc Imaging. 2016;9:e000867. https://doi.org/10.1161/CIRCIMAGING.113.000867.

20. Ishimaru S, Tsujino I, Takei T, et al. Focal uptake on ^{18}F-fluoro-2-deoxyglucose positron emission tomography images indicates cardiac involvement of sarcoidosis. Eur Heart J. 2005;26:1538–43.
21. Manabe O, et al. The effects of 18-h fasting with low-carbohydrate diet preparation on suppressed physiological myocardial (18) F-fluorodeoxyglucose (FDG) uptake and possible minimal effects of unfractionated heparin use in patients with suspected cardiac involvement sarcoidosis. J Nucl Cardiol. 2016;23:244–52.
22. Orii M, et al. Comparison of cardiac MRI and 18F-FDG positron emission tomography manifestations and regional response to corticosteroid therapy in newly diagnosed cardiac sarcoidosis with complete heart block. Heart Rhythm. 2015;12:2477–85.
23. Kandolin R, et al. Cardiac sarcoidosis: epidemiology, characteristics, and outcome over 25 years in a nationwide study. Circulation. 2015;131:624–32.
24. Ahmadian A, et al. The response of FDG uptake to immunosuppressive treatment on FDG PET/CT imaging for cardiac sarcoidosis. J Nucl Cardiol. 2017;24:413–24.
25. Waller AH, et al. Quantifying myocardial inflammation using F18-fluorodeoxyglucose positron emission tomography in cardiac sarcoidosis. J Nucl Cardiol. 2014;21:940–3.
26. Mahrholdt H, et al. Delayed enhancement cardiovascular magnetic resonance assessment of non-ischaemic cardiomyopathies. Eur Heart J. 2005;26:1461–74.
27. Kandolin R, et al. Diagnosing isolated cardiac sarcoidosis. J Intern Med. 2011;270:461–8.
28. Iannuzzi MC, et al. Sarcoidosis. N Engl J Med. 2007;357:2157–65.
29. Patel DC, et al. FDG PET-CT findings of extra-thoracic sarcoid are associated with cardiac sarcoid: A rationale for using FGD PET-CT for cardiac sarcoid evaluation. J Nucl Cardiol. 2019;26:486–92.

PET/CT for Neuroinflammation

8

Aya Ogata, Yasuyuki Kimura, Fumihiko Yasuno, Yasuomi Ouchi, and Masahiro Fujita

8.1 Role of TSPO Ligands for Neuroinflammation

Aya Ogata and Yasuyuki Kimura

Abstract Currently, PET ligands targeting TSPO, translocator protein 18 kDa, are widely used in clinical research to investigate the contribution of neuroinflammation in various neurological diseases. The uptake of TSPO ligands is increased or decreased in various diseases or conditions, and the change is positively or negatively correlated with disease status or progression. These studies revealed that activated glial cells, detected by increased TSPO binding, could exert detrimental or protective effects on the brain, which can be a target for treatment. However, considering the limitation of TSPO PET imaging, novel PET ligands targeting other molecules reflecting specific aspects of neuroinflammation need to be developed for drug development.

Keywords: Positron emission tomography, Neuroinflammation, Microglia, Translocator protein, Neurodegenerative diseases, Psychiatric diseases

8.1.1 Introduction

In this chapter, we review clinical PET imaging of TSPO in the brain. TSPO is a protein expressed on the outer membrane of mitochondria. Its expression level is low in the healthy brain but increases in lesions with neuroinflammation due to its overexpression in two major cellular components: activated microglia and astrocytes. Many PET ligands targeting TSPO have been developed and clinically used as biomarkers of neuroinflammation to image the accumulation of activated microglia and astrocytes in various diseases.

As discussed in earlier chapters, [^{11}C]PK11195 is the first PET ligand widely used to image TSPO in the brain. However, its detection sensitivity is low, and interpretation of the obtained results is challenging because of its small specific binding compared to nonspecific binding in humans [1]. A better signal-to-noise ratio and sensitivity have been achieved with second-generation PET ligands (i.e., [^{11}C]PBR28, [^{11}C]DPA713, [^{18}F]DPA714). Furthermore, interpretation of the PET imaging results is not straightforward as TSPO has three different phenotypes caused by a polymorphism of the TSPO gene and is expressed not only in microglia and astrocytes but also in neurons and vascular endothelial cells in the brain, and the cell selectivity might differ among various PET ligands for TSPO.

8.1.2 Effects of TSPO Genotype

In humans, three different phenotypes of TSPO binding have been reported: high-, mixed-, and low-affinity binders (HAB, MAB, and LAB, respectively) [2]. The difference in the binding affinity is caused by a polymorphism of the TSPO gene (rs6971) leading to an amino acid substitution (Ala147Thr). PET signal is significantly affected by the

A. Ogata · Y. Kimura (✉)
Section on Imaging Molecules, Department of Clinical and Experimental Neuroimaging, Center for Development of Advanced Medicine for Dementia, National Center for Geriatrics and Gerontology, Obu, Aichi, Japan
e-mail: a-ogata@ncgg.go.jp; yazkim@ncgg.go.jp

F. Yasuno
Department of Psychiatry, National Center for Geriatrics and Gerontology, Obu, Aichi, Japan

Y. Ouchi
Department of Brain Biofunctional Imaging, Hamamatsu University School of Medicine, Hamamatsu, Shizuoka, Japan

M. Fujita
PET Core Imaging Lab, Houston Methodist Institute for Academic Medicine, Houston, TX, USA
e-mail: mfujitamd1@hotmail.com

H. Toyama et al. (eds.), *PET/CT for Inflammatory Diseases*, https://doi.org/10.1007/978-981-15-0810-3_8

genotype; the binding potential of HABs is approximately twice that of MABs, and the distribution volume of HABs is ~50% higher than that of MABs [3]. PET ligands that are not affected by genotype are under development, but no clinical ligand has been reported at this time.

8.1.3 Quantification of TSPO PET Images

Quantification of TSPO PET has been performed invasively with a serial collection of arterial blood using the two-tissue compartmental model [4]. However, based on the recent finding that TSPO is also expressed on the vascular endothelial cells in the brain, a new model using the vascular endothelial component was proposed showing a better fit than the classical two-tissue compartmental model and a good correlation with TSPO mRNA expression in the brain [5]. Noninvasive quantification without arterial blood sampling has not done well since no reference region without TSPO expression is available in the brain. To overcome this problem, several methods were proposed to extract reference voxels devoid of TSPO expression [4, 6] or to estimate specific binding without extracting reference regions [7].

8.1.4 TSPO PET Imaging in Healthy Subjects

In healthy subjects, the uptake of [^{11}C]PK11195 is low, and it is lower in the cerebral cortex and cerebellum than in the subcortical structures, suggesting a low level of TSPO protein expression [8]. The overall pattern of the [^{11}C]PK11195 distribution in the brain does not change, but the uptake increases with age. Thus, TSPO protein expression may increase with age or the number of cells expressing these receptors may increase. The thalamus and midbrain show relatively higher increase compared with other brain regions. TSPO PET imaging was performed in healthy subjects with induced neuroinflammation. *Escherichia coli* lipopolysaccharide (also called endotoxin) was systemically injected in healthy humans. The injection significantly increased [^{11}C]PBR28 binding, reflecting an increased TSPO level on the activated microglia in the brain [9]. TSPO PET imaging has also been used to investigate the effect of anesthesia on the brain in healthy subjects. To investigate cognitively impaired patients, such as patients with severe dementia and autism, anesthesia or sedation is necessary for a PET procedure. Propofol, a widely used intravenous anesthesia, reduces the total distribution volume of [^{11}C]PBR28 in the brain, which affects the measurement of TSPO in the brain, under anesthesia [10].

8.1.5 TSPO PET Imaging in Neurodegenerative Diseases

TSPO PET imaging provides pathophysiological insights into how glia activation contributes to disease progression and neurotoxicity in various neurodegenerative diseases. In Alzheimer's disease (AD), two distinct profiles of microglial activation, detrimental and protective effects, were proposed based on the finding with TSPO PET imaging. As a detrimental effect, the binding of [^{11}C]PBR28 was high in cortical regions, especially in the parietal and temporal cortices [11]. The binding was inversely correlated with patients' cognitive performance and gray matter volume. Early-onset (<65 years old) patients showed higher binding than late-onset patients. As a protective effect, [^{18}F]DPA714 showed higher binding in AD patients than in healthy control subjects, especially at the prodromal stage [12]. The binding was positively correlated with Mini-Mental State Examination scores (higher is better) and grey matter volume. Higher binding was found in slow decliners compared to fast decliners. Thus, microglial activation seems to play a protective role in the clinical progression of the disease at these early stages. A longitudinal study clearly showed the two profiles of microglial activation. High initial [^{18}F]DPA714 binding was correlated with low subsequent increase of microglial activation and favorable clinical evolution, whereas the opposite profile was observed when initial [^{18}F]DPA714 binding was low, independent of disease severity at baseline [13]. The TSPO level is correlated with both tau aggregation and amyloid deposition, two pathological hallmarks of AD, showing the complex relationship between these processes [14]. The binding of [^{11}C]PBR28 in AD patients was correlated with tau accumulation. The correlation was stronger in AD patients than in patients with mild cognitive impairment. The binding of [^{11}C]PBR28 in AD patients was also correlated with amyloid accumulation. The correlation was stronger in patients with mild cognitive impairment than in AD patients.

In amyotrophic lateral sclerosis (ALS), a form of motor neuron disease in which upper and lower motor neurons degenerate, uptake of [^{11}C]PBR28 was increased in the motor cortices and corticospinal tracts, and the increase correlated with the patients' functional scale [15]. In another study, increase in the uptake was colocalized with the change in fractional anisotropy and cortical thinning measured with an MRI, which indicates the relationship between the glial activation and structural change in the brain [16]. The increased uptake of [^{11}C]PBR28 was also seen in the motor region of patients with primary lateral sclerosis (PLS), a form of motor neuron disease in which upper motor neurons degenerate predominantly [17]. A recent study confirmed a regional increase of [^{11}C]PBR28 uptake in the precentral and paracentral gyri in ALS and subcortical white matter in PLS [18].

In Parkinson's disease (PD), treatment with a selective and irreversible inhibitor of myeloperoxidase, AZD3421, was investigated using TSPO PET imaging to measure the reduction of neuroinflammation by the reduction of oxidative stress [19]. The distribution volume of [^{11}C]PBR28 in the nigrostriatal region was decreased by ~15% after the 8-week treatment, whereas there was no change in the placebo group.

In multiple sclerosis (MS), neuroinflammation is present and is closely linked to poor clinical outcome. The binding of [^{11}C]PBR28 was high in the cortex and cortical lesions, thalamus, hippocampus, and normal-appearing white matter [20]. White matter lesions showed a relatively modest increase. The uptake was higher in secondary-progressive MS patients than relapsing-remitting MS patients. The binding in the cortex, deep gray matter, and normal-appearing white matter correlated with a neurological disability and impaired cognitive performance.

In patients with temporal lobe epilepsy (TLE), the TSPO level is high in the regions both ipsilateral and contralateral to their seizure foci, suggesting ongoing inflammation. The uptake of [^{11}C]PBR28 and [^{11}C]DPA713 was increased in the ipsilateral temporal regions and in the contralateral hippocampus, amygdala, and temporal pole [21]. Relative [^{11}C]PBR28 and [^{11}C]DPA713 uptakes were higher in ipsilateral regions than contralateral regions of seizure foci in patients with TLE.

In patients with traumatic brain injury, TSPO PET imaging was used to assess the microglial activation and the effect of minocycline on disease progression. Patients at least 6 months after a moderate-to-severe traumatic brain injury showed increased [^{11}C]PBR28 binding in the cerebral white matter and thalamus [22]. MRI measurements of white matter damage were higher in the areas of greater [^{11}C]PBR28 binding. Minocycline treatment reduced [^{11}C]PBR28 binding in the white matter. The treatment increased plasma neurofilament light levels, a marker of neurodegeneration, suggesting that microglial activation has a reparative effect in the chronic phase of traumatic brain injury.

8.1.6 TSPO PET Imaging in Psychiatric Diseases

TSPO PET imaging is also used to investigate psychiatric diseases and pain, where slight neuroinflammation is supposed to contribute to their pathophysiology. In patients with schizophrenia and in patients with an ultra-high risk of psychosis, the uptake of [^{11}C]PBR28 was increased compared to healthy controls [23]. However, drug-naive, first-episode psychosis patients showed a significant reduction of [^{11}C]PBR28 binding in the gray matter [24]. Unmedicated major depressive disorder patients showed higher binding of [^{11}C]PBR28 in the subgenual prefrontal cortex [25]. In alcohol-dependent patients, TSPO PET imaging revealed the contribution of abnormal glial function to the disease. [^{11}C]PBR28 binding was decreased in the hippocampus [26]. The TSPO levels in the hippocampus and striatum were negatively associated with alcohol dependence severity, and the patients showed abnormal monocyte response to lipopolysaccharide stimulation [27]. Another report showed that decreased [^{11}C]PBR28 binding was observed only in MAB genotype of patients, and cholesterol levels were inversely correlated with brain [^{11}C]PBR28 binding [28]. In cocaine abusers, no significant differences were observed in [^{11}C]PBR28 distribution volume in the cortical and subcortical regions compared with healthy controls [29]. In patients with chronic low back pain, [^{11}C]PBR28 binding was increased, especially in the thalamus [30]. The binding was negatively correlated with clinical pain and circulating levels of the proinflammatory cytokine, suggesting that TSPO expression has protective effects in patients with chronic low back pain.

8.1.7 TSPO PET Imaging in Other Diseases

TSPO PET imaging has also been used to investigate the contribution of neuroinflammation in other diseases. In patients with acute ischemic stroke, uptake of [^{18}F]DPA714 was increased in and around the ischemic lesion [31]. In patients with neurocysticercosis, a major cause of epilepsy in endemic regions by the infection of the larval form of the tapeworm *Taenia solium*, [^{11}C]PBR28 binding was increased in perilesional edema or degenerating cysts, and the increase lasted for several months [32]. In symptomatic patients with human T-lymphotropic virus type 1–associated myelopathy, distribution volume of [^{11}C]PBR28 was increased across the whole brain compared to the non-symptomatic carrier [33]. This increase in the binding correlated with a marker of T-cell activation and a marker of disease severity. Cognitively healthy human immunodeficiency virus-positive individuals showed global increases in [^{11}C]PBR28 binding [34]. The binding in the hippocampus, amygdala, and thalamus was associated with poorer global cognitive performance. The effect of neuroinflammation on cognitive decline after surgery was examined using TSPO PET imaging. Patients undergoing prostatectomy under general anesthesia showed a global downregulation of [^{11}C]PBR28 binding in the gray matter 3–4 days postoperatively, recovering and upregulating after 3 months [35]. The binding change was correlated to the change in cognitive performance. Seasonal change of TSPO binding was investigated in relation to peripheral inflammation, fatigue, and sleep due to allergy. No difference in the levels of [^{11}C]PBR28 binding was observed between patients and healthy subjects [36].

8.2 Alzheimer's Disease/MCI

Fumihiko Yasuno

Abstract Positron emission tomography (PET) scans with [^{11}C]DAA1106, a potent and selective ligand for translocator protein (TSPO), were performed on Alzheimer's disease (AD)/mild cognitive impairment (MCI) subjects. MCI subjects were clinically followed for 5 years after their initial PET scans. TSPO binding was increased in widespread areas in not only AD but MCI subjects with conversion to dementia. Our findings indicated that microglial activation may occur before the onset of dementia. The detection of microglial activation may provide useful prognostic information with respect to stratifying MCI subjects at increased risk of dementia.

Keywords: Mild cognitive impairment (MCI), Alzheimer's disease (AD), Translocator protein (TSPO), Microglia, Positron emission tomography

8.2.1 Clinical Presentation

Mean %SUV images between 30 and 90 min after the injection of [^{11}C]DAA1106 of AD (male, 76-year old), MCI–AD converter (female, 76-year old), MCI–DLB converter (male, 57-year old), MCI-non-converter (male, 61-year old), and an aged normal subject (male, 67-year old).

8.2.2 Key Images

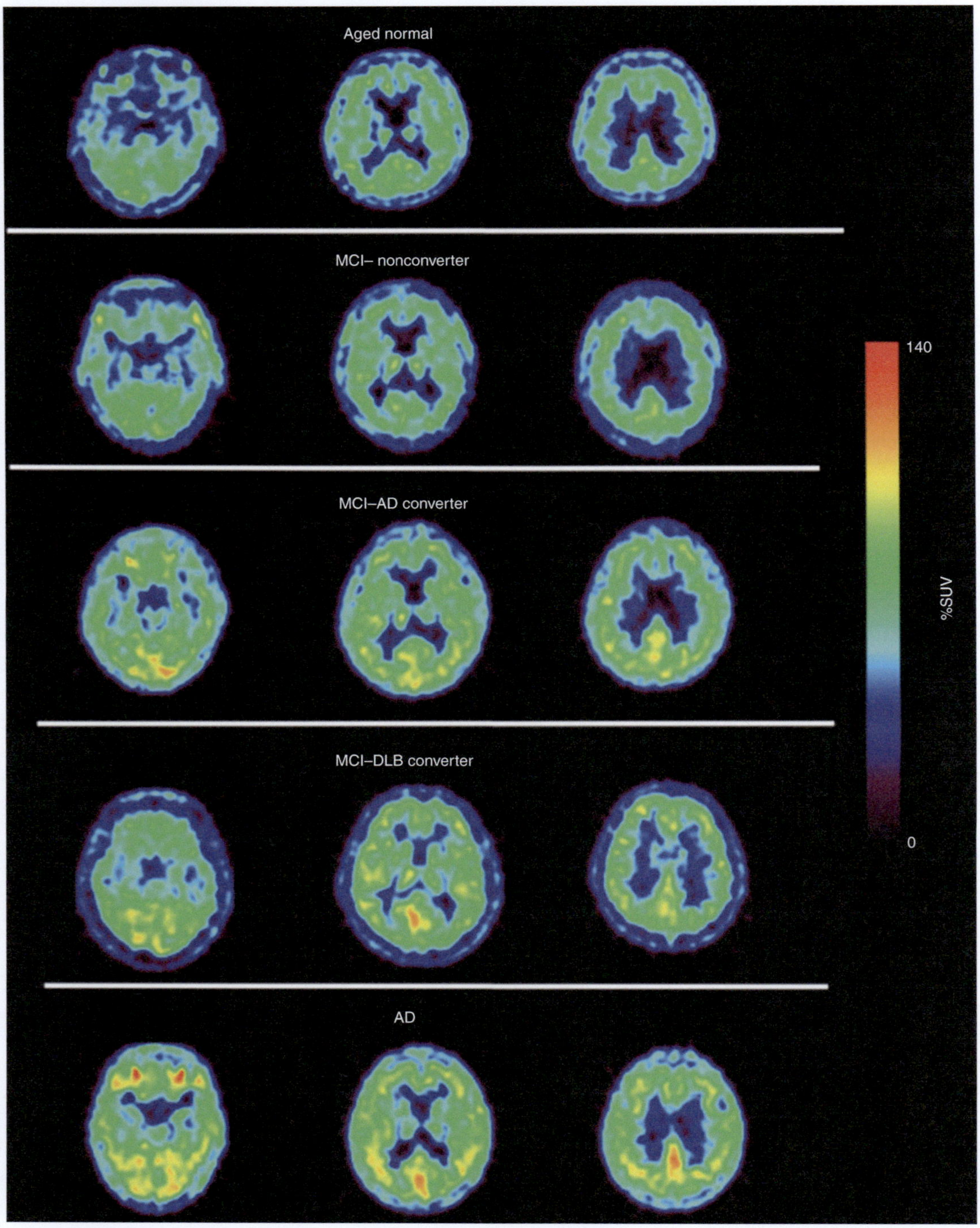

8.2.3 Technique

Patient preparation: The onset of MCI and AD was defined as the time when the earliest cognitive change was noticed by responsible caregivers, with the duration of MCI and AD ranging from 1 to 3 years. None of the subjects were taking any anti-dementia or other psychotropic medications.

Imaging device: PET scans were performed once for each subject using ECAT EXACT HR+ (CTI-Siemens, Knoxville, TN, USA), which provides 63 planes and a 15.5-cm axial field of view. Radioactivity was measured in a three-dimensional mode, and the data were reconstructed using a Hanning filter with a cutoff frequency of 0.4 (full width at half maximum = 7.5 mm). Activity was shown as % standardized uptake value (%SUV), which was normalized for injected dose and body weight. %SUV = (% injected activity/cm^3 tissue) × (g body weight). Mean %SUV images were acquired between 30 and 90 min after injection of [^{11}C]DAA1106 in a typical example of an aged normal subject and MCI and AD patients [37, 38].

8.2.4 Image Interpretation

The figure in Sect. 8.2.2 demonstrates that [^{11}C]DAA1106 binding to translocator protein (TSPO) was increased in widespread regions in AD and MCI subjects with AD and DLB converter during 5 years follow-up when compared to healthy controls. However, we found no increase of [^{11}C]DAA1106 binding in MCI subject with no conversion to dementia.

8.2.5 Differential Diagnosis

None.

8.2.6 Diagnosis and Clinical Follow-Ups

MCI subjects were followed up for 5 years after their DAA-PET scans. One non-amnesic MCI subject had converted to dementia with Lewy bodies (DLB), and multiple domain amnesic MCI subjects had converted to AD. One single-domain amnesic MCI continued to fulfill the criteria for the diagnosis of MCI.

8.2.7 Discussion

Our finding of increase of DAA binding in not only AD but MCI subjects with conversion to dementia indicated that microglial activation could occur before the onset of dementia. The detection of microglial activation may provide useful prognostic information with respect to stratifying MCI subjects at increased risk of dementia.

8.3 Alzheimer's Disease

Yasuomi Ouchi

Abstract It is known that microglial activation is present concomitant with neuronal death in Alzheimer's disease (AD). New-generation TSPO tracers have been developed to compensate for low specific binding capacity of [^{11}C](*R*)-PK11195. Here, TSPO imaging with second-generation tracer ([^{11}C]DPA713) was reported regarding changes in neuroinflammation during the course of dementia in a patient with early AD [39] . The followed-up TSPO images revealed that [^{11}C]DPA713 BP_{ND} became higher and broader in its distribution over the entire brain region in 2 years. Thus, neuroinflammation persists steadily during the early to middle stage of AD.

Keywords: Alzheimer's disease, [^{11}C]DPA713, [^{11}C]PIB, [^{18}F]FDG, Positron emission tomography

8.3.1 Clinical Presentation

A female patient in late 50s presented with memory decline that had been noticed 2 years earlier by her family. A university hospital diagnosed her with mild dementia with the scores of 22 in MMSE and 0.5 in Clinical Dementia Rating (CDR). There was no family or drug-intake history.

8.3.2 Key Images

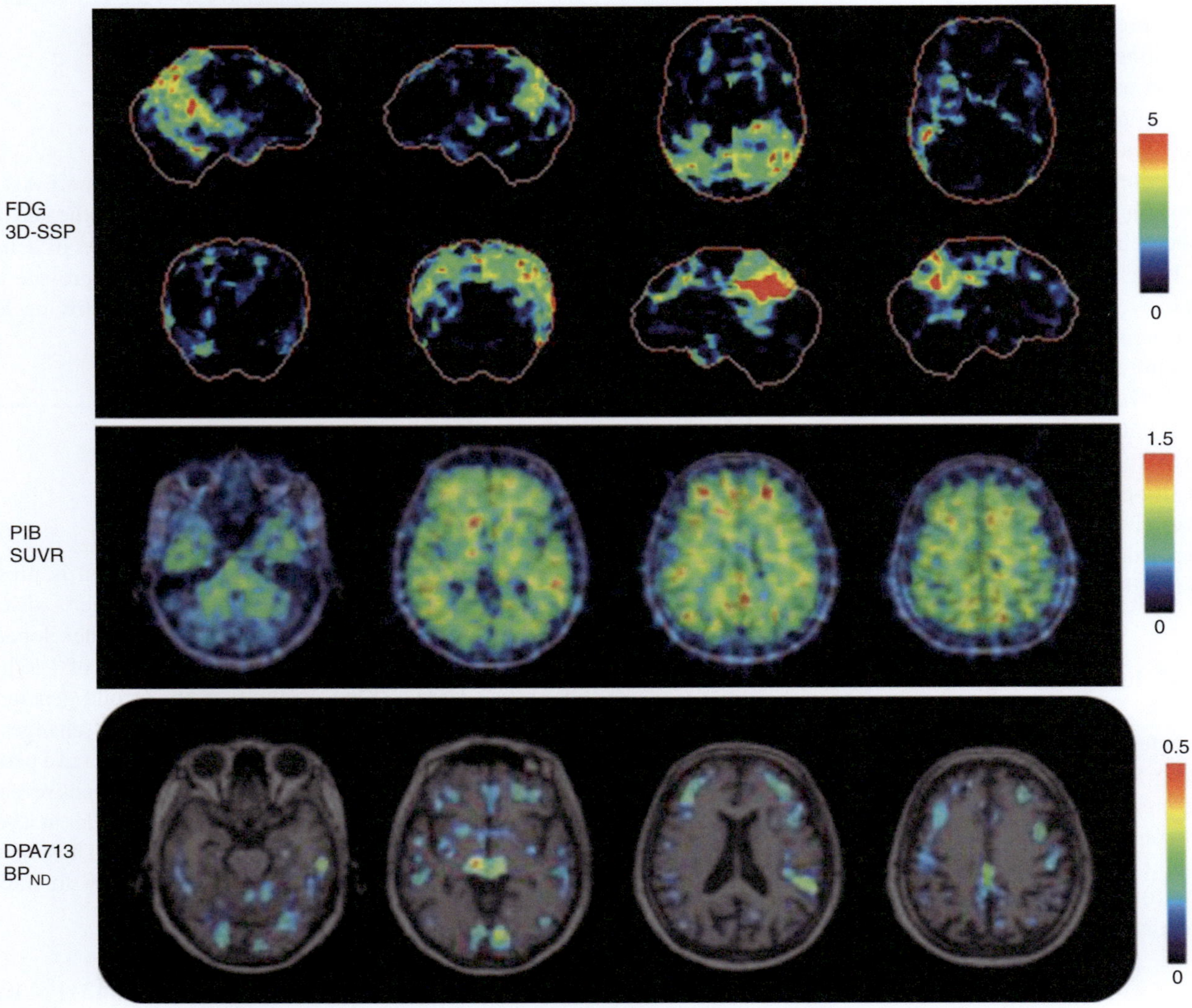

8.3.3 Technique

- Patient preparation: the patient took nothing for medication before administration of radiopharmaceutical.
- 3 MBq/kg of [^{11}C]PIB, 4 MBq/kg of [^{11}C]DPA713 and 1.5 MBq/kg of [^{18}F]FDG administered intravenously.
- Imaging device: brain-purpose PET camera (Hamamatsu Photonics KK) with a resolution of 2.9 mm FWHM.
- The binding of [^{11}C]PIB was estimated as a ratio of brain SUV count relative to the cerebellar count (SUVR). In case of [^{11}C]DPA713 binding, [^{11}C]DPA713 BP_{ND} was estimated with simplified reference tissue model.

8.3.4 Image Interpretation

The pattern of [^{18}F]FDG uptake reduction seen in the 3D-SSP images suggests Alzheimer's entity. The following amyloid imaging with [^{11}C]PIB showed marked accumulation of the tracer within the brain, indicating that the patient was strongly diagnosed with AD. TSPO imaging with [^{11}C]DPA713 showed elevation of the tracer binding entirely in the brain.

8.3.5 Differential Diagnosis

- Frontotemporal dementia
- Psychiatric disorders

8.3.6 Diagnosis and Clinical Follow-Ups

Clinical features characteristic of AD and PET findings supported AD entity [40]. The follow-up PET examination showing higher amyloid burden and typical FDG reduction characteristic of AD confirmed the diagnosis. As expected, [^{11}C]DPA713 BP_{ND} was also increased entirely in the brain.

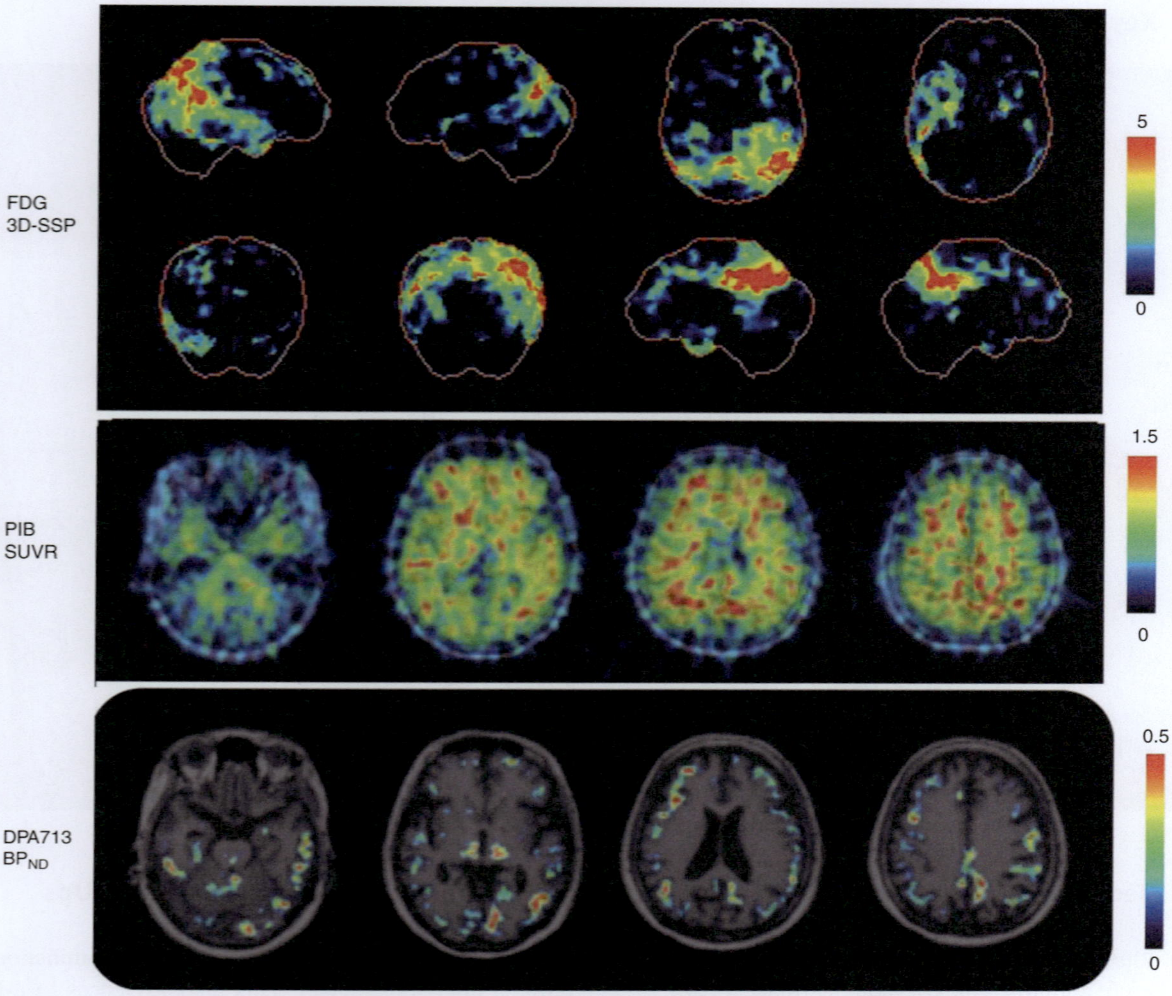

8.3.7 Discussion

While her behavioral and psychological symptoms of dementia (BPSD) did not appear, her apraxia, agnosia, aphasia, disorientation, and apathy in addition to short-term memory loss developed during the clinical course. The current finding of the broader area with higher intensity of [^{11}C] DPA713 BP_{ND} in the followed-up TSPO images confirms that persistent neuroinflammation is characteristic of AD.

8.4 Parkinson's Disease

Yasuomi Ouchi

Abstract In early drug-naïve Parkinson's disease (PD) patients, a TSPO tracer ([^{11}C](*R*)-PK11195) binding in the midbrain was reported to correlate inversely with dopamine transporter tracer ([^{11}C]CFT) binding in the putamen and that midbrain [^{11}C](*R*)-PK11195 binding was found to be positively correlated with the motor severity of parkinsonism [41–43]. Here was reported one PD patient who was scanned with [^{11}C](*R*)-PK11195 and [^{11}C]CFT to examine how these PET biomarkers changed at a stage of Hoehn–Yahr I. PET results showed that the [^{11}C]CFT binding was decreased in the striatum and that [^{11}C](*R*)-PK11195 binding was elevated in the entire brain.

Keywords: Parkinson's disease, [^{11}C](*R*)-PK11195, [^{11}C] CFT, Positron emission tomography

8.4.1 Clinical Presentation

A 65-year old man presenting with unilateral parkinsonism. Clinical examination manifested tremor, muscle stiffness in his left arm, and a difficulty in fine movement in daily chores. He did not experience any toxic environmental exposure or head injury. He did not have any relatives with PD. No drug treatment was commenced.

8.4.2 Key Images

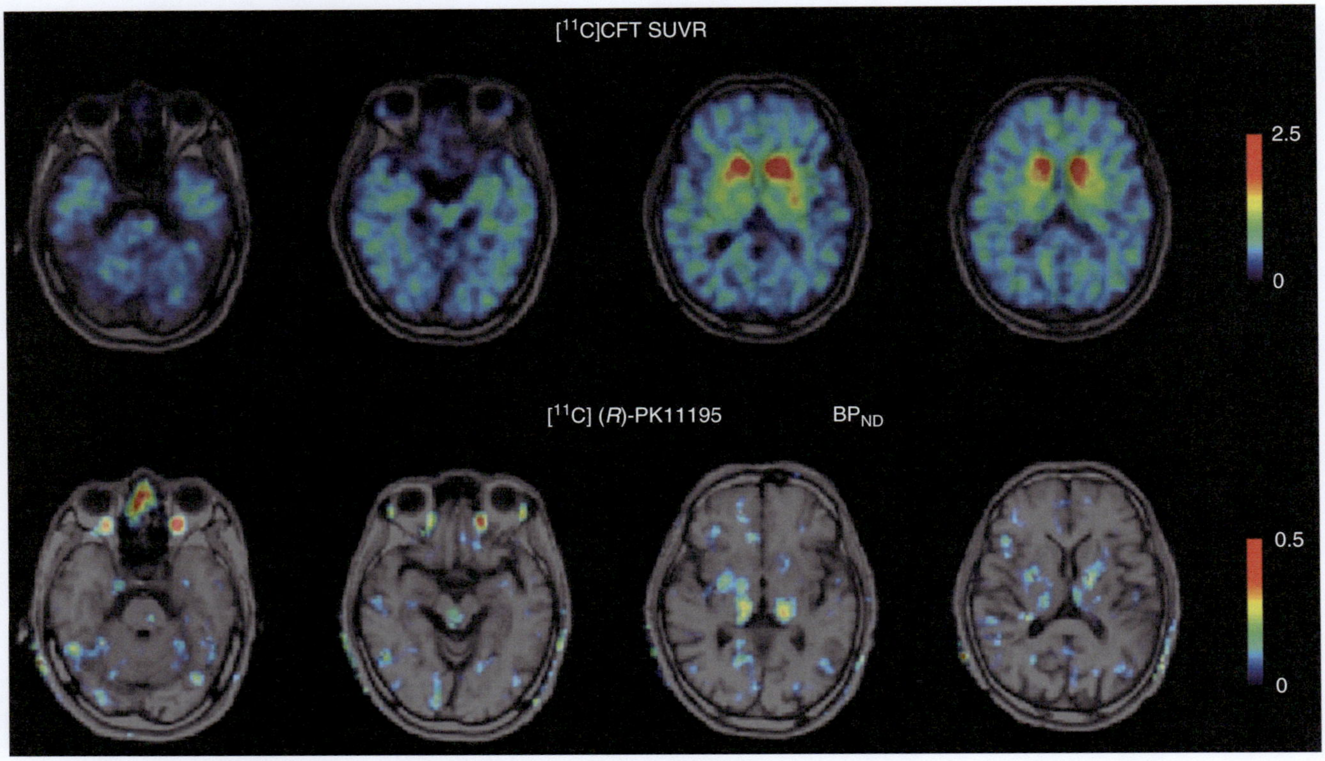

8.4.3 Technique

- Patient preparation: the patient took nothing for medication before administration of radiopharmaceutical.
- 3 MBq/kg of [^{11}C]CFT and 4 MBq/kg of [^{11}C](*R*)-PK11195 administered intravenously.
- Imaging device: brain-purpose PET camera (Hamamatsu Photonics KK) with the resolution of 2.9 mm FWHM.
- The binding of [^{11}C]CFT was estimated as a ratio of brain SUV count relative to the cerebellar count (SUVR). In case of [^{11}C](*R*)-PK11195 binding, [^{11}C](*R*)-PK11195 BP_{ND} was estimated with simplified reference tissue model.

8.4.4 Image Interpretation

PET images demonstrate the reduction of [^{11}C]CFT uptake markedly in the right putamen and mildly in the left putamen with the elevation of [^{11}C](*R*)-PK11195 binding (BP_{ND}) in the entire brain regions including the midbrain.

8.4.5 Differential Diagnosis

– Secondary parkinsonism

8.4.6 Diagnosis and Clinical Follow-Ups

A trial of L-DOPA treatment after the PET examination ameliorated his parkinsonism. This responsiveness to L-DOPA and imaging findings (above-mentioned PET finding and no abnormality in the morphological MRI) confirmed the diagnosis as PD.

8.4.7 Discussion

As reported elsewhere, since the midbrain [^{11}C](*R*)-PK11195 BP levels were positively correlated with the motor symptoms in PD [43], this patient might have comparable difficulty in handling objects with his left hand. The TSPO imaging can be used to monitor the extent of dopaminergic disorganization occurring in PD.

8.5 Multiple Sclerosis

Masahiro Fujita

Abstract Multiple sclerosis is a chronic autoimmune disease of the central nervous system which leads to demyelination and neurodegeneration. Generation of pathogenic anti-myelin T cells causes demyelination, axotomy, and eventually neuronal death [44]. This damaging process involves infiltration of peripheral immune cells, breakdown of blood–brain barrier, and activation of CNS-resident glial cells such as microglia and astrocyte. Therefore, PET imaging TSPO, a marker of microglia and astrocyte, is a useful method to monitor the activity of inflammation in multiple sclerosis.

Keywords: Blood–brain barrier, Demyelination, Autoimmune disease, Anti-myelin T cells

8.5.1 Clinical Presentation

A 39-year-old woman presented with a 15-year history of multiple sclerosis. The degree of neurological disability as measured by expanded disability status scale was 1.5 (full score is 10). The z-score of multiple sclerosis functional composite was 0.480. The patient was taking interferon-beta.

8.5.2 Key Images

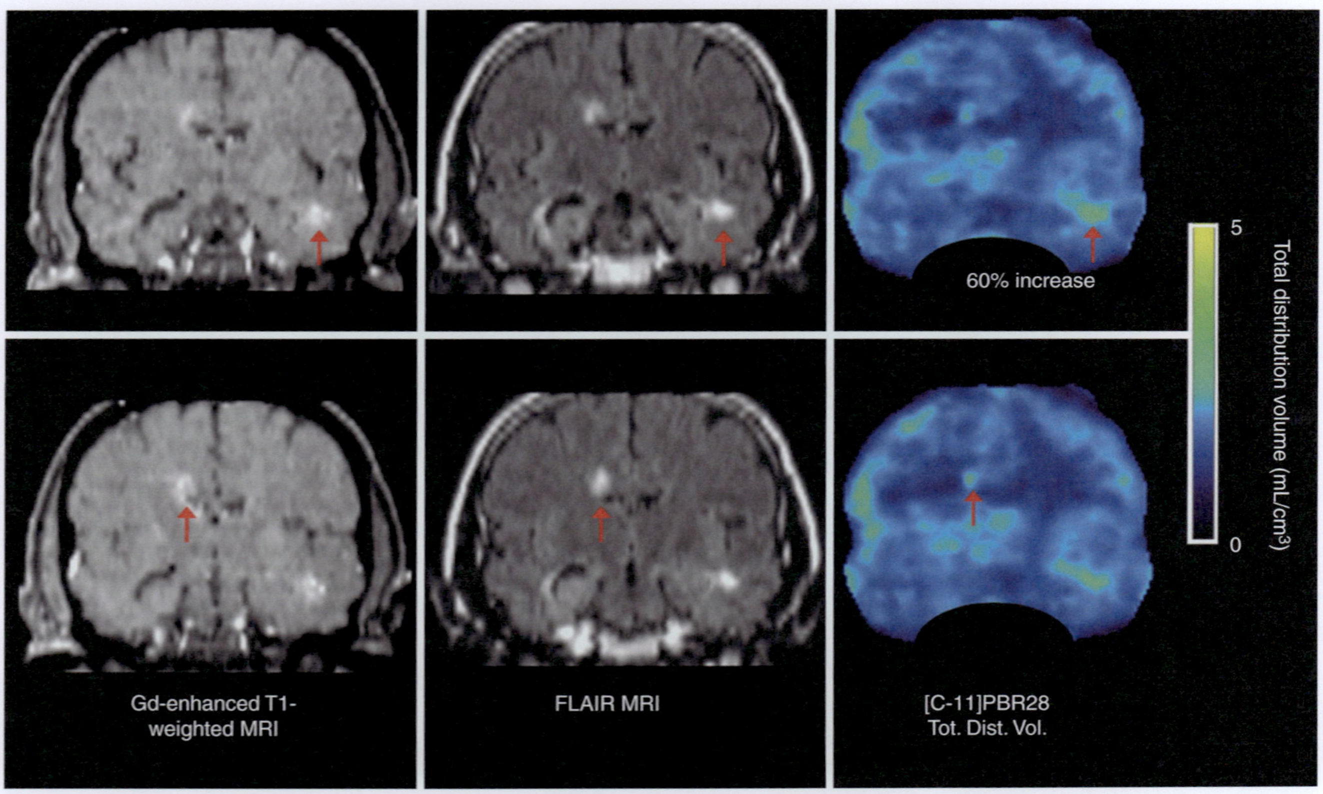

Figure from Oh, et al. 2011 with permission [46].

8.5.3 Techniques

A 3-T MRI scanner was used to acquire gadolinium-enhanced T1-weighted and fluid-attenuated inversion recovery (FLAIR) MR images. [C-11]PBR28 (~740 MBq) was intravenously administered, and a dynamic PET scan with multiple arterial sampling was performed for 120 min. Total distribution volume of [C-11]PBR28 was calculated in each voxel from brain activity and radiometabolite-corrected arterial input function using Logan plot [45].

8.5.4 Image Interpretation

Gadolinium-enhanced T1-weighted and FLAIR MR images detected the breakdown of blood–brain barrier and edema in left temporal cortex and deep white matter adjacent to the right ventricle. Parametric images representing total distribution volume of [C-11]PBR28 showed increase in TSPO in the areas with the MR changes [46].

8.5.5 Differential Diagnosis

None.

8.5.6 Diagnosis and Clinical Follow-Ups

Multiple sclerosis

8.6 Neurocysticercosis

Masahiro Fujita

Abstract Neurocysticercosis, an infection with the larval form of the tapeworm, *Taenia solium*, is one of the major causes of epilepsy in developing countries. Epilepsy in this population is mostly associated with calcified granulomas; at the time of seizure recurrence, on MRI, about a half of calcified granulomas demonstrate transient surrounding edema called perilesional edema. Surgically removed calcified granulomas associated with perilesional edema and seizures demonstrated significant inflammation with infiltration of macrophages, microglia, and activated astrocytes [47]. Therefore, perilesional edema is a result of host immunoreactions directed against parasite antigens. The host immunoreactions are detected by imaging TSPO.

Keywords: *Taenia solium*, Epilepsy, Perilesional edema, Host immunoreactions, Parasite antigens

8.6.1 Clinical Presentation

A 27-year-old woman had a long history of seizures with partial and secondary generalization. There were many calcifications on CT (not shown), and MRI documented multiple prior episodes of perilesional edema (not shown). The first [C-11]PBR28 PET scan (1/11/2008) was performed after an episode of perilesional edema around calcified granuloma in left basal ganglia that caused right face tingling.

8.6.2 Key Images

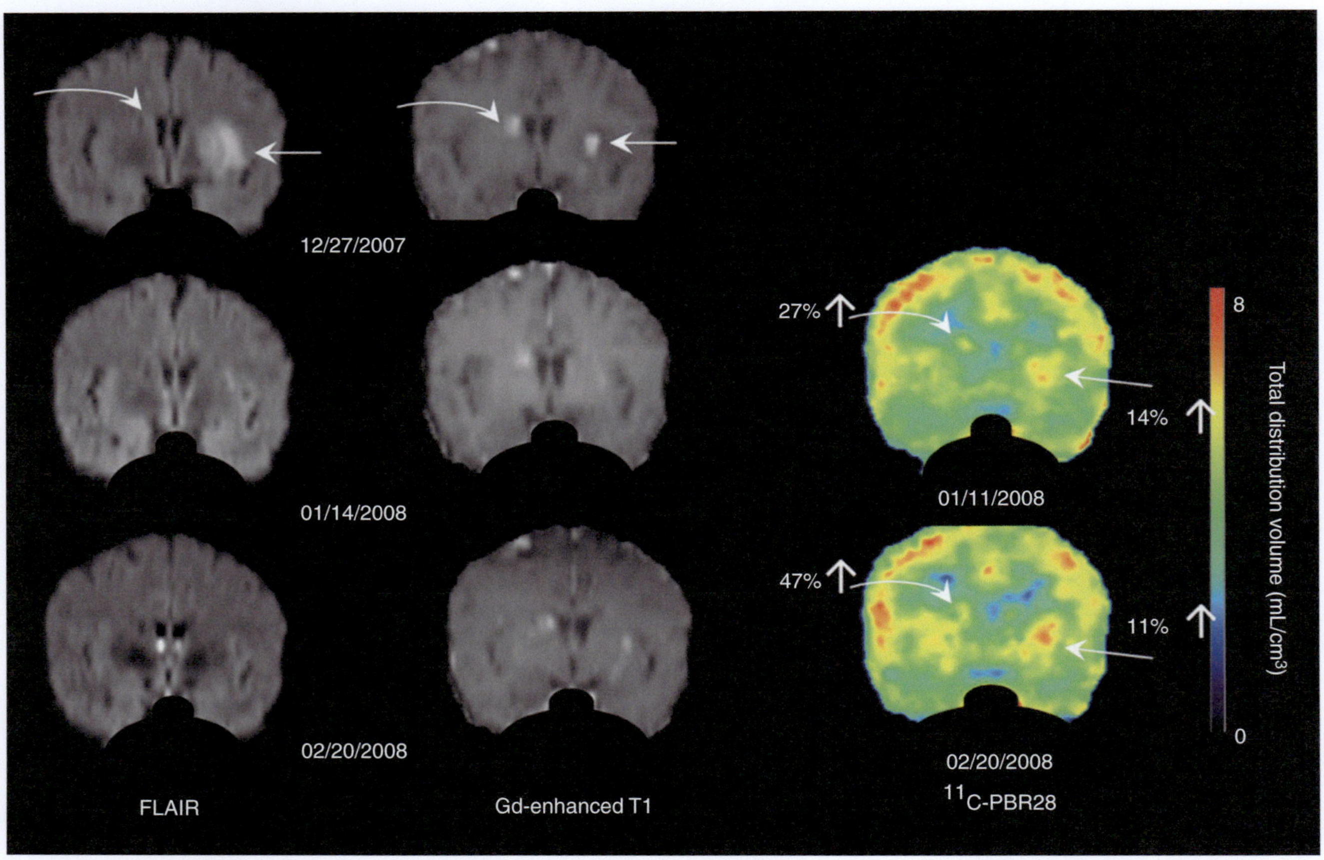

Figure used from Fujita, et al. 2013 under CC BY license [32].

8.6.3 Techniques

A 3-T MRI scanner was used to acquire FLAIR and gadolinium-enhanced T1-weighted MR images. [C-11]PBR28 (~740 MBq) was intravenously administered, and a dynamic PET scan with multiple arterial sampling was performed for 120 min. Total distribution volume of [C-11]PBR28 was calculated in each voxel from brain activity and radiometabolite-corrected arterial input function using Logan plot [45].

8.6.4 Image Interpretation

FLAIR and gadolinium-enhanced T1-weighted MR images at three time points and [C-11]PBR28 PET images obtained at two time points. Two lesions with edema and breakdown of blood–brain barrier were seen in left basal ganglia (straight arrow) and right centrum semiovale (curved arrow). Previous CT scans detected calcified cysts in both of these areas. Although perilesional edema resolved by 01/14/2008, [C-11] PBR28 uptake was still present [32].

8.6.5 Differential Diagnosis

None.

8.6.6 Diagnosis and Clinical Follow-Ups

Neurocysticercosis

References

1. Kreisl WC, Fujita M, Fujimura Y, et al. Comparison of [^{11}C]-(*R*)-PK 11195 and [^{11}C]PBR28, two radioligands for translocator protein (18 kDa) in human and monkey: implications for positron emission tomographic imaging of this inflammation biomarker. NeuroImage. 2010;49:2924–32.
2. Owen DR, Guo Q, Kalk NJ, et al. Determination of [^{11}C]PBR28 binding potential in vivo: a first human TSPO blocking study. J Cereb Blood Flow Metab. 2014;34:989–94.
3. Lavisse S, García-Lorenzo D, Peyronneau M-A, Bodini B, Thiriez C, Kuhnast B, Comtat C, Remy P, Stankoff B, Bottlaender M. Optimized quantification of Translocator protein Radioligand ^{18}F-DPA-714 uptake in the brain of genotyped healthy volunteers. J Nucl Med. 2015;56:1048–54.
4. Turkheimer F, Edison P, Pavese N, Roncaroli F, Anderson A, Hammers A, Gerhard A, Hinz R, Tai Y, Brooks DJ. Reference and target region modeling of [^{11}C]-(*R*)-PK11195 brain studies. J Nucl Med. 2007;48:158.
5. Rizzo G, Veronese M, Tonietto M, Zanotti-Fregonara P, Turkheimer FE, Bertoldo A. Kinetic modeling without accounting for the vascular component impairs the quantification of [^{11}C]PBR28 brain PET data. J Cereb Blood Flow Metab. 2014;34:1060–9.
6. García-Lorenzo D, Lavisse S, Leroy C, Wimberley C, Bodini B, Remy P, Veronese M, Turkheimer F, Stankoff B, Bottlaender M. Validation of an automatic reference region extraction for the quantification of [^{18}F]DPA-714 in dynamic brain PET studies. J Cereb Blood Flow Metab. 2017;38:333–46
7. Plavén-Sigray P, Schain M, Zanderigo F, et al. Accuracy and reliability of [^{11}C]PBR28 specific binding estimated without the use of a reference region. NeuroImage. 2019;188:102–10.
8. Kumar A, Muzik O, Shandal V, Chugani D, Chakraborty P, Chugani HT. Evaluation of age-related changes in translocator protein (TSPO) in human brain using ^{11}C-[R]-PK11195 PET. J Neuroinflammation. 2012;9:232.
9. Sandiego CM, Gallezot J-D, Pittman B, et al. Imaging robust microglial activation after lipopolysaccharide administration in humans with PET. Proc Natl Acad Sci. 2015;112:12468–73.
10. Hines CS, Fujita M, Zoghbi SS, et al. Propofol decreases in vivo binding of ^{11}C-PBR28 to translocator protein (18 kDa) in the human brain. J Nucl Med. 2013;54:64–9.
11. Kreisl WC, Lyoo CH, McGwier M, et al. In vivo radioligand binding to translocator protein correlates with severity of Alzheimer's disease. Brain. 2013;136:2228–38.
12. Hamelin L, Lagarde J, Dorothée G, et al. Early and protective microglial activation in Alzheimer's disease: a prospective study using ^{18}F-DPA-714 PET imaging. Brain. 2016;139:1252–64.
13. Hamelin L, Lagarde J, Dorothée G, et al. Distinct dynamic profiles of microglial activation are associated with progression of Alzheimer's disease. Brain. 2018;141:1855–70.
14. Dani M, Wood M, Mizoguchi R, et al. Microglial activation correlates in vivo with both tau and amyloid in Alzheimer's disease. Brain. 2018;173:44–15.
15. Zurcher NR, Loggia ML, Lawson R, et al. Increased in vivo glial activation in patients with amyotrophic lateral sclerosis: assessed with [^{11}C]-PBR28. Neuroimage Clin. 2015;7:409–14.
16. Alshikho MJ, Zurcher NR, Loggia ML, et al. Glial activation colocalizes with structural abnormalities in amyotrophic lateral sclerosis. Neurology. 2016;87:2554–61.
17. Paganoni S, Alshikho MJ, Zurcher NR, et al. Imaging of glia activation in people with primary lateral sclerosis. Neuroimage Clin. 2017;17:347–53.
18. Alshikho MJ, Zurcher NR, Loggia ML, et al. Integrated magnetic resonance imaging and [^{11}C]-PBR28 positron emission tomographic imaging in amyotrophic lateral sclerosis. Ann Neurol. 2018;83:1186–97.
19. Jucaite A, Svenningsson P, Rinne JO, et al. Effect of the myeloperoxidase inhibitor AZD3241 on microglia: a PET study in Parkinson's disease. Brain. 2015;138:2687–700.
20. Herranz E, Giannì C, Louapre C, et al. Neuroinflammatory component of gray matter pathology in multiple sclerosis. Ann Neurol. 2016;80:776–90.
21. Gershen LD, Zanotti-Fregonara P, Dustin IH, et al. Neuroinflammation in temporal lobe epilepsy measured using positron emission tomographic imaging of Translocator protein. JAMA Neurol. 2015;72:882–16.
22. Scott G, Zetterberg H, Jolly A, et al. Minocycline reduces chronic microglial activation after brain trauma but increases neurodegeneration. Brain. 2017;141:459–71.
23. Bloomfield PS, Selvaraj S, Veronese M, et al. Microglial activity in people at ultra high risk of psychosis and in schizophrenia: an [^{11}C]PBR28 PET brain imaging study. Am J Psychiatry. 2016;173:44–52.
24. Collste K, Plavén-Sigray P, Fatouros-Bergman H, et al. Lower levels of the glial cell marker TSPO in drug-naive first-episode

psychosis patients as measured using PET and [^{11}C]PBR28. Mol Psychiatry. 2017;22:850–6.

25. Richards EM, Zanotti-Fregonara P, Fujita M, et al. PET radioligand binding to translocator protein (TSPO) is increased in unmedicated depressed subjects. EJNMMI Res. 2018;8:57.
26. Kalk NJ, Guo Q, Owen D, et al. Decreased hippocampal translocator protein (18 kDa) expression in alcohol dependence: a [^{11}C] PBR28 PET study. Transl Psychiatry. 2017;7:e996.
27. Hillmer AT, Sandiego CM, Hannestad J, et al. In vivo imaging of translocator protein, a marker of activated microglia, in alcohol dependence. Mol Psychiatry. 2017;22:1759–66.
28. Kim SW, Wiers CE, Tyler R, et al. Influence of alcoholism and cholesterol on TSPO binding in brain: PET [^{11}C]PBR28 studies in humans and rodents. Neuropsychopharmacology. 2018;43:1–8.
29. Narendran R, Lopresti BJ, Mason NS, Deuitch L, Paris J, Himes ML, Kodavali CV, Nimgaonkar VL. Cocaine abuse in humans is not associated with increased microglial activation: an 18-kDa Translocator protein positron emission tomography imaging study with [^{11}C]PBR28. J Neurosci. 2014;34:9945–50.
30. Loggia ML, Chonde DB, Akeju O, et al. Evidence for brain glial activation in chronic pain patients. Brain. 2015;138:604–15.
31. Ribeiro M-J, Vercouillie J, Debiais S, Cottier J-P, Bonnaud I, Camus V, Banister S, Kassiou M, Arlicot N, Guilloteau D. Could ^{18}F-DPA-714 PET imaging be interesting to use in the early post-stroke period? EJNMMI Res. 2014;4:28.
32. Fujita M, Mahanty S, Zoghbi SS, Ferraris Araneta MD, Hong J, Pike VW, Innis RB, Nash TE. PET reveals inflammation around calcified *Taenia solium* granulomas with perilesional edema. PLoS One. 2013;8:e74052–11.
33. Dimber R, Guo Q, Bishop C, et al. Evidence of brain inflammation in patients with human T-Lymphotropic virus type 1-associated myelopathy (HAM): a pilot, multimodal imaging study using ^{11}C-PBR28 PET, MR T1-weighted, and diffusion-weighted imaging. J Nucl Med. 2016;57:1905–12.
34. Vera JH, Guo Q, Cole JH, et al. Neuroinflammation in treated HIV-positive individuals. Neurology. 2016;86:1425–32.
35. Forsberg A, Cervenka S, Jonsson Fagerlund M, et al. The immune response of the human brain to abdominal surgery. Ann Neurol. 2017;81:572–82.
36. Tamm S, Cervenka S, Forsberg A, et al. Evidence of fatigue, disordered sleep and peripheral inflammation, but not increased brain TSPO expression, in seasonal allergy: a [^{11}C]PBR28 PET study. Brain Behav Immun. 2018;68:146–57.
37. Yasuno F, et al. Increased binding of peripheral benzodiazepine receptor in Alzheimer's disease measured by positron emission tomography with [^{11}C]DAA1106. Biol Psychiatry. 2008;64(10):835–41.
38. Yasuno F, et al. Increased binding of peripheral benzodiazepine receptor in mild cognitive impairment-dementia converters measured by positron emission tomography with [^{11}C]DAA1106. Psychiatry Res Neuroimaging. 2012;203(1):67–74.
39. Yokokura M, et al. Depiction of microglial activation in aging and dementia: positron emission tomography with [^{11}C]DPA713 versus [^{11}C](*R*)PK11195. J Cereb Blood Flow Metab. 2017;37(3):877–89.
40. Hanseeuw BJ, et al. PET staging of amyloidosis using striatum. Alzheimers Dement. 2018;14(10):1281–92.
41. Ouchi Y, et al. Microglial activation and dopamine terminal loss in early Parkinson's disease. Ann Neurol. 2005;57:168–75.
42. Gerhard A, et al. In vivo imaging of microglial activation with [^{11}C] (*R*)-PK11195 PET in idiopathic Parkinson's disease. Neurobiol Dis. 2006;21:404–12.
43. Ouchi Y, et al. Neuroinflammation in the living brain of Parkinson's disease. Parkinsonism Relat Disord. 2009;15:200–4.
44. Ransohoff RM. How neuroinflammation contributes to neurodegeneration. Science. 2016;353:777–83.
45. Logan J, Fowler JS, Volkow ND, Wolf AP, Dewey SL, Schlyer DJ, MacGregor RR, Hitzemann R, Bendriem B, Gatley SJ, Christman DR. Graphical analysis of reversible radioligand binding from time-activity measurements applied to [N-^{11}C-methyl]-(−)-cocaine PET studies in human subjects. J Cereb Blood Flow Metab. 1990;10(5):740–7.
46. Oh U, Fujita M, Ikonomidou VN, Evangelou IE, Matsuura E, Harberts E, Fujimura Y, Richert ND, Ohayon J, Pike VW, Zhang Y, Zoghbi SS, Innis RB, Jacobson S. Translocator protein PET imaging for glial activation in multiple sclerosis. J Neuroimmune Pharmacol. 2011;6:354–61.
47. Nash TE, Bartelt LA, Korpe PS, Lopes B, Houpt ER. Calcified neurocysticercosis, perilesional edema, and histologic inflammation. Am J Trop Med Hyg. 2014;90(2):318–21.

Index

H. Toyama et al. (eds.), *PET/CT for Inflammatory Diseases*, https://doi.org/10.1007/978-981-15-0810-3

MIX
Papier aus verantwortungsvollen Quellen
Paper from responsible sources
FSC® C105338

If you have any concerns about our products,
you can contact us on
ProductSafety@springernature.com

In case Publisher is established outside the EU,
the EU authorized representative is:
Springer Nature Customer Service Center GmbH
Europaplatz 3, 69115 Heidelberg, Germany

Printed by Libri Plureos GmbH
in Hamburg, Germany